Lecture Notes in Mathematics

Edited by A. Dold and B. Eckmann

Subseries: USSR

Adviser: L. D. Faddeev, Leningrad

1211

M. B. Sevryuk

Reversible Systems

Springer-Verlag

Berlin Heidelberg New York London Paris Tokyo

Author

Mikhail B. Sevryuk

Consulting Editor

Vladimir I. Arnol'd
Leningrad Branch of V. A. Steklov
Mathematical Institute
Fontanka 27, 191011 Leningrad, D-11, USSR

ISBN 3-540-16819-2 Springer-Verlag Berlin Heidelberg New York
ISBN 0-387-16819-2 Springer-Verlag New York Berlin Heidelberg

Printed in Germany

Printing and binding: Druckhaus Beltz, Hemsbach/Bergstr.
2146/3140-543210

TABLE OF CONTENTS

INTRODUCTION

1°. In this work we prove the existence of Kolmogorov tori of weakly reversible dynamical systems with discrete and continuous time both in the phase space of systems close to reversible integrable ones and near elliptic equilibria.

A simplest example of a weakly reversible system (with discrete time) is a plane annulus mapping A which is transformed into its inverse by a diffeomorphism $G : A^{-1} = GAG^{-1}$. For instance, the twist rotation $(\tau, \varphi) \mapsto (\tau, \varphi + \tau)$ is transformed into the inverse rotation by the plane reflection $(\tau, \varphi) \mapsto (\tau, -\varphi)$.

The twist rotation is integrable in the sense that it leaves invariant the circles $\tau = const$.

We prove that every analytic annulus mapping sufficiently close to the twist rotation and transformed into its inverse by a diffeomorphism sufficiently close to the reflection admits a family of invariant curves close to the circles $\tau = const$ and parametrized by their rotation numbers belonging to some Cantor set.

A similar "twist theorem" has been proved by A.N.Kolmogorov (see [14]) for analytic symplectic (area-preserving) annulus diffeomorphisms and by J.Moser for smooth symplectic annulus diffeomorphisms [24] and for reversible (transformed into their inverses by involutions) flows with a multidimensional phase space [5, 6 (Chapter V)]. Our result is different from the Moser theorem in the following point. We do not require the mapping G to be an involution (but we prove that it is an involution).

In a more general Kolmogorov-Moser twist theorem one requires (instead of symplecticity) that every closed curve $\tau = \tau(\varphi)$ lying in the annulus intersects its image. Examples show (see § 1.5) that the weak reversibility (and even the reversibility) does not imply this "intersection property". The reversible diffeomorphism of the example in § 1.5 does not look like the twist rotation at all. I don't know whether there exist reversible (or weakly reversible) diffeomorphisms arbitrarily C^0 - close to the twist rotation for which the intersection property fails.

Our proof follows the main lines and stages of the proof of the Kolmogorov-Moser theorem on symplectic annulus mappings close to the twist rotation. The only considerable difference is that of the homological equations for weakly reversible diffeomorphisms and vectorfields. These equations are new and in the continuous time case show the expedience of introducing a new variant of cohomology for appropriate algebraical systems (see § 1.9).

The greatest part of the sequel has arisen from an attempt to explain some strange properties of the periodic solutions of the equation

$$u^{IV} + K_1 u'' + K_2 u + (u')^2 = 0 \qquad (*)$$

(K_1 and K_2 are parameters) that were revealed in numerical experiments (see [1, 2, 36]).

Let us proceed to more precise descriptions.

2°. An autonomous system of differential equations associated with a vectorfield V is called a reversible system (see [1, 2, 3, 6 (Chapter II , § 2,c)]) if there exists a phase space involution G (a mapping whose square is the identity mapping) transforming this system into the system with reversed time direction (i.e. transforming the field V into the opposite one: $G_* V = -V$). Such a field V is also called reversible with respect to G . An example is the motion of particles under interaction forces (that may be non-potential) not depending on the velocities. Here the phase space involution changes the signs of all the velocities.

There is a very close similarity between the behaviour of solutions of reversible systems and that of Hamiltonian ones (see [1,2]). In particular, the KAM-theory dealing with the preservation of quasi-periodic motions under a small perturbation of a nondegenerate integrable Hamiltonian system and with the existence of quasi-periodic motions near an elliptic Hamiltonian equilibrium (see [12, 13, 16, 17] and [5, 6 (Chapter II , § 3), 7, 11 (Chapter III), 15, 18 (Appendix 8), 19 (Chapter 4, § 19), 20 (Chapter 4, §§ 19,21), 21 (Lecture 3), 22 (§ 36), 28] as well, for more information see [40,41, 42, 43]) can be mutatis mutandis transferred to the class of reversible systems.

The definition of integrable reversible systems in $\mathbb{R}^{2m}$ is similar to that of integrable Hamiltonian systems with m degrees of freedom. A reversible system of differential equations in $\mathbb{R}^{2m}$ is said to be integrable if its phase space is foliated into m-dimensional tori invariant under both the phase flow of the system and the reversing involution such that the system induces on these tori quasi-periodic motions. A standard example of an integrable reversible system is $\dot{x}=\omega(y)$, $\dot{y}=0$, where $x \pmod{2\pi}$ are angular coordinates on an m-dimensional torus T^m and y varies over some domain in $\mathbb{R}^m$. Here the reversing involution is $(x,y)\mapsto(-x,y)$.

Consider a nondegenerate integrable system reversible with respect to involution G (in our example the nondegeneracy means that the Jacobian determinant $\partial\omega/\partial y$ is everywhere different from zero) and a small perturbation of this system still reversible with respect to G . It turns out that the majority of invariant tori of the integrable system does not disintegrate under such a perturbation but only undergoes a slight deformation so that the deformed tori are invariant under both the phase flow of the perturbed system and G . More precisely, those tori do not disintegrate on which the frequencies of the quasi-periodic motion are rationally independent (i.e. linearly independent over the field $\mathbb{Q}$) and can not be approximated by rationally dependent numbers overfast. On deformed tori called Kolmogorov ones the perturbed system induces the quasi-periodic motions with the same frequencies.

As far as I know, this result was first announced by J.Moser in [4] (ibidem the applications were discussed) and proved by him in [5 (see §§ 5, 6]. The point in the proof [5] is that the perturbation of an integrable reversible system is not only small but depends on a small parameter ε ($\varepsilon = 0$ corresponds to the unperturbed system). The theorem on the existence of Kolmogorov tori without this restriction can be found, e.g., in [6 (Chapter V), 7 (Section 5)] .

As well as in the Hamiltonian case, the theorem on the preservation of quasi-periodic motions under small perturbations of an integrable reversible system (the global KAM-theorem) admits a local version: the existence of quasi-periodic motions near an elliptic equilibrium of a reversible system (here the nearness to an equilibrium is to be substituted for the smallness of a perturbation). The local KAM-theory of reversible systems was developed by Yu.N.Bibikov and V.A.Pliss, see [8, 9, 10, 11 (Chapter III)] . More precisely, these papers contain the proof of the existence of invariant tori in any neighbourhood of an elliptic equilibrium of an analytic system of differential equations whenever these equations satisfy certain conditions, virtually equivalent to the reversibility (in some cases these conditions are fulfilled for Hamiltonian systems, too). The paper [9] deals with non-autonomous systems with the right hand side depending on time periodically. Non-autonomous periodic in time reversible equations are considered in Chapter 4 of the present paper.

3°. One may propose the following three avenues of generalization of the reversible KAM-theorem.

A. Reversible dynamical systems with discrete time (reversible diffeomorphisms).

A self-bijection A of a set D is called reversible if there exists an involution $G : D \to D$ transforming A into its inverse: $A^{-1} = GAG$. For example, the phase flow mapping of a reversible system of differential equations at any fixed time is reversible (with respect to the same involution).

The detailed consideration of notions of reversible mappings and reversible vectorfields can be found, e.g., in [1, 2, 3].

Although reversible diffeomorphisms often appear in several different branches of mathematics (see [1]) and are intimately connected with reversible differential equations, the discrete time version of the reversible KAM-theorem was first (as far as I know) announced in 1984 in [1] (for reversible plane diffeomorphisms near elliptic fixed points). In [2] this theorem was announced for any dimension in both local and global situations.

Note that the discrete time version of the Hamiltonian KAM-theorem (Kolmogorov tori of symplectic diffeomorphisms) is well known (see [6 (Chapter II, § 4), 18 (Appendix 8), 20 (Appendix 34, see also Chapter 4, §§ 19-21 and Appendix 28), 21 (Lecture 3), 22 (§§ 32-34), 24, 26, 27, 28]).

B. Weakly reversible dynamical systems.

Many properties of the reversible objects can be extended to all vectorfields (mappings) that are transformed into opposite (resp. inverse) ones by some phase space diffeomorphism that is possibly not an involution. Such vectorfields (resp. mappings) are called weakly reversible ones [2]. Thus, a vectorfield V and the differential equation associated with this field as well are weakly reversible with respect to a diffeomorphism G of the phase space D if $G_* V = -V$; a diffeomorphism $A : D \to D$ is weakly reversible with respect to another diffeomorphism $G : D \to D$ if $A^{-1} = GAG^{-1}$ (equivalently $AGA = G$).

A vectorfield or mapping reversed by some diffeomorphism G is reversed also by the diffeomorphism G^{-1}. If a vectorfield is weakly reversible with respect to some phase space diffeomorphism then the phase flow mapping of this field at any fixed time is also weakly reversible with respect to the same diffeomorphism (and conversely).

It turns out that the reversible KAM-theory can be generalized to weakly reversible dynamical systems.

Consider a nondegenerate analytic integrable vectorfield V (resp. a mapping A) reversible with respect to an analytic involution G and its small smooth perturbation V' (resp. A') weakly reversible with respect to a smooth diffeomorphism G' (not required to be an involution) that is close to G . Then there exist Kolmogorov tori invariant under V' and G' (resp. A' and G'). Moreover, the restriction of G' to any Kolmogorov torus is an involution. If the perturbation is small enough so that the measure of the union of Kolmogorov tori is positive then this ensures that G' is an involution-provided G' is analytic. Thus, if all the objects involved are analytic then a small weakly reversible perturbation of a nondegenerate integrable reversible vectorfield (resp. mapping) is actually always reversible.

A similar statement is true for the local situation, i.e. near an elliptic equilibrium (resp. fixed point) of a weakly reversible vectorfield (resp. mapping) provided this equilibrium (resp. fixed point) is kept fixed by the reversing diffeomorphism.

The expedience of generalizing the conception of reversibility to that of weak reversibility was pointed out in [1] . The results of the weakly reversible KAM-theory mentioned above were announced in [2] in detail.

C. The "proper degeneracy".

Up to now we confined ourselves to the situations when the phase space was of even dimension $2m$ and both the fixed point manifold of the involution and each invariant torus had the middle dimension m . It turns out that the reversible (but not the weakly reversible

KAM-theory (both global and local) can be extended to the case of the so called "proper degeneracy". This term means that the dimension of invariant tori is less than $N/2$ whereas the dimension of the fixed point manifold of the reversing involution is greater than $N/2$, where N is the dimension of the phase space. Moreover, N may be odd.

In a phase space D with coordinates $x=(x_1,\dots,x_m)\in T^m$ (x is defined $\mathrm{modd}\ 2\pi$), $y=(y_1,\dots,y_m)$ and $\eta=(\eta_1,\dots,\eta_K)$ (y and η vary over some domains in spaces $\mathbb{R}^m$ and $\mathbb{R}^K$ respectively) consider the vectorfield V associated with the differential equation

$$\dot{x}=y\ ,\quad \dot{y}=0\ ,\quad \dot{\eta}=0$$

and the mapping

$$A:(x,y,\eta)\mapsto(x+y,y,\eta).$$

They are reversible with respect to the involution

$$G:(x,y,\eta)\mapsto(-x,y,\eta).$$

Then D is foliated into invariant under V, A, and G m-dimensional tori $y=\mathrm{const}, \eta=\mathrm{const}$, on which both V and A determine quasi-periodic motions whose frequencies depend on y only, so tori with the same frequencies are organized into K-parameter families (the parameter being η).

It turns out that the majority of these families does not disintegrate under small perturbations of the field V (of the mapping A) preserving the reversibility, but only undergoes a slight deformation. Thus, in the phase space of the perturbed field (mapping), there exist manifolds of dimension $m+K$ foliated into m-dimensional tori invariant under both the flow (mapping) and the reversing involution, the motion on the tori being quasi-periodic with frequencies being constants on every $(m+K)$-dimensional manifold.

Note that weakly reversible perturbations do not, in general, preserve invariant tori in this situation because they allow a shift along $(m+K)$-dimensional manifolds foliated into invariant under the unperturbed system tori with the same frequencies. The shift maps (almost) every torus onto another one. For instance, the vectorfield V_ε associated with the differential equation

$$\dot{x}=y\,,\ \dot{y}=0\,,\ \dot{z}_1=e^{-\frac{1}{\varepsilon}}\sin\frac{z_1}{\varepsilon}\,,\ \dot{z}_2=0,\dots,\dot{z}_K=0$$

is weakly reversible with respect to the mapping

$$G_\varepsilon:(x,y,z_1,z_2,\dots,z_K)\mapsto(-x,y,z_1+\pi\varepsilon\,,z_2,\dots,z_K)$$

($\varepsilon>0$ is a small parameter). The phase flow mapping A_ε of the field V_ε at time 1 has the form

$$A_\varepsilon:(x,y,z_1,z_2,\dots,z_K)\mapsto(x+y\,,y,z_1+F_\varepsilon(z_1),z_2,\dots,z_K)$$

where $F_\varepsilon(z_1)=0$ iff $z_1/(\varepsilon\pi)\in\mathbb{Z}$ and $F_\varepsilon\to 0$ as $\varepsilon\to 0$. It is also weakly reversible with respect to G_ε.

The described KAM-result and the corresponding local statement as well were announced in [2]. The geometrical situation of organizing quasi-periodic motions of the same frequencies into smooth families first appeared in [1] (in investigating a neighbourhood of a symmetric periodic motion of a reversible system with the four-dimensional phase space). Kolmogorov tori near symmetric periodic solutions of reversible differential equations are considered in Chapter 3.

4°. The most intricate technique is used in Chapter 1 of this paper, where the proof of the global KAM-theorem for both diffeomorphism and vectorfields is presented: in the case of the "proper degeneracy" - for reversible perturbations whereas in the "classical" case of Kolmogorov tori of middle dimension - for weakly reversible perturbations.

The proofs are based on the standard (proposed in 1954 by A.N. Kolmogorov [12]) method of constructing an infinite sequence of Newton approximations - of changes of variables whose definition domains contract to desired deformed tori.

All objects will be assumed to be analytic. The cases of C^{∞}-perturbations and perturbations of a finite smoothness are considered in [7] (but only for continuous time, reversible (not weakly reversible) perturbations and invariant tori of middle dimension). One can find the technique for the C^{∞}-case or for the finite smoothness case in the Hamiltonian KAM-theory in [7, 23, 24, 25, 26, 27, 28], see [17 (Chapter VI, § 5)] as well.

For each frequency vector, we shall construct its own infinite sequence of changes of variables whose definition domains shrink down to the desired Kolmogorov torus (or the family of Kolmogorov tori in the "proper degeneracy" case) with this frequency vector. In order to prove that the measure of the union of Kolmogorov tori is positive one has to control how much sequences of changes of variables corresponding to various frequency vectors differ. We follow most closely [22 (§§ 32-34)] . At the same time we correct the inadvertence of all Moser's proofs [22, 24] in the convergence analysis (see § 1.4).

At every iteration step it is necessary to solve a certain homological equation. It is to establish its solvability that the weak reversibility of the objects in question is used. An obstruction for this solvability is the one-dimensional cohomology of an appropriate algebraic system (in particular, in the discrete time case this system is the group generated by the unperturbed diffeomorphism and the involution reversing it). This cohomology is therefore trivial. Moreover, the case when one perturbs not only an integrable reversible vectorfield or diffeomorphism but also the reversing involution turns out to have a more adequate cohomological interpretation than the case when the reversing involution does not undergo the perturbation.

In Chapter 2, by means of the Poincaré-Dulac-Birkhoff normal forms theory, we prove local theorems on Kolmogorov tori near elliptic equilibria. In contrast to many papers devoted to the local KAM-theory [8, 9, 10, 11 (Chapter III)] in which all results are established directly, here these theorems are proved by reducing to global statements.

Chapter 3 considers periodic motions of reversible vectorfields and Kolmogorov tori in neighbourhoods of these motions. In Chapter 4, the KAM-theory is extended to non-autonomous differential equations.

Let us put together all the KAM-theorems considered in this paper.

A. Global theorems.

a) For diffeomorphisms (Chapter 1, Part 1 (§§1.1-1.6), Theorem 1.1).

b) For autonomous differential equations (Chapter 1, Part 2 (§§ 1.7-1.11), Theorem 1.2).

c) For non-autonomous differential equations (Chapter 4, § 4.2, Theorem 4.1).

B. Local theorems.

a) Near fixed points of diffeomorphisms (Chapter 2, §§ 2.2-2.4, 2.8-2.9, Theorem 2.9).

b) Near equilibria of autonomous differential equations (Chapter 2, §§ 2.5-2.7, 2.10, Theorem 2.11).

c) Near equilibria of non-autonomous differential equations (Chapter 4, § 4.3, Theorem 4.2).

d) Near symmetric periodic solutions of autonomous differential equations (Chapter 3, Theorem 3.2).

e) Near symmetric periodic solutions of non-autonomous differential equations (Chapter 4, § 4.3, Theorem 4.3).

5°. Chapter 5 is devoted to the structure of resonance zones between Kolmogorov tori of reversible diffeomorphisms and vectorfields close to integrable ones.

EXAMPLE. Consider again the twist rotation of an annulus: $(\tau,\varphi)\mapsto(\tau,\varphi+\tau)$. Under a small reversible perturbation of this mapping, invariant circles $\tau=C=\mathrm{const}$ with C irrational and badly approximable by rational numbers do not disintegrate but only undergo a slight deformation. At the same time invariant circles $\tau=2\pi p/q$ (where $p\in\mathbb{Z}$, $q\in\mathbb{N}$, p and q are relatively prime) generally break up under a small perturbation of the twist rotation. Indeed, let us suppose that the perturbed mapping admits a close invariant curve on which it is the rotation through the angle $2\pi p/q$ (for an appropriate choice of the angular coordinate). Then the q-th iteration of the perturbed mapping leaves every point of this curve fixed. A generic plane mapping has no curves of fixed points (even under the condition of reversibility). Consequently, in general the invariant circle $\tau=2\pi p/q$ disintegrates under a small reversible perturbation of the rotation $(\tau,\varphi)\mapsto(\tau,\varphi+\tau)$. All invariant circles close to $\tau=2\pi p/q$ also disintegrate, and on the space of their decay there appears the so called resonance zone.

Nevertheless, it turns out that the q-th iteration A^q of a reversible mapping A sufficiently close to the rotation $(\tau,\varphi)\mapsto(\tau,\varphi+\tau)$ always has at least $2q$ fixed points situated near the circle $\tau=2\pi p/q$ (as a rule, the number of these points equals $2q$ exactly). In the resonance zone, the diffeomorphism A^q differs only slightly from the mapping at time 1 of the phase flow of a vectorfield invariant under the rotation through the angle $2\pi/q$, this vectorfield being simultaneously reversible and Hamiltonian. The typical behaviour of the mapping in the resonance zone is the following one. The points fixed under A^q are situated approximately at the apices of a regular $2q$-gon. The reversing reflection $(\tau, \varphi) \mapsto (\tau, -\varphi)$ maps the set of these points onto itself. At q points, the linearization of A^q is a rotation (elliptic points), at the other q points, it is a hyperbolic rotation (hyperbolic points). Besides that, in a neighbourhood of each of these $2q$ points there acts some involution leaving the point fixed and reversing A^q. Hence in neighbourhoods of elliptic points one can apply the local version of the KAM-theorem for reversible mappings to A^q, and for every elliptic point this theorem provides a family of close curves surrounding this point which are invariant under A^q. The motions along these curves under the action of the mapping A^q are called phase oscillations (since it is the "phase" φ that varies mainly). Between the trajections of phase oscillations, there lie resonance zones of the mapping A^q (one may call them resonance zones "of the second order"), and so on.

Thus, the behaviour of a reversible mapping close to the rotation $(\tau, \varphi) \mapsto (\tau, \varphi + \tau)$ is extremely similar to that of a symplectic (area-preserving) mapping close to the twist rotation.

The majority of the results just exposed can be generalized (mutatis mutandis) to higher dimensions. For instance, consider in $\mathbb{R}^{2m}$ an integrable nondegenerate reversible diffeomorphism $(x,y) \mapsto (x+y, y)$, where $x (\mathrm{modd}\ 2\pi)$ are angular coordinates on T^m and y varies over some domain in $\mathbb{R}^m$. Then the invariant torus $y = 2\pi p/q$, where $p = (p_1, \ldots, p_m) \in \mathbb{Z}^m$, $q \in \mathbb{N}$ and the greatest common divisor of numbers $p_1, \ldots, p_m, q$ equals 1, generally disintegrates under a small reversible perturbation of this diffeomorphism, but the q-th iteration of the perturbed mapping has at least $2^m q$ fixed points.

Similar results also hold for perturbations of integrable reversible vectorfields.

6°. In a neighbourhood of the origin in $\mathbb{R}^{2m}$ consider a reversible vectorfield for which 0 is an elliptic equilibrium. In the nonresonant case (when the eigenfrequencies $\omega_1, \ldots, \omega_m$ of the linearization are rationally independent) this field can be reduced to the formal normal form

$$R_1(r_1^2,\ldots,r_m^2)\frac{\partial}{\partial \varphi_1}+\ldots+R_m(r_1^2,\ldots,r_m^2)\frac{\partial}{\partial \varphi_m},$$

where $(r_1, \varphi_1, \ldots, r_m, \varphi_m)$ is a polypolar coordinate system in a neighbourhood of $0 \in \mathbb{R}^{2m}$ and $R_1, \ldots, R_m$ are formal power series in m variables. The constant terms of these series are $\omega_1, \ldots, \omega_m$. The reversing involution changes the signs of all the angular coordinates $\varphi_1, \ldots, \varphi_m$ (see § 2.5, Proposition 2.12 or § 2.6, Proposition 2.14).

Let us suppose that both the initial vectorfield and the change of variables reducing this field to a normal form are analytic. Then a whole neighbourhood of 0 in $\mathbb{R}^{2m}$ consists of invariant tori of various dimensions. More precisely, through the origin there pass m two-dimensional surfaces $(r_1=\ldots=r_{j-1}=r_{j+1}=\ldots=r_m=0,\ j=1,\ldots,m)$ foliated into close phase curves, $m(m-1)/2$ four-dimensional surfaces filled with close phase curves and invariant 2-tori (these surfaces are given by the following: $m-2$ of the m polar radii $r_1, \ldots, r_m$ are assumed to equal 0), ..., m surfaces of dimension $2m-2$ $(r_j=0,\ j=1,\ldots,m)$ filled with invariant tori of dimensions $\leq m-1$, and the space outside the surfaces $r_j=0$ is foliated into m-dimensional invariant tori. The motions on invariant tori of all dimensions are quasiperiodic.

But for $m>1$ the series giving the normalizing change of variables diverge as a rule and, consequently, the true phase portrait of a reversible field near an equilibrium is immeasurably more complicated. According to the local KAM-theorem, if $R_1, \ldots, R_m$ satisfy a certain nondegeneracy condition then near O this field possesses a Cantor family of m-dimensional invariant tori on which quasiperiodic motions with rationally independent frequencies are induced. What can one say on invariant tori of smaller dimensions?

To my knowledge, the question on invariant tori of a reversible field (near an equilibrium) of intermediate dimensions d, where $2 \leq d \leq m-1$, was not as yet given attention to. As far as passing through O two-dimensional surfaces foliated into close phase curves of this field are concerned, it turns out that these surfaces are not influenced by the divergence of the normalizing change of variables. Namely, through a nonresonant equilibrium of the field there always pass m smooth two-dimensional surfaces, each of which is foliated into close phase curves invariant under the reversing involution. These surfaces are tangent at O to the corresponding two-dimensional invariant planes of the linearization. The period of cycles on the surface, tangent at O to the invariant plane with eigenvalues $\pm i\omega_j$, tends to $2\pi/\omega_j$ as the initial conditions tend to the equilibrium [3].

This analogue of the Lyapunov theorem for Hamiltonian systems is proved in § 6.1 (Theorems 6.2 and 6.3). For its validity, the absolute absence of resonances among frequencies $\omega_1, \ldots, \omega_m$, i.e. their rational independence, is not a necessary condition. It suffices that none of the ratios $\omega_i/\omega_j, 1 \leq i, j \leq m, i \neq j$, be a natural number.

The main part of Chapter 6 is devoted to close trajectories of resonant reversible systems (whose linearizations have an eigenfrequency being an integer multiple of another one). Furthermore, we study not only the surfaces foliated into close phase curves of resonant fields but also the bifurcations of these surfaces as a field passes through the resonance. Otherwise speaking, the resonant field is assumed to be embedded in a one-parameter family of reversible fields depending on a small parameter ε (the value $\varepsilon=0$ corresponds to the resonance).

In 1984, the pattern of these bifurcations was considered by V.I. Arnol'd. He guessed the answer for resonance $1:1$.

Let us formulate the main results for the simplest case of a four-dimensional phase space (Theorems 6.5 and 6.8 describe the case of an arbitrary number of degrees of freedom).

Consider a family of reversible fields in $\mathbb{R}^4$ with an equilibrium at 0, which depend on a small parameter $\varepsilon\in\mathbb{R}$ (we assume that the reversing involution is the same for all ε and that the two-dimensional plane Fix of its fixed points passes through 0). Let for $\varepsilon=0$ the eigenvalues of the linearization of the field at 0 be $\pm i\omega$, $\pm iN\omega$, where $N\in\mathbb{N}$.

Then for sufficiently small ε in a neighbourhood of 0 the field has an invariant two-dimensional surface $\mathcal{M}_\varepsilon$ foliated into closed trajectories invariant under the involution with periods close to $2\pi/\omega$. This surface intersects the plane Fix along a curve Γ_ε. Points of the curve Γ_ε are being characterized by the following: the field's trajectories, starting at these points, in a time close to π/ω (but not earlier on) intersect Fix again (at points which necessarily belong to Γ_ε again). Call Γ_ε the return curve.

Consider the germ of the diagram

$$\Pi \xrightarrow{i} \mathbb{R}^3 \xrightarrow{\rho} \mathbb{R} \qquad (**)$$

where $\Pi=\{(P,\varepsilon)\in Fix\times\mathbb{R} \mid P\in\Gamma_\varepsilon\}$, $i:\Pi\hookrightarrow Fix\times\mathbb{R}=\mathbb{R}^3$

is the natural embedding, $\rho : (P, \varepsilon) \mapsto \varepsilon$. The surface Π (call it the return surface) consists of return curves for various values of the parameter ε , more precisely, its sections by the level planes $\rho = \varepsilon$ of the coordinate function ρ are return curves Γ_ε .

THEOREM 1. For generic families of fields, one can choose such a coordinate system (u, v, w) in $\mathbb{R}^3$ in which the equation of the return surface takes the form $v^2 = u^2 w$ for $N=1$ and $vw + u^N = 0$ for $N \geqslant 2$.

Otherwise speaking, generically the return surface is the Whitney umbrella for $N=1$ and the singularity of type A_{N-1} for $N \geqslant 2$ (in particular, for $N=2$ it is a cone), see [37 (Chapter I , § 1,1.9 and Chapter II , § 17, 17.1)] .

The functions ρ in the diagrams (**) corresponding to families of fields are not in general position regarding the return surfaces (expect for $N=2$).

EXAMPLE. All smooth curves lying on the Whitney umbrella $\{ v^2 = u^2 w, \ w \geqslant 0 \}$ and passing through its vertex 0 have a common tangent at 0 (namely, the axis u). It turns out that for diagrams coming from generic families of fields, the derivative of the function ρ at 0 along this tangent vanishes.

Consider all diagrams of the above form (**) with two-dimensional Π and smooth i and ρ . Call two diagrams $(\Pi_\nu, i_\nu, \rho_\nu)$, $\nu = 1, 2$, equivalent whenever there exist such diffeomorphisms $D : \mathbb{R}^3 \to \mathbb{R}^3$, $\Delta : \Pi_1 \to \Pi_2$, $d : \mathbb{R} \to \mathbb{R}$ preserving 0 (where d is assumed to be linear, i.e. to be the multiplication by a nonzero constant) that the diagram

$$\begin{array}{ccccc}
\Pi_1 & \xhookrightarrow{i_1} & \mathbb{R}^3 & \xrightarrow{\rho_1} & \mathbb{R} \\
\downarrow \Delta & & \downarrow D & & \downarrow d \\
\Pi_2 & \xhookrightarrow{i_2} & \mathbb{R}^3 & \xrightarrow{\rho_2} & \mathbb{R}
\end{array}$$

is commutative, i.e. $Di_1 = i_2\Delta$, $d\rho_1 = \rho_2 D$.

THEOREM 2. Every diagram (**) corresponding to a generic family of fields is equivalent to one of the standard diagrams. There are two standard diagrams for $N \neq 3$, while for $N = 3$ the standard diagram depends on one module, i.e. they form a one-parameter family.

The standard diagrams are the following ones.

$N=1$	$\Pi = \{v^2 = u^2 w\}$ $\rho_\pm(u,v,w) = w \pm u^2$
$N=2$	$\Pi = \{vw + u^2 = 0\}$ $\rho_\pm(u,v,w) = v \pm w$
$N=3$	$\Pi = \{vw + u^3 = 0\}$ $\rho_\theta(u,v,w) = w - uv\cos\theta - v^2\sin\theta$ (where $\theta \bmod 2\pi \in \mathbb{R}$, $4\cos^3\theta + 27\sin^2\theta \neq 0$)
$N \geq 4$	$\Pi = \{vw + u^N = 0\}$ $\rho_\pm(u,v,w) = w + u^2 \pm v^2$

The precise formulations are given in Theorems 6.6, 6.9, 6.10, and 6.11.

EXAMPLE. The standard diagrams for resonance $1:1$ (i.e. for $N=1$) describe the **fibrations** of the return surface into return curves shown in figures 1 and 2.

In fig.1, the Whitney umbrella $v^2 = u^2 w$ is dissected by the level surfaces of function $\rho = w + u^2$. In this case near 0 return curves exist only for one value of $\operatorname{sgn} \varepsilon$ and look like a figure-of-eight. Closed trajectories of the initial vectorfield in $\mathbb{R}^4$ intersect the figure-of-eight at points nearly symmetric with respect to the origin. The surface $\mathcal{M}_\varepsilon$ composed of these closed trajectories has the topology of a sphere with two identified points corresponding to the origin O (at O, $\mathcal{M}_\varepsilon$ self-intersects transversally). Taking identified points of the sphere as northern and southern poles, one can imagine $\mathcal{M}_\varepsilon$ by considering parallels closed phase curves and one of meridians the return curve (i.e. the intersection of $\mathcal{M}_\varepsilon$ and Fix). Since the poles are identified, this meridian looks like a figure-of-eight.

In paper [36 (§ 3)] , such a sphere with two identified points was found by means of computing several first terms of the series giving a solution of the reversible differential equation (*) with K_1 close to 2 and $K_2 = 1$. It is an attempt to explain the results of these computations that V.I.Arnol'd's programme of the investigation of resonant reversible systems has arisen from.

In fig. 2, the same umbrella is dissected by the level surfaces of function $\rho = w - u^2$.

As a direct consequence of Theorem 2, we can obtain normal forms for return curves.

THEOREM 3. One can reduce the equation of the collection of return curves for generic families of fields to the following form:

$N=1$	$(\varepsilon \pm \xi^2)\xi^2 = \eta^2$
$N=2$	$\eta(\varepsilon - \eta) \pm \xi^2 = 0$
$N=3$	$\eta(\varepsilon + \eta\xi\cos\theta + \eta^2\sin\theta) + \xi^3 = 0$ (where $\theta \bmod 2\pi \in \mathbb{R}$, $4\cos^3\theta + 27\sin^2\theta \neq 0$)
$N \geq 4$	$\eta(\varepsilon \pm \eta^2 - \xi^2) + \xi^N = 0$

by choosing suitable smoothly depending on ε coordinates ξ, η on Fix with the origin at 0 (and by multiplying ε by a suitable nonzero constant to equal ± 1 for $N=1$ and to be 1 for $2 \leq N \leq 3$).

The normal forms for the bifurcations of the surfaces $\mathcal{M}_\varepsilon$ have not as yet been found.

The results of the present paper were announced in [2] .

7°. The author is very grateful to Professor V.I.Arnol'd for raising the problems, helpful advices and the literature information (in particular, allowing to read through the manuscript of [1]). It was he who put forward the idea of an explicit cohomological interpretation of reversibility. Without his countenance this paper would not have been written.

8°. Fix some notations.

Whenever F is a smooth mapping, TF denotes the mapping tangent to F and $T_z F$ denotes the differential of F at point z. For diffeomorphism G and vectorfield V the expression $G_* V$ denotes the vectorfield whose value at any point z is

$$T_{G^{-1}(z)} G(V(G^{-1}(z))) .$$

In other words,

$$G_* V = TG \circ V \circ G^{-1} .$$

The weak reversibility condition $G_* V = -V$ may be rewritten in the form $TG \circ V = -V \circ G$.

The meaning of the expression $G_* V$ for formal G and V is also clear.

The symbol id denotes the identity mapping. We denote by $\mathbb{R}_+$ (resp. $\mathbb{Z}_+$) the set of nonnegative real numbers (resp. integers).

Whenever $N \in \mathbb{N}$ and $w=(w_1,\ldots,w_N) \in \mathbb{C}^N$ (in particular, $w \in \mathbb{R}^N$ or $w \in \mathbb{Z}^N$), $|w|$ denotes the norm

$$|w| = \sum_{i=1}^{N} |w_i| .$$

Let $\tilde{D}$ be an arbitrary domain in $\mathbb{C}^m \times \mathbb{C}^s$. We shall call a function $\tilde{D} \longrightarrow \mathbb{C}^N$ normal in $\tilde{D}$ if it is holomorphic, 2π - periodic in the first m arguments and real-valued on $D=\tilde{D}\cap\mathbb{R}^{m+s}$.

Whenever $z = x + iy$ is one of the (local) complex coordinates on a complex manifold, $w\partial/\partial z$ (where $w = u + iv$) will always denote the vectorfield $u\partial/\partial x + v\partial/\partial y$. We adopt this agreement to simplify some formulas. It is unusual (usually $w\partial/\partial z$ $=(w/2)\partial/\partial x-(iw/2)\,\partial/\partial y$) but our notation is compatible with the differentials: if $F:\mathbb{C}\to\mathbb{C}$ is a holomorphic function then the differential $T_\xi F$ maps vector $w\partial/\partial z$ (at point $\xi\in\mathbb{C}$) to the vector $F'(\xi)\,w\,\partial/\partial z$. If a function $F:\mathbb{C}\to\mathbb{C}$ is not holomorphic then $T_\xi F$ maps $w\partial/\partial z$ to $(F_z(\xi)w+F_{\bar z}(\xi)\bar w)\,\partial/\partial z$, where $F_z=\frac{1}{2}(F_x-iF_y)$, $F_{\bar z}=\frac{1}{2}(F_x+iF_y)$.

For $u=(u_1,\ldots,u_N)\in\mathbb{R}^N$ and $\gamma\in\mathbb{R}$, we set γu $=(\gamma u_1,\ldots,\gamma u_N)$. For $\mathcal{U}\subset\mathbb{R}^N$ and $v\in\mathbb{R}^N$, we set $\gamma\mathcal{U}=\{\gamma u\,|\,u\in\mathcal{U}\}$ and $\gamma\,\mathcal{U}+v=\{\gamma u+v\,|\,u\in\mathcal{U}\}$.

We never refer to formulas "from one chapter to another". Thus in each chapter we number formulas occupying a separate line in the following way: (1), (2), (3),... (but not (1.1), (1.2), (1.3),... in Chapter 1, (2.1), (2.2), (2.3),... in Chapter 2, etc).

The mark X denotes the end of a proof.

9°. Point out some other notations used in Chapters 1 - 5. All constructions in these chapters depend on the constants $m\in\mathbb{N}$ and $K\in\mathbb{Z}_+$ assumed to be fixed. T^m denotes the m-dimensional torus $(S^1)^m=(\mathbb{R}/2\pi\mathbb{Z})^m$. In §§ 2.3 and 2.6 we use the constant

$n \in \mathbb{Z}_+$ whose role is similar to that of m .

Throughout Chapters 1 - 5 the indices j, t (for $k \geqslant 1$) and τ have the ranges from 1 to m , from 1 to k and from 1 to 3 respectively.

In Chapter 1 the indices l and i have the ranges from 0 to 4 and from 1 to 2 respectively.

In §§ 2.3 and 2.6 the index r has the range from 1 to n .

In §§ 5.2 - 5.3 the index ψ has the range from 2 to 3.

In these parts of the paper, any relation containing the letters j, t, τ, l, i, r or ψ as indices is to be understood as the assertion that this relation is valid for all the values of the corresponding indices (except when stated otherwise).

CHAPTER 1

KOLMOGOROV TORI OF PERTURBATIONS OF INTEGRABLE REVERSIBLE DIFFEOMORPHISMS AND VECTORFIELDS

Part 1

The discrete time case: Kolmogorov tori of perturbations of reversible diffeomorphisms

§ 1.1. Preliminaries

Let $K>0$, $\varepsilon>0$. A number $\omega\in\mathbb{R}^m$ is called a number of type $\mathfrak{M}_m(K,\varepsilon)$ if for all $q\in\mathbb{Z}^m\setminus\{0\}$ and $p\in\mathbb{Z}$ the following inequality holds

$$\left|\frac{(q,\omega)}{2\pi}-p\right|\geqslant\frac{K}{|q|^{m+\varepsilon}}.$$

The following lemma is well known from the Diophantine approximations theory.

ω-LEMMA 1. Let $C>0$, $R>0$ and let $B_R\subset\mathbb{R}^m$ be a ball of radius R. Then for each fixed ε, $T>0$

$$\frac{\operatorname{mes}\{\omega\in B_R\,|\,\omega \text{ is of type } \mathfrak{M}_m(Rc,\varepsilon)\}}{\operatorname{mes} B_R}\rightrightarrows 1\ (c\to 0)$$

uniformly with respect to $R\in(0,T)$ and to all balls B_R.

Now consider a domain $D\subset\mathbb{R}^{2m+k}$ and smooth diffeomorphisms $A,G:D\to D$ such that $AGA=G$ and D is smoothly foliated into m-dimensional tori, which are invariant under the actions of A and G. Suppose that one has chosen in D a coordinate system (x, w) where $x=(x_1,\dots,x_m)$ are angular coordinates on T^m defined $\mathrm{mod}\, 2\pi$ and $w=(w_1,\dots,w_{m+k})$ are coordinates on a domain in the space $\mathbb{R}^{m+k}$, such that these tori are given by equalities $w=\mathrm{const}$, and

$$A:(x,w)\mapsto(x+\omega(w),w),\quad G:(x,w)\mapsto(F(x,w),w) \qquad (1)$$

(i.e. the action of A is quasiperiodic on each torus).

A diffeomorphism A defined by the formula (1) is called slightly integrable, or integrable in a generalized sense (for $k=0$ - integrable).

PROPOSITION 1.1. Assume that the rank of the mapping $w\mapsto\omega(w)$ is equal to m everywhere. Then G is an involution and in a neighbourhood of each torus $w=\overset{0}{w}=\mathrm{const}$ one can choose a coordinate system (x', y, η) (where $x'\in T^m$, $y\in\mathbb{R}^m$, $\eta\in\mathbb{R}^k$), in which the tori under consideration are given by equalities $y=\mathrm{const}$, $\eta=\mathrm{const}$, and

$$A:(x',y,\eta)\longmapsto(x'+y,y,\eta),\quad G:(x',y,\eta)\longmapsto(-x',y,\eta). \qquad (2)$$

PROOF. Since the rank of the mapping $w\mapsto\omega(w)$ is equal to m at the point $\overset{0}{w}$ it follows that by the Implicit Function Theorem in a neighbourhood of $\overset{0}{w}$ one can choose coordinates (y,η) (where $y\in\mathbb{R}^m$, $\eta\in\mathbb{R}^k$), in which this mapping takes the form $(y,\eta)\mapsto y$. In coordinates (x,y,η)

$$A:(x,y,\eta)\mapsto(x+y,y,\eta),\quad G:(x,y,\eta)\mapsto(F'(x,y,\eta),y,\eta).$$

Write down the Fourier series expansion for $F'(x,y,\eta)+x=\tilde F(x,y,\eta)$:

$$\tilde F(x,y,\eta)=\sum_{q\in\mathbb{Z}^m}F_q(y,\eta)e^{i(q,x)}.$$

$AGA = G$ implies $F'(x+y, y, \eta)+y = F'(x,y,\eta)$, i.e. $\tilde{F}(x,y,\eta) = \tilde{F}(x+y, y, \eta)$. Therefore $F_q(y,\eta)(e^{i(q,y)}-1) \equiv 0$. If $q \neq 0$ then this follows that $F_q(y,\eta) = 0$ for all y such that $y_1, \dots, y_m, \pi$ are rationally independent, whence by the continuity $F_q(y,\eta) = 0$ for all y and η. Thus, $\tilde{F}(x,y,\eta) = F_0(y,\eta)$ depends on y and η only. Setting $x' = x - \frac{1}{2} F_0(y,\eta)$ we obtain (2). The mapping G in (2) is obviously an involution. χ

Our purpose is to investigate the preservation of invariant tori under small reversible (weakly reversible, if $\kappa = 0$) perturbations of the pair (2) of diffeomorphisms A and G. All mappings we shall consider will be analytic and, moreover, have been already extended into the complex space. In order that it would be more convenient for us to obtain local results for the future we will consider the mapping $(x', y, \eta) \longmapsto (x' + \gamma y, y, \eta)$, where $\gamma \in (0,1]$, instead of the mapping A in (2), but in addition to that suppose that the real part of a domain, over which the coordinate y varies, contains a unit ball.

§ 1.2. Principal theorem

THEOREM 1.1. Let $\Omega \subset \mathbb{R}^m$ be a closed ball of radius 1 and $D_* \subset \mathbb{C}^m$ be a complex neighbourhood of Ω. Let $\tau_0, \tilde{\tau}_0 \in (0,1]$. Let also $B_R(b)$ be a closed ball in $\mathbb{R}^\kappa$ with an arbitrary centre b and radius R. Denote by D the following domain in $\mathbb{C}^{2m+\kappa}$:

$$D = \{x \in \mathbb{C}^m \mid |\operatorname{Im} x_j| < \tau_0\} \times \{y \in \mathbb{C}^m \mid y \in D_*\} \times \{\eta \in \mathbb{C}^\kappa \mid |\eta_t - b_t| < R + \tilde{\tau}_0\}.$$

Suppose that $\gamma, c \in (0,1]$ are fixed and on D the following mappings are given:

$$A : \begin{array}{l} x \\ y \\ \eta \end{array} \longmapsto \begin{array}{l} x + \gamma y + \overset{1}{f}(x, y, \eta) \\ y + \overset{2}{f}(x, y, \eta) \\ \eta + \overset{3}{f}(x, y, \eta) \end{array} \qquad G : \begin{array}{l} x \\ y \\ \eta \end{array} \longmapsto \begin{array}{l} -x + \overset{1}{\alpha}(x, y, \eta) \\ y + \overset{2}{\alpha}(x, y, \eta) \\ \eta + \overset{3}{\alpha}(x, y, \eta) \end{array} \tag{3}$$

where $\overset{\tau}{f}$ and $\overset{\tau}{\alpha}$ are normal in D functions.

Assume that $AGA = G$ throughout D, where AGA is defined, and if $\kappa > 0$ then in addition $G^2 = id$ throughout D, where G^2 is defined.

Introduce the notation $\Omega_{\gamma, c} = \{ \omega \in \gamma \Omega \mid \omega$ is of type $\mathfrak{M}_m(\gamma c, 1)\}$.

Then for each $\varepsilon > 0$ there exists $\delta > 0$, depending only on ε, D and c but not on γ, such that if on D $|\overset{\tau}{f}| < \gamma\delta$ and $|\overset{\tau}{\alpha}| < \gamma\delta$ then for each $\omega \in \Omega_{\gamma, c}$ the mappings A and G have a common invariant $(m+\kappa)$-dimensional manifold

$$x = \varphi + \overset{1}{\Phi}_{\omega}(\varphi, \chi), \; y = \gamma^{-1}\omega + \overset{2}{\Phi}_{\omega}(\varphi, \chi), \; \eta = \chi + \overset{3}{\Phi}_{\omega}(\varphi, \chi) \tag{4}$$

where $\overset{\tau}{\Phi}_{\omega}$ are normal in

$$\{ \varphi \in \mathbb{C}^m \mid |\operatorname{Im} \varphi_j| < \tfrac{\tau_0}{2} \} \times \{ \chi \in \mathbb{C}^{\kappa} \mid |\chi_t - b_t| < R + \tfrac{\tilde{\tau}_0}{2} \} \tag{5}$$

functions, such that diffeomorphisms of the manifold (4) induced by the mappings A and G are $(\varphi, \chi) \longmapsto (\varphi + \omega, \chi)$ and $(\varphi, \chi) \longmapsto (-\varphi, \chi)$ respectively (so that (4) is foliated into invariant under A and G spaces $\chi = const$) and the following inequality holds

$$|\overset{\tau}{\Phi}_{\omega}| < \varepsilon . \tag{6}$$

Moreover, for every two ω^1 and ω^2 in $\Omega_{\gamma,c}$ the following estimate holds

$$|\Phi^{\tau}_{\omega^1} - \Phi^{\tau}_{\omega^2}| < \gamma^{-1}|\omega^1 - \omega^2|\varepsilon . \tag{7}$$

REMARK. By factorization by the period lattice $(2\pi\mathbb{Z})^m$ one would convert spaces $\{x = \mathrm{const}\} \cap \{y \in \mathbb{R}^m\}$ into m-dimensional tori, on which the action of A is quasiperiodic, and the real part of the manifold (4) into an $(m+\varkappa)$-dimensional cylinder over an m-dimensional torus.

COROLLARY 1. Let us consider x and y to vary over T^m. Then for sufficiently small δ the measure μ of the union of the real invariant cylinders is arbitrarily close to $\mu_0 = \mathrm{mes}(T^m \times \Omega \times B_R(b))$ uniformly in γ (i.e. $\mu\mu_0^{-1} \rightrightarrows 1$).

Indeed, fix $\varepsilon > 0$, $c \in (0,1]$ and consider the mapping

$$F : T^m \times (\gamma^{-1}\Omega_{\gamma,c}) \times B_R(b) \to T^m \times \mathrm{Re}\, D_* \times \{\eta \in \mathbb{R}^{\varkappa} \mid |\eta_t - b_t| < R + \tilde{\tau}_0\}$$

defined by

$$F : (y, \omega, x) \mapsto (y + \Phi^1_{\gamma\omega}(y,x), \omega + \Phi^2_{\gamma\omega}(y,x), x + \Phi^3_{\gamma\omega}(y,x)).$$

By ω-lemma 1 $(\mathrm{mes}\,\gamma\Omega)^{-1}\,\mathrm{mes}\,\Omega_{\gamma,c} \rightrightarrows 1 \, (c \to 0)$ uniformly in $\gamma \in (0,1]$.

According to Theorem 1.1 for sufficiently small ε F has the form $id + F_0$ where F_0 satisfies a Lipschitz inequality with an arbitrarily small (uniformly in γ) constant (indeed, a Lipschitz inequality for ω is asserted by (7) and one for y and x follows from (6) with Cauchy's estimates of derivatives of a holomorphic function by the function itself). Now it remains to apply the following lemma.

LEMMA. Let S be a subset of $\mathbb{R}^N$ of a finite measure and a mapping $F: S \to \mathbb{R}^N$ be of the form $id + F_0$, where F_0 satisfies a Lipschitz inequality with constant $\nu < 1$. Then

$$\left(\frac{1-\nu}{1+\nu}\right)^N mes\, S \leq mes\, F(S) \leq (1+2\nu)^N mes\, S.$$

PROOF. Consider an arbitrary ball $B_R(b) \subset \mathbb{R}^N$ of radius R. Suppose that $Q = B \cap S \neq \emptyset$. Fix $w_0 \in Q$. For each $w \in Q$ one has the equality $F(w) = w + F_0(w_0) + F_0(w) - F_0(w_0)$. But $\|w - w_0\| \leq 2R$ which implies that $\|F_0(w) - F_0(w_0)\| \leq 2R\nu$. Thus, $F(Q)$ lies in the ball with centre $b + F_0(w_0)$ and radius $R(1+2\nu)$. This implies the right inequality.

Furthermore, on account of $\nu < 1$, F is injective. Consider $F^{-1}: F(S) \to S$, let $F_1(w) = F^{-1}(w) - w$ $(w \in F(S))$. As is easy to verify, F_1 satisfies a Lipschitz inequality with constant $\nu(1-\nu)^{-1}$. Now the left inequality can be obtained by the same reasoning as the right one. This completes the proof of the Lemma and, consequently, of Corollary 1. X

COROLLARY 2. For $\kappa = 0$ for sufficiently small δ $\sigma^2 = id$ throughout D where σ^2 is defined.

This corollary follows from the fact that σ is holomorphic and the measure of the union of the real invariant cylinders is positive for sufficiently small δ (see Corollary 1), since $\sigma^2 = id$ on these cylinders.

The main part of the proof of Theorem 1.1 is contained in the following lemma, which is used for constructing the infinite sequence of changes of variables (one at every iteration step).

All numbers $C_1, C_2, \ldots$ in the formulation and the proof of the lemma are positive constants, whose values are irrelevant. These constants depend on m and $\varkappa$ only.

§ 1.3. Main lemma

MAIN LEMMA 1. Fix $\gamma, c \in (0,1]$ and $\omega^1, \omega^2 \in \mathbb{R}^m$ of type $\mathfrak{M}_m(\gamma c, 1)$. Let $\rho, r, \tilde{\rho}, \tilde{r}, \sigma, s, d, d'$ be positive numbers such that $\rho < r \leq 1$, $\tilde{\rho} < \tilde{r} \leq 1$, $3\sigma < s < 1/4 \min\{r-\rho, \tilde{r}-\tilde{\rho}\}$, $6d < s$. In addition assume that

$$\Theta = \frac{C_1}{c^2} \frac{1}{(r-\rho)^{4m+2}} \frac{d}{s} < \frac{1}{15}.$$

Let domains D_l^i $(l \in \mathbb{Z}_+, 0 \leq l \leq 4, i \in \{1;2\})$ in $\mathbb{C}^{2m+\varkappa}$ be defined as follows

$$D_l^i = \{x \in \mathbb{C}^m \mid |\operatorname{Im} x_j| < r - \frac{r-\rho}{4} l\}$$

$$\times \{y \in \mathbb{C}^m \mid |y_j - \gamma^{-1} \omega_j^i| < s - \frac{s-\sigma}{4} l\} \times \{\eta \in \mathbb{C}^\varkappa \mid |\eta_t - b_t| < R + \tilde{r} - \frac{\tilde{r}-\tilde{\rho}}{4} l\}$$

where $b \in \mathbb{R}^\varkappa$ and $R > 0$ are fixed. Then $D_l^i \subset D_{l-1}^i$ (for $1 \leq l \leq 4$) and $D_0^i \subset \mathbb{C}^{2m+\varkappa}$.

Let A_i and B_i be mappings defined on D_0^i by the formulas (3) in which the functions f^τ and α^τ (they, as before, are assumed to be normal) are equipped with the lower index i.

Suppose that on D_0^i the following inequalities hold:

$$|f_i^\tau| < \gamma d, \quad |\alpha_i^\tau| < \gamma d. \tag{8}$$

Since $d < s/6$ and $\sigma < s/3$, one has $d + (s+\sigma)/2 < s < (r-\rho)/4$, $d < (s-\sigma)/4$ and $d < (\tilde{r}-\tilde{\rho})/4$. Therefore $A_i D_2^i \subset D_1^i$ and

$G_i D_1^i \subset D_0^i$. Thus, $A_i G_i A_i$ is defined on D_2^i.

Assume that $A_i G_i A_i = G_i$ on D_2^i (the weak reversibility condition), and if $\kappa > 0$ then assume in addition that $G_i^2 = id$ on D_1^i.

Denote by $\Delta\omega$ the difference $\Delta\omega = \omega^2 - \omega^1$ and by $\Lambda : D_0^1 \to D_0^2$ the mapping $\Lambda : (x, y, \eta) \longmapsto (x, y + \gamma^{-1}\Delta\omega, \eta)$.

Let the following inequalities hold on D_0^1 :

$$|\overset{\tau}{f}_2 \circ \Lambda - \overset{\tau}{f}_1| < |\Delta\omega| d', \quad |\overset{\tau}{\alpha}_2 \circ \Lambda - \overset{\tau}{\alpha}_1| < |\Delta\omega| d'. \tag{9}$$

The lemma states that by all these assumptions there exists a mapping $\mathcal{U}_i$ on D_1^i of the form

$$\mathcal{U}_i : (x, y, \eta) \mapsto (x + \overset{1}{\psi}_i(x, y, \eta),\ y + \overset{2}{\psi}_i(x, y, \eta),\ \eta + \overset{3}{\psi}_i(x, y, \eta)) \tag{10}$$

possessing the following properties.

a) Functions $\overset{\tau}{\psi}_i$ are normal in D_1^i and satisfy the inequality

$$|\overset{\tau}{\psi}_i| < \Theta s = \frac{C_1}{c^2} \frac{d}{(r-\rho)^{4m+2}} \tag{11}$$

on D_1^i and the inequality

$$|\overset{\tau}{\psi}_2 \circ \Lambda - \overset{\tau}{\psi}_1| < \frac{C_2}{\gamma c^2} \frac{|\Delta\omega|}{(r-\rho)^{4m+2}} \left(d' + \frac{d}{c(r-\rho)^{m+2}} \right) \tag{12}$$

on D_1^1.

b) $\mathcal{U}_i D_4^i \subset D_3^i$ and $\mathcal{U}_i^{-1} D_2^i \subset D_1^i$ (with $A_i D_3^i \subset D_2^i$ and $G_i D_3^i \subset D_2^i$ this implies that $\mathcal{U}_i^{-1} A_i \mathcal{U}_i D_4^i \subset D_1^i$ and $\mathcal{U}_i^{-1} G_i \mathcal{U}_i D_4^i \subset D_1^i$).

c) On D_4^i the mappings $\mathcal{U}_i^{-1} A_i \mathcal{U}_i$ and $\mathcal{U}_i^{-1} G_i \mathcal{U}_i$ have the form

$$\mathcal{U}_i^{-1} A_i \mathcal{U}_i : \begin{array}{l} x \\ y \mapsto \\ \eta \end{array} \begin{array}{l} x + \gamma y + \overset{1}{h}_i(x,y,\eta) \\ y + \overset{2}{h}_i(x,y,\eta) \\ \eta + \overset{3}{h}_i(x,y,\eta) \end{array} \qquad \mathcal{U}_i^{-1} B_i \mathcal{U}_i : \begin{array}{l} x \\ y \mapsto \\ \eta \end{array} \begin{array}{l} -x + \overset{1}{\beta}_i(x,y,\eta) \\ y + \overset{2}{\beta}_i(x,y,\eta) \\ \eta + \overset{3}{\beta}_i(x,y,\eta) \end{array} \tag{13}$$

where functions $\overset{\tau}{h}_i$ and $\overset{\tau}{\beta}_i$ are normal in $\overset{i}{D}_4$ and satisfy the inequalities

$$|\overset{\tau}{h}_i| < \gamma C_*, \quad |\overset{\tau}{\beta}_i| < \gamma C_* \tag{14}$$

on $\overset{i}{D}_4$ and the inequalities

$$|\overset{\tau}{h}_2 \circ \Lambda - \overset{\tau}{h}_1| < |\Delta\omega| C_{**}, \quad |\overset{\tau}{\beta}_2 \circ \Lambda - \overset{\tau}{\beta}_1| < |\Delta\omega| C_{**} \tag{I5}$$

on $\overset{1}{D}_4$, where

$$C_* = \frac{C_3}{c^2} \frac{d}{(r-\rho)^{4m+3}} \left(\frac{d}{s} + s \right), \; C_{**} = \frac{C_4}{c^5} \frac{d + d'}{(r-\rho)^{9m+7}} \left(\frac{d}{s} + s \right).$$

We will not carry out the proof of Main Lemma 1 in this section completely, namely, we shall not verify inequalities (12) and (15) (and, accordingly, not use inequalities (9)). Otherwise speaking, we will fulfil an iteration step only for one frequency vector ω . The proof of the estimate (12) showing how much changes of variables $\mathcal{U}_1$ and $\mathcal{U}_2$, corresponding to two various frequency vectors $\overset{1}{\omega}$ and $\overset{2}{\omega}$, differ (this estimate is necessary for the following proof of (7), i.e. for estimating the measure of resonance zones between invariant tori), as well as the verification of inequalities (15) (necessary for carrying out the next iteration step) are postponed by us to § 1.6. All the particular features of the reversible KAM-theory (among them, the cohomological interpretation of the existence of a change of variables greatly diminishing the perturbation) are exposed at full length by consideration of one frequency vector ω of type $\mathfrak{M}_m$.

Accordingly we will drop the index i everywhere in this section.

A. OPERATOR L.

Let W be an arbitrary set, $\tau' > 0$, and let $\mathfrak{N}$ denote the space of holomorphic and 2π-periodic in x functions $F: \{x \in \mathbb{C}^m \mid |\mathrm{Im}\, x_j| < \tau'\} \times W \to \mathbb{C}$. Denote by $\langle\ \rangle$ the average operator with respect to x:

$$\langle F \rangle(w) = (2\pi)^{-m} \int_{0 \le x_j \le 2\pi} \cdots \int F(x,w)\,dx .$$

Let $\mathfrak{N}_0 = \{F \in \mathfrak{N} \mid \langle F \rangle = 0\}$. Define the operator $L: \mathfrak{N}_0 \to \mathfrak{N}_0$ by the equality

$$(LF)(x+\omega, w) - (LF)(x,w) \equiv F(x,w).$$

Estimate LF by F. Suppose $F \in \mathfrak{N}_0$ and $|F| < C_0$ for all x and w. Let

$$F(x,w) = \sum_{q \ne 0} F_q(w) e^{i(q,x)} .$$

Then

$$(LF)(x,w) = \sum_{q \ne 0} \frac{F_q(w)}{e^{i(q,\omega)} - 1} e^{i(q,x)} .$$

In the equality $F_q = (2\pi)^{-m} \int F e^{-i(q,x)}\,dx$ shift the m-dimensional cube of integration $\{0 \leq x_j \leq 2\pi\}$ by the vector $(\pm i\tau'', \pm i\tau'', \dots, \pm i\tau'')$, where $0 < \tau'' < \tau'$. Then, with τ'' tending to τ', we obtain $|F_q| < C_0 e^{-|q|\tau'}$ for all $q \in \mathbb{Z}^m \setminus \{0\}$. Furthermore, ω is of type $\mathfrak{M}_m(\gamma c, 1)$, which implies easily that

$$\left| e^{i(q,\omega)} - 1 \right| \geq \frac{4\gamma c}{|q|^{m+1}}.$$

Now, given an arbitrary $\rho' \in (0, \tau')$, for $|\operatorname{Im} x_j| < \rho'$ we have

$$|LF| < C_0 \sum_{q \neq 0} \frac{|q|^{m+1}}{4\gamma c} e^{|q|(\rho' - \tau')}$$

$$\leq C_0 \frac{2^m}{4\gamma c} \sum_{|q|=1}^{\infty} |q|^{2m} e^{|q|(\rho'-\tau')} \leq \frac{C_5 C_0}{\gamma c} \frac{1}{(\tau' - \rho')^{2m+1}}.$$

B. HOMOLOGICAL EQUATIONS.

Main Lemma 1 asserts that by means of a fit change of variables $\mathcal{U}$, close to the identity map, we can greatly diminish the difference of perturbed mappings A and G from unperturbed ones

$$A_0 : (x, y, \eta) \mapsto (x + \gamma y, y, \eta), \quad G_0 : (x, y, \eta) \mapsto (-x, y, \eta).$$

In this item we will formulate and prove an infinitesimal analogue of this statement.

Consider the torus in $\{(x, y, \eta)\} = T^m \times \mathbb{R}^m \times \mathbb{R}^\kappa \subset (\mathbb{C}/2\pi\mathbb{Z})^m \times \mathbb{C}^m \times \mathbb{C}^\kappa$ given by the equalities $y = \gamma^{-1}\omega$, $\eta = \eta^0$. Let Z be the space of deformation fields of this torus, i.e. the space of all vectorfields on its neighbourhood in $T^m \times \mathbb{R}^m \times \mathbb{R}^\kappa$ analytic in $x \in T^m$ and (generally speaking) discontinuous in $(y,\eta)\in\mathbb{R}^m\times\mathbb{R}^k$ which is factorized by the following equivalence relation: two fields are equivalent if and only if they coincide on our torus. Elements of Z depend only on the coordinate $x\in T^m$. Since the torus under consideration is invariant under A_0 and G_0, these mappings act on Z according to formulas $A_0:\zeta\mapsto(A_0)_*\zeta$, $G_0:\zeta\mapsto(G_0)_*\zeta$, where $\zeta\in Z$.

Components of a field ζ on $T^m\times\mathbb{R}^m\times\mathbb{R}^k$ (or of an element ζ of Z) will be denoted by ζ^1, ζ^2, and ζ^3 (projections onto T^m, $\mathbb{R}^m$, and $\mathbb{R}^k$ respectively).

For the future all fields ought to be considered as elements of Z.

For an arbitrary function F on T^m symbols F_-, F_ω, and $F_{-\omega}$ will denote the following functions

$$F_-(x)=F(-x),\ F_\omega(x)=F(x+\omega),\ F_{-\omega}(x)=F(-x-\omega).$$

Assume A_0 and G_0 to be included into curves A_ε and G_ε so that $A_\varepsilon G_\varepsilon A_\varepsilon=G_\varepsilon$ for all ε. For $k>0$ assume in addition that $G_\varepsilon^2=id$ for all ε.

Define the fields $a,g\in Z$ by

$$a(x+\omega)=\frac{d}{d\varepsilon}A_\varepsilon(x,\gamma^{-1}\omega,\eta^0)_{|\varepsilon=0},$$

$$g(-x)=\frac{d}{d\varepsilon}G_\varepsilon(x,\gamma^{-1}\omega,\eta^0)_{|\varepsilon=0}.$$

Then the equality

$$\frac{d}{d\varepsilon}A_\varepsilon G_\varepsilon A_{\varepsilon\,|\varepsilon=0}=\frac{d}{d\varepsilon}G_{\varepsilon\,|\varepsilon=0} \qquad (16)$$

means that

$$(A_0)_*(G_0)_* a + (A_0)_* g + a - g = 0 \tag{17}$$

i.e.

$$-\overset{1}{a}_\omega + \gamma \overset{2}{a}_\omega + \overset{1}{g}_{-\omega} + \gamma \overset{2}{g}_{-\omega} + \overset{1}{a}_- - \overset{1}{g}_- = 0,$$

$$\overset{2}{a}_\omega + \overset{2}{g}_{-\omega} + \overset{2}{a}_- - \overset{2}{g}_- = 0, \quad \overset{3}{a}_\omega + \overset{3}{g}_{-\omega} + \overset{3}{a}_- - \overset{3}{g}_- = 0 . \tag{18}$$

PROPOSITION. There exists a curve of diffeomorphisms $\mathcal{U}_\varepsilon$ (where $\mathcal{U}_0 = id$) such that

$$\frac{d}{d\varepsilon} A_\varepsilon \mathcal{U}_{\varepsilon}{}_{|\varepsilon=0} = \frac{d}{d\varepsilon} \mathcal{U}_\varepsilon A_{0}{}_{|\varepsilon=0} ,$$

$$\frac{d}{d\varepsilon} G_\varepsilon \mathcal{U}_{\varepsilon}{}_{|\varepsilon=0} = \frac{d}{d\varepsilon} \mathcal{U}_\varepsilon G_{0}{}_{|\varepsilon=0} . \tag{19}$$

It is this proposition that means that by a normalizing change of variables the perturbation can be eliminated up to the second order of smallness.

PROOF. (19) may be transcribed in the form

$$\begin{cases} (A_0)_* \, u + a - u = 0 & (20_1) \\ (G_0)_* \, u + g - u = 0 & (20_2) \end{cases}$$

where

$$u = \frac{d}{d\varepsilon} \mathcal{U}_{\varepsilon}{}_{|\varepsilon=0} .$$

The equations (20) are called the homological equations of the original problem. We will show that on condition (17) (in the case $\varkappa > 0$ - in combination with the condition $G_\varepsilon^2 = id$) they are solvable.

Study the equation $(A_0)_* u + \tilde{u} - u = 0$, where $\tilde{u}$ is a known field and u is an unknown one. Transcribe it for every component separately:

$$\overset{1}{u} + \gamma \overset{2}{u} + \overset{\sim 1}{u}_\omega - \overset{1}{u}_\omega = 0, \quad \overset{2}{u} + \overset{\sim 2}{u}_\omega - \overset{2}{u}_\omega = 0, \quad \overset{3}{u} + \overset{\sim 3}{u}_\omega - \overset{3}{u}_\omega = 0 .$$

A solution exists if and only if $\langle \tilde{u}^2 \rangle = 0$ and $\langle \tilde{u}^3 \rangle = 0$. In this case all possible solutions are given by formulas

$$\overset{2}{u} = -\gamma^{-1} \langle \overset{\sim 1}{u} \rangle + L(\overset{\sim 2}{u}_\omega), \quad \overset{1}{u} = L(\gamma \overset{2}{u} + \overset{\sim 1}{u}_\omega) + K_1 , \tag{21}$$

$$\overset{3}{u} = L(\overset{\sim 3}{u}_\omega) + K_3 ,$$

$K_1 \in \mathbb{R}^m$ and $K_3 \in \mathbb{R}^k$ being arbitrary constants.

(18) implies that $\langle \overset{2}{a} \rangle = 0$ and $\langle \overset{3}{a} \rangle = 0$. Therefore (20_1) is solvable.

Verify that if u is a solution of (20_1) then $(G_0)_* u + g$ is a solution of (20_1) too. We have to show that $(A_0)_* (G_0)_* u + (A_0)_* g + a - (G_0)_* u - g = 0$. By (17) this equality is equivalent to $(A_0)_* (G_0)_* u - (G_0)_* u - (A_0)_* (G_0)_* a = 0$. But $(A_0)_* (G_0)_* (u - (A_0)_* u - a) = 0$ because u is a solution of (20_1). In view of $A_0 G_0 A_0 = G_0$ we obtain the desired relation.

Thus, if u is a solution of (20_1) then $(G_0)_* u + g$ is a solution of (20_1) too. If, besides that, the following equalities hold

$$\begin{cases} \langle \overset{1}{u} \rangle = \langle \overset{1}{((G_0)_* u)} + \overset{1}{g} \rangle & (22_1) \\ \langle \overset{3}{u} \rangle = \langle \overset{3}{((G_0)_* u)} + \overset{3}{g} \rangle & (22_2) \end{cases}$$

then on account of (21) $u = (G_0)_* u + g$, i.e. u is a solution of (20_2). Note that $(G_0)_* u = (-\overset{1}{u}_-, \overset{2}{u}_-, \overset{3}{u}_-)$. Hence (22_1) is equivalent to $\langle \overset{1}{u} \rangle = \frac{1}{2}\langle \overset{1}{g} \rangle$ and (22_2) is equivalent to $\langle \overset{3}{g} \rangle = 0$.

Let $\kappa > 0$. Then the equality

$$\frac{d}{d\varepsilon} \sigma^2_{\varepsilon}\Big|_{\varepsilon=0} = 0 \tag{23}$$

means that

$$(\sigma_0)_* g + g = 0 \tag{24}$$

i.e. $\overset{1}{g}_- = \overset{1}{g}, \overset{2}{g}_- = -\overset{2}{g}, \overset{3}{g}_- = -\overset{3}{g}$. This follows that $\langle \overset{3}{g} \rangle = 0$ (and $\langle \overset{2}{g} \rangle = 0$), so that (22_2) is valid.

Thus, (20) has solutions

$$\overset{2}{u} = -\gamma^{-1}\langle \overset{1}{a} \rangle + L\overset{2}{a}_\omega, \quad \overset{1}{u} = \frac{1}{2}\langle \overset{1}{g} \rangle + L(\gamma \overset{2}{u} + \overset{1}{a}_\omega),$$
$$\overset{3}{u} = K_3 + L\overset{3}{a}_\omega, \tag{25}$$

$K_3 \in \mathbb{R}^\kappa$ being an arbitrary constant.

If $\kappa = 0$ then a solution of (20) is unique. X

REMARK. The solvability of (20_2) in combination with $\sigma_0^2 = id$ implies that (24) holds, i.e. (23) is valid. Indeed, if u is a solution of (20_2) then $(\sigma_0)_* g + g = (\sigma_0)_*(u - (\sigma_0)_* u) + u - (\sigma_0)_* u = 0$. Thus, while for $\kappa > 0$ one has to require (in addition to (16)) that the curves A_ε and σ_ε satisfy (23), for $\kappa = 0$ this condition is not only needless, but even follows from the equality (16) meaning that A_ε is weakly reversible with respect to σ_ε.

C. COHOMOLOGIC INTERPRETATION.

Let Π be the group of diffeomorphisms generated by A_0 and σ_0 which acts on Z by linear isomorphisms (the homomorphism $\Pi \to \mathrm{Aut}\, Z$ is defined by $A_0 \mapsto (A_0)_*$, $\sigma_0 \mapsto (\sigma_0)_*$). Π is an arithmetical progression's symmetry group. It can be included into the short exact sequence $0 \to \mathbb{Z} \to \Pi \to \mathbb{Z}_2 \to 0$ and is one of three nonisomorphic expansions of $\mathbb{Z}$ by means of $\mathbb{Z}_2$ (the other two possible expansions are abelian groups $\mathbb{Z} \oplus \mathbb{Z}_2$ and $\mathbb{Z}$).

In this item Z will be considered as a $\mathbb{Z}$-module, although it is equipped with the $\mathbb{R}$-module structure.

The action of Π on Z equips Z with the Π-module structure.

It turns out that the solvability of homological equations (20) on conditions (17) and (24) (for the case $\kappa=0$ (24) is a consequence of (17)) is equivalent to

$$H^1(\Pi, Z)=0$$

where the cohomology has the usual meaning, see, e.g. [38 (Chapter 4, § 5)] .

Indeed, as is easy to verify, all one-dimensional cocycles $F:\Pi\to Z$ have the form

$$F(A_0^n)=\sum_{p=0}^{n-1}(A_0^p)_* a-\sum_{p=n}^{-1}(A_0^p)_* a$$

$$F(A_0^n G_0)=(A_0^n)_* g+F(A_0^n) \tag{26}$$

$(n\in\mathbb{Z})$, where a and g are arbitrary elements of Z satisfying relations (17) and (24). At the same time the equations (20) mean that the cocycle F given by such a way is the coboundary of the element $u\in Z$. Thus $H^1(\Pi, Z)=0$ is equivalent to the solvability of (20) on conditions (17) and (24).

D. WEAK REVERSIBILITY CONDITION .

Return to the perturbed mappings A and G defined on D_0 . First of all observe that by Cauchy's formula

$$\left|\frac{\partial f^\tau}{\partial x_j}\right|<\frac{4\gamma d}{(\tau-\rho)\ell}<\frac{\gamma d}{s\ell}\ ,\qquad \left|\frac{\partial f^\tau}{\partial y_j}\right|<\frac{4\gamma d}{(s-\sigma)\ell}<\frac{6\gamma d}{s\ell}\ ,$$

$$\left|\frac{\partial f^{\tau}}{\partial \eta_t}\right| < \frac{4\gamma d}{(\tilde{\tau}-\tilde{\rho})\ell} < \frac{\gamma d}{s\ell}$$

on D_ℓ , where $1 \leqslant \ell \leqslant 4$, and exactly the same estimates are valid for derivatives of α^{τ}.

For an arbitrary function F defined on D_0 symbols F_-, F_ω, and $F_{-\omega}$ will denote the following functions

$$F_-(x,y,\eta) = F(-x,y,\eta),$$

$$F_\omega(x,y,\eta) = F(x+\omega,y,\eta), \; F_{-\omega}(x,y,\eta) = F(-x-\omega,y,\eta).$$

The mapping GA has the form

$$GA : (x,y,\eta) \mapsto (-x-\gamma y-\overset{1}{f}+\overset{1}{\alpha}\circ A,\; y+\overset{2}{f}+\overset{2}{\alpha}\circ A,\; \eta+\overset{3}{f}+\overset{3}{\alpha}\circ A)$$

and the equality $AGA = G$ may be written down in the following way

$$\begin{cases} \gamma\overset{2}{f}-\overset{1}{f}+\gamma\overset{2}{\alpha}\circ A+\overset{1}{\alpha}\circ A+\overset{1}{f}\circ GA=\overset{1}{\alpha} \\ \overset{2}{f}+\overset{2}{\alpha}\circ A+\overset{2}{f}\circ GA=\overset{2}{\alpha} \\ \overset{3}{f}+\overset{3}{\alpha}\circ A+\overset{3}{f}\circ GA=\overset{3}{\alpha} . \end{cases}$$

Let $(x,y,\eta) \in D_3$. Then $GA(x,y,\eta) \in D_1$, which implies that on D_3

$$|\overset{\tau}{f}\circ GA-\overset{\tau}{f}_{-\omega}| < \left(m\left(\sigma+\frac{s-\sigma}{4}\right)+2d\right)\frac{4\gamma^2 d}{\tau-\rho}+\frac{12\gamma^2 d^2}{s}+\frac{8\gamma^2 d^2}{\tilde{\tau}-\tilde{\rho}}$$

$$< C_6\,\gamma^2 d\left(\frac{d}{s}+\frac{s}{\tau-\rho}\right).$$

Besides that, $A(x,y,\eta)\in D_2$, and therefore on D_3

$$|\overset{\tau}{\alpha}\circ A-\overset{\tau}{\alpha}_\omega|$$

$$<\left(m\left(\sigma+\frac{s-\sigma}{4}\right)+d\right)\frac{2\gamma^2 d}{\tau-\rho}+\frac{3\gamma^2 d^2}{s}+\frac{2\gamma^2 d^2}{\tilde{\tau}-\tilde{\rho}}<C_7\gamma^2 d\left(\frac{d}{s}+\frac{s}{\tau-\rho}\right).$$

Thus, on D_3

$$\begin{cases}\gamma\overset{2}{f}-\overset{1}{f}+\gamma\overset{2}{\alpha}_\omega+\overset{1}{\alpha}_\omega+\overset{1}{f}_{-\omega}-\overset{1}{\alpha}=\overset{1}{\delta}\\ \overset{2}{f}+\overset{2}{\alpha}_\omega+\overset{2}{f}_{-\omega}-\overset{2}{\alpha}=\overset{2}{\delta}\\ \overset{3}{f}+\overset{3}{\alpha}_\omega+\overset{3}{f}_{-\omega}-\overset{3}{\alpha}=\overset{3}{\delta}\end{cases}\tag{27}$$

where

$$|\overset{\tau}{\delta}|<C_8\gamma^2 d\left(\frac{d}{s}+\frac{s}{\tau-\rho}\right).$$

E. INVOLUTIVITY PROPERTY OF σ FOR $\kappa>0$.

The relation $\sigma^2=id$ can be transcribed in the form

$$\begin{cases}-\overset{1}{\alpha}+\overset{1}{\alpha}\circ\sigma=0\\ \overset{2}{\alpha}+\overset{2}{\alpha}\circ\sigma=0\\ \overset{3}{\alpha}+\overset{3}{\alpha}\circ\sigma=0\end{cases}.$$

For later use we will need only an estimate of $\langle\overset{3}{\alpha}\rangle$ on D_2. Let $(x,y,\eta)\in D_2$. Then $\sigma(x,y,\eta)\in D_1$, and on D_2 we obtain

$$|\overset{\tau}{\alpha}\circ\sigma-\overset{\tau}{\alpha}_-|<\gamma^2 d^2\left(\frac{4}{\tau-\rho}+\frac{6}{s}+\frac{4}{\tilde{\tau}-\tilde{\rho}}\right).$$

Consequently on D_2 $\overset{3}{\alpha}+\overset{3}{\alpha}_-=\overset{4}{\delta}$, where $|\overset{4}{\delta}|<2C_9\gamma^2 d^2 s^{-1}$, and $|\langle \alpha^3 \rangle| < C_9 \gamma^2 d^2 s^{-1}$.

F. MAPPING $\mathcal{U}$.

Following (25), we set

$$\begin{cases} \psi^2 = -\gamma^{-1} \langle f^1 \rangle + L(f^2 - \langle f^2 \rangle) \\ \psi^1 = \frac{1}{2} \langle \alpha^1 \rangle + L(\gamma \psi^2 + f^1) \\ \psi^3 = L(f^3 - \langle f^3 \rangle) \end{cases} \tag{28}$$

and define $\mathcal{U}$ by $\mathcal{U} : (x, y, \eta) \mapsto (x + \psi^1, y + \psi^2, \eta + \psi^3)$.

$\mathcal{U}$ is defined on D_0, but we estimate ψ^τ only on D_1.

In virtue of the estimates in the item A

$$|\psi^2| < d + \frac{2C_5 d}{c} \left(\frac{16}{\tau - \rho} \right)^{2m+1}$$

on the domain

$$D_{0.25} = \left\{ (x, y, \eta) \in D_0 \mid |\operatorname{Im} x_j| < \tau - \frac{\tau - \rho}{16} \right\} .$$

Now on the domain

$$D_{0.5} = \left\{ (x, y, \eta) \in D_0 \mid |\operatorname{Im} x_j| < \tau - \frac{\tau - \rho}{8} \right\}$$

we can estimate ψ^1 and ψ^3 :

$$|\psi^1| < \frac{\gamma d}{2} + \frac{2C_5 d}{c} \left(\frac{16}{\tau - \rho} \right)^{2m+1} \left(1 + \frac{C_5}{c} \left(\frac{16}{\tau - \rho} \right)^{2m+1} \right),$$

$$|\psi^3| < \frac{2C_5 d}{c} \left(\frac{8}{\tau - \rho} \right)^{2m+1} .$$

Finally on the domain $D_{0.5}$ we obtain the estimate

$$|\psi^{\tau}| < \frac{C_1}{c^2}\,\frac{d}{(\tau-\rho)^{4m+2}} = \Theta s\,.$$

By Cauchy's formula on D_1

$$\left|\frac{\partial\psi^{\tau}}{\partial x_j}\right| < \frac{8\Theta s}{\tau-\rho} < 2\Theta\,,$$

$$\left|\frac{\partial\psi^{\tau}}{\partial y_j}\right| < \frac{4\Theta s}{s-\sigma} < 6\Theta\,,\quad \left|\frac{\partial\psi^{\tau}}{\partial \eta_t}\right| < \frac{4\Theta s}{\tilde{\tau}-\tilde{\rho}} < \Theta.$$

G. THE INVERSE OF $\mathcal{U}$.

First of all verify that $\mathcal{U}D_4 \subset D_3$. We have to show that $\Theta s < \frac{1}{4}\min\{\tau-\rho,\, s-\sigma,\, \tilde{\tau}-\tilde{\rho}\}$. On account of $\Theta < \frac{1}{6}$ this is true, as $s < \frac{1}{4}\min\{\tau-\rho,\ \tilde{\tau}-\tilde{\rho}\}$ and $s/6 < (s-\sigma)/4$.

Prove that $\mathcal{U}^{-1}$ is defined on D_2 and maps D_2 into D_1. Let $w=(x,y,\eta)\in D_2$. Find $\tilde{w}=(\tilde{x},\tilde{y},\tilde{\eta})\in D_1$ such that $w=\mathcal{U}\tilde{w}$. If a point $\tilde{w}$ exists then it is obviously unique.

Construct an infinite sequence of points $w^n=(x^n,y^n,\eta^n)$, $n\in\mathbb{Z}_+$, in the following way. Set $w^0=w$ and then by induction $w^{n+1}=w+w^n-\mathcal{U}(w^n)$.

We wish to show that w^n is defined and lies in $D_1\setminus O(\partial D_1)$, $O(\partial D_1)$ being some neighbourhood of ∂D_1 in $\mathbb{C}^{2m+k}$, for all $n\in\mathbb{Z}_+$. Introduce the notation

$$\Delta_n = \max\{\,|x^{n+1}-x^n|,\,|y^{n+1}-y^n|,\,|\eta^{n+1}-\eta^n|\,\}.$$

Fix $n\in\mathbb{Z}_+$. Suppose that $w^p\in D_1$ for all p, $0\le p\le n$, and prove that $w^{n+1}\in D_1$. For all p, $1\le p\le n$,

$$\Delta_p < 2\Theta|x^{p} - x^{p-1}| + 6\Theta|y^{p} - y^{p-1}| + \Theta|\eta^{p} - \eta^{p-1}| \leq 9\Theta\Delta_{p-1}.$$

By $\Delta_0 < \Theta s$ and $\Theta(1-9\Theta)^{-1} < 1/6$ (for $\Theta < 1/15$) this implies that

$$\max\{|x^{n+1} - x|, |y^{n+1} - y|, |\eta^{n+1} - \eta|\}$$

$$< \Theta s \sum_{p=0}^{n} (9\Theta)^{p} < \frac{\Theta s}{1-9\Theta} < \frac{s}{6} < \frac{1}{4} \min\{r-\rho, s-\sigma, \tilde{r}-\tilde{\rho}\},$$

i.e. $w^{n+1} \in D_1$.

Thus, $w^{n} \in D_1 \setminus O(\partial D_1)$ for all $n \in \mathbb{Z}_+$. Now in virtue of $\Delta_p < 9\Theta\Delta_{p-1} < 3/5\,\Delta_{p-1}$ the sequence (w^{n}) tends to a point $\tilde{w}$, as $n \to \infty$. The point $\tilde{w}$ is the desired one. It is obvious that it depends on w holomorphically.

H. ESTIMATE OF $\mathcal{U}^{-1}A\,\mathcal{U}$.

Let for $(x, y, \eta) \in D_4$ the mapping $\tilde{A} = \mathcal{U}^{-1}A\,\mathcal{U}$ be written in the form (13). Transcribe the equality $\mathcal{U}\tilde{A} = A\,\mathcal{U}$ in a more detailed way:

$$h^{1} = \psi^{1} - \psi^{1}\circ\tilde{A} + \gamma\psi^{2} + f^{1}\circ\mathcal{U}, \quad h^{2} = \psi^{2} - \psi^{2}\circ\tilde{A} + h^{2}\circ\mathcal{U},$$

$$h^{3} = \psi^{3} - \psi^{3}\circ\tilde{A} + h^{3}\circ\mathcal{U}.$$

Represent h^{τ} as $h^{\tau} = h^{\tau,1} + h^{\tau,2} + h^{\tau,3}$, where

$$h^{1,1} = f^{1} + \psi^{1} - \psi^{1}_{\omega} + \gamma\psi^{2}, \; h^{2,1} = \psi^{2} - \psi^{2}_{\omega} + f^{2}, \; h^{3,1} = \psi^{3} - \psi^{3}_{\omega} + f^{3},$$

$$h^{\tau,2} = f^{\tau}\circ\mathcal{U} - f^{\tau}, \; h^{\tau,3} = \psi^{\tau}_{\omega} - \psi^{\tau}\circ\tilde{A}.$$

By the definition of ψ^{τ} we have $h^{1,1} = 0$, $h^{2,1} = \langle f^{2}\rangle$, $h^{3,1} = \langle f^{3}\rangle$. By (27) $\langle f^{2}\rangle = 1/2\,\langle \delta^{2}\rangle$ and $\langle f^{3}\rangle = 1/2\,\langle \delta^{3}\rangle$. Thus,

$$|h^{\tau,1}| < \frac{1}{2} C_8 \gamma^2 d\left(\frac{d}{s} + \frac{s}{\tau-\rho}\right).$$

Furthermore,

$$|h^{\tau,2}| < \Theta s \gamma d\left(\frac{4}{3(\tau-\rho)} + \frac{2}{s} + \frac{4}{3(\tilde{\tau}-\tilde{\rho})}\right) < \frac{8}{3}\gamma d\Theta,$$

$$|h^{\tau,3}| < \frac{8\Theta s}{\tau-\rho}(m\gamma\sigma + |h^1|) + 6\Theta|h^2| + \Theta|h^3|$$

$$< \frac{8m\gamma}{3}\,\frac{\Theta s^2}{\tau-\rho} + 2\Theta|h^1| + 6\Theta|h^2| + \Theta|h^3|.$$

Recalling the definition of Θ we obtain the system of equations

$$|h^\tau| = 2\Theta|h^1| + 6\Theta|h^2| + \Theta|h^3| + \varepsilon_\tau$$

where numbers ε_τ satisfy the inequalities

$$\varepsilon_\tau < \frac{C_{10}\gamma}{c^2}\,\frac{d}{(\tau-\rho)^{4m+3}}\left(\frac{d}{s} + s\right).$$

The solution of these equations is

$$\begin{cases} |h^1| = \dfrac{1}{1-9\Theta}\left((1-7\Theta)\varepsilon_1 + 6\Theta\varepsilon_2 + \Theta\varepsilon_3\right) \\[2ex] |h^2| = \dfrac{1}{1-9\Theta}\left(2\Theta\varepsilon_1 + (1-3\Theta)\varepsilon_2 + \Theta\varepsilon_3\right) \\[2ex] |h^3| = \dfrac{1}{1-9\Theta}\left(2\Theta\varepsilon_1 + 6\Theta\varepsilon_2 + (1-8\Theta)\varepsilon_3\right). \end{cases}$$

With $\Theta < 1/15$ this provides the desired estimate of h^τ.

I. Estimate of $\mathcal{U}^{-1}\mathcal{G}\mathcal{U}$.

Let for $(x, y, \eta) \in D_4$ the mapping $\tilde{\mathcal{G}} = \mathcal{U}^{-1}\mathcal{G}\mathcal{U}$ be written in the form (13). Transcribe the equality $\mathcal{U}\tilde{\mathcal{G}} = \mathcal{G}\mathcal{U}$ in a more detailed way:

$$\beta^1 = -\psi^1 \circ \tilde{\mathcal{G}} - \psi^1 + \alpha^1 \circ \mathcal{U}, \quad \beta^2 = -\psi^2 \circ \tilde{\mathcal{G}} + \psi^2 + \alpha^2 \circ \mathcal{U}, \quad \beta^3 = -\psi^3 \circ \tilde{\mathcal{G}} + \psi^3 + \alpha^3 \circ \mathcal{U}.$$

Represent β^τ as $\beta^\tau = \beta^{\tau,1} + \beta^{\tau,2} + \beta^{\tau,3}$, where

$$\beta^{1,1} = -\psi^1_- - \psi^1 + \alpha^1, \quad \beta^{2,1} = -\psi^2_- + \psi^2 + \alpha^2, \quad \beta^{3,1} = -\psi^3_- + \psi^3 + \alpha^3,$$

$$\beta^{\tau,2} = \alpha^\tau \circ \mathcal{U} - \alpha^\tau, \quad \beta^{\tau,3} = \psi^\tau_- - \psi^\tau \circ \tilde{\mathcal{G}}.$$

Firstly estimate $\beta^{\tau,1}$. By the definition (28) of ψ^1 we have $\psi^1_\omega - \psi^1 = \gamma\psi^2 + f^1$ (it is equivalent to $\psi^1_{-\omega} - \psi^1_- = -\gamma\psi^2_{-\omega} - f^1_{-\omega}$) and $2\langle\psi^1\rangle = \langle\alpha^1\rangle$ (whence $\langle\beta^{1,1}\rangle = 0$). Therefore $\beta^{1,1} = LI$,where

$$I = \gamma\psi^2_{-\omega} + f^1_{-\omega} - \gamma\psi^2 - f^1 + \alpha^1_\omega - \alpha^1.$$

Represent I in the form $I = I^1 + I^2 + I^3$, where

$$I^1 = \gamma(\psi^2_- - \psi^2 - \alpha^2 + \langle\alpha^2\rangle),$$

$$I^2 = \gamma\psi^2_{-\omega} - \gamma\psi^2_- + \gamma\alpha^2 + f^1_{-\omega} - f^1 + \alpha^1_\omega - \alpha^1, \quad I^3 = -\gamma\langle\alpha^2\rangle.$$

$\langle I^1\rangle = 0$, consequently the definition (28) of ψ^2 easily implies that $I^1 = \gamma L(\langle\delta^2\rangle - \delta^2)$ and $I^2 = \gamma\langle f^2\rangle - \gamma f^2_{-\omega} + \gamma\alpha^2 + f^1_{-\omega} - f^1 + \alpha^1_\omega - \alpha^1 = (\gamma/2)\langle\delta^2\rangle - \gamma\delta^2 + \delta^1$. Finally, $I^3 = (\gamma/2)\langle\delta^2\rangle - \langle\delta^1\rangle$ (for the definition of δ^τ see (27)).

As is easy to verify, $\beta^{2,1} = -\gamma^{-1}(I^1 + I^3)$. To estimate $\beta^{3,1}$ for

$\varkappa > 0$ we represent $\beta^{3,1}$ as $\beta^{3,1} = I^4 + \langle \alpha^3 \rangle$, where $I^4 = -\psi^3_- + \psi^3 + \alpha^3 - \langle \alpha^3 \rangle$. The definition (28) of ψ^3 in combination with $\langle I^4 \rangle = 0$ implies $I^4 = L(\delta^3 - \langle \delta^3 \rangle)$.

Now we can apply the estimates of quantities δ^τ on D_3, obtained in the item D, and the estimate of $\langle \alpha^3 \rangle$ (for $\varkappa > 0$) on $D_2 \supset D_4$, obtained in the item E.

The functions I^2 and I^3 can be estimated immediately. To estimate the functions I^4 on D_4 and I^1 on

$$\{(x,y,\eta) \in D_3 \,\|\, |\operatorname{Im} x_j| < \rho + \frac{r-\rho}{8}\} = D_{3.5}$$

one has to use properties of the operator L established in the item A. Now $|\beta^{2,1}| \leq \gamma^{-1}(|I^1| + |I^3|)$ and $|\beta^{3,1}| \leq |I^4| + |\langle \alpha^3 \rangle|$ have been estimated. Possessing the estimate of I on $D_{3.5}$ and appealing to the item A again we obtain an estimate of $\beta^{1,1}$. Realizing this programme explicitly we find

$$|\beta^{\tau,1}| < \frac{C_{11}\gamma}{c^2} \frac{d}{(r-\rho)^{4m+3}} \left(\frac{d}{s} + s\right).$$

Analogously to the item H $|\beta^{\tau,2}| < 8/3 \, \gamma d \Theta$ and $|\beta^{\tau,3}| < 2\Theta|\beta^1| + 6\Theta|\beta^2| + \Theta|\beta^3|$, after which the desired estimate of β^τ can be obtained by the same reasoning as that of h^τ.

This completes the proof of Main Lemma 1 (without (12) and (15)).

REMARK. $\alpha^\tau = 0$ does not imply $\beta^\tau = 0$, since $\sigma = \sigma_0$ does not imply $\gamma f^2 - f^1 + f^1_{-\omega} = 0$, $f^2 + f^2_{-\omega} = 0$, $f^3 + f^3_{-\omega} = 0$ (i.e. $\delta^\tau = 0$). If for $\alpha^\tau = 0$ we want β^τ to equal 0 too, i.e. $\mathcal{U}$ to commute with σ_0, we have to require ψ^2 and ψ^3 to be even and ψ^1 to be odd with respect to x. This can be secured by setting

$$\begin{cases} \psi^2 = -\gamma^{-1}\langle f^1\rangle + \frac{1}{2} L(f^2 - f^2_{-\omega}) \\ \psi^1 = \frac{1}{2} L(\gamma\psi^2 + \gamma\psi^2_{-\omega} + f^1 + f^1_{-\omega}) \\ \psi^3 = \frac{1}{2} L(f^3 - f^3_{-\omega}) \end{cases} \tag{29}$$

instead of (28).

All the estimates and their proofs are similar to those for (28).

An infinitesimal analogue to this remark is the following one. Rewrite the equations (17) and (20) for $g=0$:

$$(A_0)_* (G_0)_* a + a = 0 , \tag{30}$$

$$\begin{cases} (A_0)_* u + a - u = 0 \\ (G_0)_* u - u = 0 . \end{cases} \tag{31}$$

In virtue of (30) the system of equations (31) can be transcribed in the form

$$\begin{cases} (A_0)_* u - u + \frac{1}{2}(a - (A_0)_* (G_0)_* a) = 0 \\ (G_0)_* u - u = 0 . \end{cases} \tag{32}$$

It is easy to verify that (32) has a solution (unique, if $\varkappa=0$) independently whether (30) is valid.

§ 1.4. Termination of the proof of the principal theorem

Fix a constant $s_* \in (0,1]$ such that for each $\omega' \in \Omega$

$$\{y \in \mathbb{C}^m \mid |y_j - \omega'_j| < 2s_*\} \subset D_* .$$

Let arbitrary $\varepsilon > 0$ be fixed. Introduce into consideration the following three constants:

$$T_0 = \max\{1, C_3 c^{-2} \tau_0^{-4m-3} 2^{8m+7}, C_4 c^{-5} \tau_0^{-9m-7} 2^{18m+16}\}, \tag{33}$$

an appropriate constant $d_* \in (0,1]$ depending only on $\tau_0, \tilde{\tau}_0$ and c (we shall not present its precise value) and constant

$$d_0 = \min\{d_*, s_*^{3/2}, \varepsilon^{3/2}\}. \tag{34}$$

If the constant d_* is small enough then one can take the number $d_0 s_*$ as the desired constant δ of the formulation of Theorem 1.1.

Indeed, suppose on D $|f^\tau| < \gamma d_0 s_*$ and $|\alpha^\tau| < \gamma d_0 s_*$.

Define sequences $(d_n), (s_n), (\tau_n)$, and $(\tilde{\tau}_n)$ of positive numbers $(n \in \mathbb{Z}_+)$ in the following way:

$$d_n = T_0^n d_{n-1}^{4/3} \ (n \in \mathbb{N}), \tag{35}$$

$$s_n = d_n^{2/3} \ (n \in \mathbb{Z}_+), \tag{36}$$

$$\tau_n = \frac{\tau_0}{2}(1 + 2^{-n}), \quad \tilde{\tau}_n = \frac{\tilde{\tau}_0}{2}(1 + 2^{-n}) (n \in \mathbb{N}) \tag{37}$$

(for $n = 0$ equalities (37) are identities).

The sequences (τ_n) and $(\tilde{\tau}_n)$ obviously decrease, and $\tau_n \to \tau_0/2$, $\tilde{\tau}_n \to \tilde{\tau}_0/2$ $(n \to \infty)$. Observe that $\tau_n - \tau_{n+1} = \tau_0 2^{-n-2}$, $\tilde{\tau}_n - \tilde{\tau}_{n+1} = \tilde{\tau}_0 2^{-n-2}$.

Set $e_n = T_0^{3n+12} d_n$ for all $n \in \mathbb{Z}_+$, then by (35) $e_{n+1} = e_n^{4/3}$. If $d_* \geq d_0$ is sufficiently small (namely, $d_* < T_0^{-12}$) then $e_0 < 1$. Therefore (e_n) decreases and tends to 0 as

$n \to \infty$. The sequences $(d_n) = (e_n T_0^{-3n-12})$ and (s_n) possess the same property (because of $T_0 \geq 1$ and (36)).

Now using Main Lemma 1 we for each $\omega \in \Omega_{\gamma,C}$ are able to construct a suitable infinite sequence of changes of variables normalizing A and G . To have an opportunity to compare at every iteration step changes of variables, corresponding to different ω's , we carry out the iteration process simultaneously for two frequency vectors in $\Omega_{\gamma,C}$.

Thus, let us fix arbitrary $\omega^1, \omega^2 \in \Omega_{\gamma,C}$.

Define domains $D^i_{(n)}$ $(n \in \mathbb{Z}_+)$ in $\mathbb{C}^{2m+\kappa}$ in the following way:

$$D^i_{(n)} = \{x \in \mathbb{C}^m \mid |\mathrm{Im}\, x_j| < \tau_n\} \times \{y \in \mathbb{C}^m \mid |y_j - \gamma^{-1}\omega^i_j| < s_n\}$$

$$\times \{\eta \in \mathbb{C}^\kappa \mid |\eta_t - b_t| < R + \tilde{\tau}_n\}.$$

Furthermore, let

$$D^i_\infty = \{(x, \gamma^{-1}\omega^i, \eta) \in \mathbb{C}^{2m+\kappa} \mid |\mathrm{Im}\, x_j| < \frac{\tau_0}{2},\ |\eta_t - b_t| < R + \frac{\tilde{\tau}_0}{2}\}.$$

The properties of sequences $(\tau_n), (\tilde{\tau}_n)$ and (s_n) proved above imply that $D^i_{(0)} \supset D^i_{(1)} \supset D^i_{(2)} \supset \ldots$ and

$$\bigcap_{n=0}^{\infty} D^i_{(n)} = D^i_\infty .$$

Besides that, $d_0 \leq s_*^{3/2}$ implies $s_0 \leq s_*$, whence $D^i_{(0)} \subset D$.

Denote by $\Delta\omega$ the difference $\Delta\omega = \omega^2 - \omega^1$ and by $\Lambda : D^1_{(0)} \to D^2_{(0)}$ the mapping $\Lambda : (x, y, \eta) \mapsto (x, y + \gamma^{-1}\Delta\omega, \eta)$.

Set $A^{(0)}_i = A$ and $G^{(0)}_i = G$. For all $n \in \mathbb{Z}_+$ we apply Main

Lemma 1 to domains $D^{i}_{(n)}$ and mappings $A^{(n)}_i$ and $\mathcal{B}^{(n)}_i$ defined on them, setting $\tau=\tau_n$, $\rho=\tau_{n+1}$, $\tilde{\tau}=\tilde{\tau}_n$, $\tilde{\rho}=\tilde{\tau}_{n+1}$, $s=s_n$, $\sigma=s_{n+1}$, $d=d'=d_n$ in this lemma, supposing that

$$|f^{(n),\tau}_i|<\gamma d_n\,,\quad |\alpha^{(n),\tau}_i|<\gamma d_n \tag{38}$$

on $D^{i}_{(n)}$ and

$$|f^{(n),\tau}_2\circ\Lambda-f^{(n),\tau}_1|<|\Delta\omega|d_n\,,\ |\alpha^{(n),\tau}_2\circ\Lambda-\alpha^{(n),\tau}_1|<|\Delta\omega|d_n \tag{39}$$

on $D^{1}_{(n)}$ and preparing the next iteration step by setting

$$A^{(n+1)}_i=(\mathcal{U}^{(n)}_i)^{-1}A^{(n)}_i\,\mathcal{U}^{(n)}_i\,,\ \mathcal{B}^{(n+1)}_i=(\mathcal{U}^{(n)}_i)^{-1}\mathcal{B}^{(n)}_i\,\mathcal{U}^{(n)}_i$$

where $\mathcal{U}^{(n)}_i : D^{i}_{(n+1)}\to D^{i}_{(n)}$.

We have to check the assumptions of Main Lemma 1, i.e. inequalities

$$\tau_{n+1}<\tau_n\le 1\ ,\ \tilde{\tau}_{n+1}<\tilde{\tau}_n\le 1,$$

$$3s_{n+1}<s_n<2^{-n-6}\min\{\tau_0,\tilde{\tau}_0\}\,,\ 6d_n<s_n, \tag{40}$$

$$\Theta_n=C_1c^{-2}\tau_0^{-4m-2}2^{(4m+2)(n+2)}d_n s_n^{-1}<1/15\,.$$

The first two inequalities in (40) are obvious. In view of (36) we have to verify

$$3d_{n+1}^{2/3}<d_n^{2/3}<2^{-n-6}\min\{\tau_0,\tilde{\tau}_0\}\ ,\ d_n^{1/3}<1/6\ ,$$

$$C_1c^{-2}\tau_0^{-4m-2}2^{(4m+2)(n+2)}d_n^{1/3}<1/15$$

or

$$d_n > 3^{3/2} d_{n+1}, \; d_n^{2/3} < 2^{-n-6} \min\{r_0, \tilde{r}_0\}, \; d_n < \frac{1}{216},$$

$$d_n^{1/3} < \frac{1}{15} C_1^{-1} c^2 r_0^{4m+2} 2^{-(4m+2)(n+2)} . \tag{41}$$

Since

$$d_n = e_0^{(4/3)^n} T^{-3n-12},$$

where $e_0 = T_0^{12} d_0$, for sufficiently small $d_* \geq d_0$ all inequalities (41) hold.

Besides that, we have to prove the inequalities (38) and (39) (by induction). For $n = 0$ inequality (38) is valid, since $s_* \leq 1$. By Cauchy's formula on the domain

$$\{x \in \mathbb{C}^m \,|\, |\mathrm{Im}\, x_j| < r_0\} \times \bigcup_{\omega' \in \Omega} \{y \in \mathbb{C}^m \,|\, |y_j - \omega'_j|$$

$$\leq s_*\} \times \{\eta \in \mathbb{C}^\kappa \,|\, |\eta_t - b_t| < R + \tilde{r}_0\}$$

estimates

$$\left|\frac{\partial f^\tau}{\partial y_j}\right| < \gamma d_0 \quad \text{and} \quad \left|\frac{\partial \alpha^\tau}{\partial y_j}\right| < \gamma d_0$$

hold. Therefore inequality (39) is also valid for $n = 0$.

For passage from n to $n+1$ we have to verify that

$$C_3 c^{-2} r_0^{-4m-3} 2^{(4m+3)(n+2)} (d_n^{4/3} + d_n^{5/3}) \leq d_{n+1}$$

and

$$2C_4 c^{-5} \tau_0^{-9m-7} 2^{(9m+7)(n+2)} (d_n^{4/3} + d_n^{5/3}) \le d_{n+1}$$

according to (14) and (15).

Since $d_n \le d_0 \le d_* \le 1$, in view of (35) it suffices to establish

$$2C_3 c^{-2} \tau_0^{-4m-3} 2^{(4m+3)(n+2)} \le T_0^{n+1} ,$$

$$4C_4 c^{-5} \tau_0^{-9m-7} 2^{(9m+7)(n+2)} \le T_0^{n+1} ,$$

but these two inequalities hold because of (33).

Set $\varphi_i^{(n)} = \mathcal{U}_i^{(0)} \circ \mathcal{U}_i^{(1)} \circ \dots \circ \mathcal{U}_i^{(n)}$. The mapping $\varphi_i^{(n)}$ is defined on $D^i_{(n+1)}$. Let on $D^i_{(n+1)}$

$$\varphi_i^{(n)} : \begin{array}{l} x \longmapsto x + H_i^{(n),1}(x, y, \eta) \\ y \longmapsto y + H_i^{(n),2}(x, y, \eta) \\ \eta \longmapsto \eta + H_i^{(n),3}(x, y, \eta) . \end{array}$$

$H_i^{(n),\tau}$ are normal in $D^i_{(n+1)}$ functions. Estimate $H_i^{(n),\tau}$ on $D^i_{(n+1)}$ and $H_2^{(n),\tau} \circ \Lambda - H_1^{(n),\tau}$ on $D^1_{(n+1)}$.

It is clear that $H_i^{(0),\tau} = \psi_i^{(0),\tau}$. Let $n \ge 1$. The equality $\varphi_i^{(n)} = \varphi_i^{(n-1)} \circ \mathcal{U}_i^{(n)}$ implies that on $D^i_{(n+1)}$

$$H_i^{(n),\tau} = \psi_i^{(n),\tau} + H_i^{(n-1),\tau} \circ \mathcal{U}_i^{(n)} . \tag{42}$$

By (11) $|\psi_i^{(n),\tau}| < \Theta_n s_n < s_n/15$ on $D^i_{(n+1)}$. Consequently one can obtain by induction that on $D^i_{(n+1)}$

$$| H_i^{(n),\tau} | < \frac{1}{15}\sum_{p=0}^{n} s_p < \frac{s_0}{15}\sum_{p=0}^{n}\frac{1}{3^p} < \frac{s_0}{10} . \qquad (43)$$

Estimate the derivatives of $H_i^{(n),\tau}$ on $D^i_{(n+1)}$. Let

$$\rho_n^1 = \max_{\tau,i,j} \sup_{D^i_{(n+1)}} \left| \frac{\partial H_i^{(n),\tau}}{\partial x_j} \right| ,$$

$$\rho_n^2 = \max_{\tau,i,j} \sup_{D^i_{(n+1)}} \left| \frac{\partial H_i^{(n),\tau}}{\partial y_j} \right| ,$$

$$\rho_n^3 = \max_{\tau,i,t} \sup_{D^i_{(n+1)}} \left| \frac{\partial H_i^{(n),\tau}}{\partial \eta_t} \right| .$$

Show by induction that for all $n \geq 0$

$$\rho_n^1 + \rho_n^2 + \rho_n^3 < \prod_{p=0}^{n} (1 + 9\Theta_p) - 1 . \qquad (44)$$

For $n = 0$, the inequality (44) is fulfilled, since

$$\left| \frac{\partial \psi_i^{(n),\tau}}{\partial x_j} \right| < 2\Theta_n , \quad \left| \frac{\partial \psi_i^{(n),\tau}}{\partial y_j} \right| < 6\Theta_n , \quad \left| \frac{\partial \psi_i^{(n),\tau}}{\partial \eta_t} \right| < \Theta_n$$

on $D^i_{(n+1)}$ for all n (see § 1.3,F).

Let $n \geq 1$. Since $\mathcal{U}_i^{(n)} D^i_{(n+1)} \subset D^i_{(n)}$ it follows that (42) implies

$$\left|\frac{\partial H_i^{(n),\tau}}{\partial x_j}\right| < 2\Theta_n + (1+2\Theta_n)\overset{1}{P}_{n-1} + 2\Theta_n \overset{2}{P}_{n-1} + 2\Theta_n \overset{3}{P}_{n-1},$$

$$\left|\frac{\partial H_i^{(n),\tau}}{\partial y_j}\right| < 6\Theta_n + 6\Theta_n \overset{1}{P}_{n-1} + (1+6\Theta_n)\overset{2}{P}_{n-1} + 6\Theta_n \overset{3}{P}_{n-1},$$

$$\left|\frac{\partial H_i^{(n),\tau}}{\partial z_t}\right| < \Theta_n + \Theta_n \overset{1}{P}_{n-1} + \Theta_n \overset{2}{P}_{n-1} + (1+\Theta_n)\overset{3}{P}_{n-1}$$

on $D^i_{(n+1)}$.

Thus, $\overset{1}{P}_n + \overset{2}{P}_n + \overset{3}{P}_n < (1+9\Theta_n)(\overset{1}{P}_{n-1} + \overset{2}{P}_{n-1} + \overset{3}{P}_{n-1}) + 9\Theta_n$. We have proved the inequality (44) for all n. Note that (44) implies

$$\overset{1}{P}_n + \overset{2}{P}_n + \overset{3}{P}_n < \left(\frac{8}{5}\right)^n - 1$$

for all n.

Introduce the notation

$$Q_n = C_2 c^{-2} \tau_0^{-4m-2}\, 2^{(4m+2)(n+2)}\left(1 + c^{-1}\tau_0^{-m-2}\, 2^{(m+2)(n+2)}\right),$$

$n \geq 0$. Note that by $c \leq 1$ and $\tau_0 \leq 1$

$$Q_n < C_2 c^{-3} \tau_0^{-5m-4}\, 2^{(5m+4)(n+2)+1}.$$

Now in view of (12) and (42) one has on $D^1_{(n+1)}$

$$|H_2^{(n),\tau}\circ\Lambda - H_1^{(n),\tau}| \leq |\Psi_2^{(n),\tau}\circ\Lambda - \Psi_1^{(n),\tau}|$$

$$+|H_2^{(n-1),\tau}\circ\mathcal{U}_2^{(n)}\circ\Lambda - H_2^{(n-1),\tau}\circ\Lambda\circ\mathcal{U}_1^{(n)}| + |H_2^{(n-1),\tau}\circ\Lambda\circ\mathcal{U}_1^{(n)} - H_1^{(n-1),\tau}\circ\mathcal{U}_1^{(n)}|$$

$$<\gamma^{-1}|\Delta\omega|Q_n d_n(1+\overset{1}{P}_n+\overset{2}{P}_n+\overset{3}{P}_n)+\sup_{D^1_{(n)}}|H_2^{(n-1),\tau}\circ\Lambda - H_1^{(n-1),\tau}|$$

for $n\geq 1$. Besides, in view of (12) on $D^1_{(1)}$

$$|H_2^{(0),\tau}\circ\Lambda - H_1^{(0),\tau}| < \gamma^{-1}|\Delta\omega|Q_0 d_0 .$$

If $d_*\geq d_0$ is small enough then for all $n\in\mathbb{Z}_+$ the inequality

$$d_n^{1/3} < C_2^{-1} c^3 \tau_0^{5m+4}\, 2^{-(5m+4)(n+2)-4n-3}\, 5^n$$

holds. It implies

$$Q_n d_n(1+\overset{1}{P}_n+\overset{2}{P}_n+\overset{3}{P}_n) < \left(\frac{8}{5}\right)^n Q_n d_n < \frac{s_n}{2^{n+2}} \leq \frac{s_0}{2^{n+2}} .$$

Consequently, if d_* is small enough then on $D^1_{(n+1)}$

$$|H_2^{(n),\tau}\circ\Lambda - H_1^{(n),\tau}| < \gamma^{-1}|\Delta\omega|s_0\sum_{p=0}^{n}\frac{1}{2^{p+2}} < \frac{1}{2}\gamma^{-1}|\Delta\omega|s_0 \tag{45}$$

for all $n\in\mathbb{Z}_+$.

Up to now, we followed the constructions of [22 (§ 32)]. Prove the convergence of $\varphi_{\mathcal{J}_i}^{(n)}$ on D^i_∞ as $n\to\infty$. We remark that there is an inadvertence in the convergence analysis in [22, 24].

Namely, it is maintained in [22, 24] (for $m=1$, $\kappa=0$ and using the notations different from ours) that the convergence of $\mathcal{G}_i^{(n)}$ follows from

$$\sum_{n=0}^{\infty} \sup_{D_\infty^i} |\Psi_i^{(n),\tau}| < \infty .$$

But the fact is that this is not sufficient because by (42) $|H_i^{(n),\tau} - H_i^{(n-1),\tau}|$ is bounded from above not by $|\Psi_i^{(n),\tau}|_1$ but by

$$|\Psi_i^{(n),\tau}|_1 + \left|\frac{\partial H_i^{(n-1),\tau}}{\partial x_j}\right|_2 |\Psi_i^{(n),1}|_1 + \left|\frac{\partial H_i^{(n-1),\tau}}{\partial y_j}\right|_2 |\Psi_i^{(n),2}|_1 + \left|\frac{\partial H_i^{(n-1),\tau}}{\partial \eta_t}\right|_3 |\Psi_i^{(n),3}|_1 ,$$

where

$$|\,|_1 = \sup_{D_\infty^i} |\,| , \quad |\,|_2 = \max_j \sup_{\mathcal{U}_i^{(n)} D_\infty^i} |\,| , \quad |\,|_3 = \max_t \sup_{\mathcal{U}_i^{(n)} D_\infty^i} |\,| .$$

$\mathcal{U}_i^{(n)} D_\infty^i \subset \mathcal{U}_i^{(n)} D_{(n+1)}^i \subset D_{(n)}^i$, therefore by (11) and (44) on D_∞^i

$$|H_i^{(n),\tau} - H_i^{(n-1),\tau}| < \Theta_n s_n (1 + \rho_n^1 + \rho_n^2 + \rho_n^3) < \frac{s_n}{15}\left(\frac{8}{5}\right)^n .$$

One sees

$$\sum_{n=1}^{\infty} \left(\frac{8}{5}\right)^n s_n < \infty$$

since

$$s_n = e_0^{(2/3)(4/3)^n} T_0^{-2n-8}$$

decay faster than a geometrical progression. Thus, $H_i^{(n),\tau}$ converge on D_∞^i to normal functions to be denoted by $\Phi_{\omega^i}^\tau$. These functions depend on two arguments x and η only. The manifold (4) is the desired one. Furthermore, by (43) $|\Phi_{\omega^i}^\tau| \leq s_0/10$ and by (45) $|\Phi_{\omega^2}^\tau - \Phi_{\omega^1}^\tau| \leq \frac{1}{2}\gamma^{-1}|\Delta\omega| s_0$. Since $s_0 = d_0^{2/3} \leq \varepsilon$, the inequalities (6) and (7) hold.

This completes the proof of Theorem 1.1.

REMARK. All statements of Theorem 1.1 remain true (up to obvious slight modifications of some formulas) if the mapping A on D has the form

$$A: \begin{array}{l} x \\ y \\ \eta \end{array} \longmapsto \begin{array}{l} x+\theta+\gamma y+f^1(x,y,\eta) \\ y+f^2(x,y,\eta) \\ \eta+f^3(x,y,\eta) \end{array}$$

differing from (3) by the presence of a constant $\theta \in \mathbb{R}^m$.

Replacing the coordinate y by $\tilde{y} = y + \gamma^{-1}\theta$ we reduce the mapping A to the form (3).

§ 1.5. Reversible diffeomorphisms of a plane

The case $m=1$, $\kappa=0$ of Theorem 1.1 ought to be considered more narrowly. On a plane $\mathbb{R}^2$ introduce polar coordinates (x,y), $x \bmod 2\pi$ and y being an angular coordinate and a polar radius, respectively. Let $D \subset \mathbb{R}^2$ be an annulus with center at the origin. As is well known, the existence of invariant circles of a diffeomorphism $A: D \to D$, sufficiently close to the twist rotation

$A_0 : (x,y) \to (x+\theta+\gamma y, y)$, follows from the so called intersection property: every closed curve $y = y(x)$ lying in the annulus intersects its A-image (see [21 (Lecture 3), 22 (§§ 32-34), 24, 26]). A symplectic (area-preserving) diffeomorphism A possesses the intersection property automatically.

We show now that the weak reversibility (and even the reversibility) does not imply, generally speaking, the intersection property. For convenience we give an appropriate example in Cartesian coordinates (u,v) . Let the rectangle with apices (u_0, v_0), $(-u_0, v_0)$, $(-u_0,-v_0)$, $(u_0,-v_0)$ be denoted by $[u_0, v_0]$. Consider the domain D bounded by two rectangles $[\pi,\pi]$ and $[3\pi, 3\pi]$ (that is homeomorphic to an annulus) and the function $F: \mathbb{R} \to \mathbb{R}$, $F(t) = t+\sin t$. Let $F^{-1}: \mathbb{R} \to \mathbb{R}$ denote the inverse of F . Setting $A(u,v) = (F(u), F^{-1}(v))$, $G(u,v) = (v,u)$ we obtain the desired mappings A and G . Indeed, it is obvious that $G^2 = id$ and $GAG = A^{-1}$. On the other hand, A maps the rectangle $\Gamma = [3\pi/2, 5\pi/2]$ onto the rectangle $\Gamma' = [3\pi/2-1, F^{-1}(5\pi/2)]$ lying strictly inside Γ (since $F(5\pi/2) = 5\pi/2+1$ and, consequently, $F^{-1}(5\pi/2) < 5\pi/2$).

Of course, in this example the mapping A does not look like a twist rotation at all. I don't know whether there exist reversible (or weakly reversible) diffeomorphisms arbitrarily close to a twist rotation, for which the intersection property fails. Seemingly such diffeomorphisms do not exist. Formulate this conjecture in an exact manner.

CONJECTURE. Let the smooth mapping A given on an annulus $D = S^1 \times (a,b)$ be weakly reversible with respect to a smooth diffeomorphism $G: D \to S^1 \times \mathbb{R}$, A and G being of the form

$$A: \begin{pmatrix} x \\ y \end{pmatrix} \mapsto \begin{pmatrix} x+\theta+\gamma y+f^1(x,y) \\ y+f^2(x,y) \end{pmatrix} \qquad G: \begin{pmatrix} x \\ y \end{pmatrix} \mapsto \begin{pmatrix} -x+\alpha^1(x,y) \\ y+\alpha^2(x,y) \end{pmatrix}$$

where $\gamma > 0$, $\theta \in S^1$, x is an angular coordinate on S^1 and y is a coordinate on $(a,b) \subset \mathbb{R}$.

Then for each fixed γ there exists a positive δ depending on the interval (a,b) but not on the angle θ, such that if $|f^\tau| < \delta$ and $|\alpha^\tau| < \delta$ on D then A possesses the intersection property.

Remark that in any case the intersection property of the mapping A does not provide us with Kolmogorov circles, common for A and G.

§ 1.6. Appendix

In this section we prove inequalities (12) and (15) of Main Lemma 1. We shall use notations of the items A, D-F, H-I of § 1.3.

A'. Operators L^i.

Let sets W, $\mathfrak{M}$, $\mathfrak{M}_0$ and the operator L, as well as the number $\omega \in \mathbb{R}^m$, be equipped with the upper index $i \in \{1;2\}$. Given a bijection $\Lambda_0 : W^1 \longrightarrow W^2$, denote by Λ the mapping $\Lambda : (x, w) \mapsto (x, \Lambda_0(w))$, where $x \in \mathbb{C}^m$, $|\operatorname{Im} x_j| < \tau'$, and $w \in W^1$.

Let $F^i \in \mathfrak{M}_0^i$. Estimate $(L^2F^2)\circ\Lambda - L^1F^1$ by F^1, F^2 and $F^2\circ\Lambda - F^1$. Suppose $|F^i| < C_0$ and $|F^2\circ\Lambda - F^1| < |\Delta\omega|\, C_0'$. Then

$$|F_q^i| < C_0 e^{-|q|\tau'} \quad \text{and} \quad |F_q^2\circ\Lambda_0 - F_q^1| < |\Delta\omega|\, C_0' e^{-|q|\tau'}$$

for all $q \in \mathbb{Z}^m \setminus \{0\}$, where $F_q^i(w)$ denote coefficients of the Fourier series expansions for F^i, $w \in W^i$. In view of

$$|e^{i(q,\omega^i)} - 1| \geqslant \frac{4\gamma C}{|q|^{m+1}}$$

we have

$$\left| \frac{F_q^2 \circ \Lambda_0}{e^{i(q,\omega^2)}-1} - \frac{F_q^1}{e^{i(q,\omega^1)}-1} \right|$$

$$\leq |F_q^1| \frac{|e^{i(q,\omega^1)} - e^{i(q,\omega^2)}|}{|e^{i(q,\omega^2)}-1| \, |e^{i(q,\omega^1)}-1|} + \frac{|F_q^2 \circ \Lambda_0 - F_q^1|}{|e^{i(q,\omega^2)}-1|}$$

$$\leq \left(\frac{C_0 |\Delta\omega| |q|^{2m+3}}{16\gamma^2 c^2} + \frac{C_0' |\Delta\omega| |q|^{m+1}}{4\gamma c} \right) e^{-|q|\tau'} .$$

Hence, for $|\operatorname{Im} x_j| < \rho' < \tau'$

$$|(\overset{2}{L}\overset{2}{F}) \circ \Lambda - \overset{1}{L}\overset{1}{F}|$$

$$< \frac{C_{12} C_0 |\Delta\omega|}{\gamma^2 c^2} \frac{1}{(\tau'-\rho')^{3m+3}} + \frac{C_5 C_0' |\Delta\omega|}{\gamma c} \frac{1}{(\tau'-\rho')^{2m+1}} .$$

D'. Weak reversibility condition.

Return to the perturbed mappings A_i and G_i defined on D_0^i. From now on, $\Lambda : D_0^1 \to D_0^2$, $\Lambda : (x, y, \eta) \mapsto (x, y + \gamma^{-1}\Delta\omega, \eta)$.

Adopt the following notation agreement. For any functions F_1 and F_2 defined on D_0^1 and D_0^2 respectively we will denote the difference $F_2 \circ \Lambda - F_1$ on D_0^1 by ΔF.

We equip the functions δ^τ in (27) with the lower index i. The goal of this item is to estimate $\Delta\delta^\tau$. To do it we need the following lemma.

Δ-LEMMA. Let F_i be a normal function in $D_{l_1}^i$ and K_i be a mapping $K_i : D_l^i \longrightarrow D_{l_1}^i$ of the form

$$K_i : \begin{array}{ccc} x & & \mu x + \nu \gamma y + u_i^1(x,y,\eta) \\ y & \longmapsto & y + u_i^2(x,y,\eta) \\ \eta & & \eta + u_i^3(x,y,\eta) \end{array}$$

where μ_i and ν_i are real numbers and u_i^τ are normal functions.

Let $\xi_i : D_0^i \to D_0$, $\xi_i : (x,y,\eta) \mapsto (\mu_i x + \nu_i \omega, y, \eta)$ and

$$* F_i(x,y,\eta) = F_i(x+\nu\Delta\omega, y, \eta) - F_i(x,y,\eta),\ (x,y,\eta) \in D_{\ell_1}^i .$$

Then on D_ℓ^1

$$|\Delta(F\circ K - F\circ\xi)|$$

$$\leqslant \left(\left| \frac{\partial * F_1}{\partial x_j} \right| + \left| \frac{\partial * F_1}{\partial y_j} \right| + \left| \frac{\partial * F_1}{\partial \eta_t} \right| + \left| \frac{\partial \Delta F}{\partial x_j} \right| + \left| \frac{\partial \Delta F}{\partial y_j} \right| + \left| \frac{\partial \Delta F}{\partial \eta_t} \right| \right) |u_i^\tau|$$

$$+ \left(\left| \frac{\partial * F_1}{\partial x_j} \right| + \left| \frac{\partial \Delta F}{\partial x_j} \right| \right) |\nu| \gamma m s + \left| \frac{\partial F_1}{\partial x_j} \right| |\Delta u^1| + \left| \frac{\partial F_1}{\partial y_j} \right| |\Delta u^2| + \left| \frac{\partial F_1}{\partial \eta_t} \right| |\Delta u^3| \quad (46)$$

where we dropped on the right hand side the symbols of taking suprema over definition domains of all the functions involved and maxima over indices i, j, t, τ lest the inequality would be immense.

PROOF. We have

$$|\Delta(F\circ K - F\circ\xi)| = |F_2\circ K_2\circ\Lambda - F_2\circ\xi_2\circ\Lambda - F_1\circ K_1 + F_1\circ\xi_1|$$

$$\leqslant |F_1\circ\zeta\circ K_1 - F_1\circ K_1 - F_1\circ\hat{\xi} + F_1\circ\xi_1| \quad (47)$$

$$+ |F_2\circ K_2\circ\Lambda - F_1\circ\Lambda^{-1}\circ K_2\circ\Lambda - F_2\circ\xi_2\circ\Lambda + F_1\circ\hat{\xi}|$$

$$+ |F_1\circ\Lambda^{-1}\circ K_2\circ\Lambda - F_1\circ\zeta\circ K_1| ,$$

where

$$\hat{\xi} : \overset{1}{D}_0 \to \overset{1}{D}_0 , \quad \hat{\xi} : (x,y,\eta) \mapsto (\mu x + \nu \overset{2}{\omega}, y, \eta),$$

$$\zeta : \overset{1}{D}_0 \to \overset{1}{D}_0 , \quad \zeta : (x,y,\eta) \mapsto (x + \nu \Delta\omega, y, \eta).$$

Estimate three terms of the right hand side of (47) separately. In view of $*F_1 = F_1 \circ \zeta - F_1$ and $\hat{\xi} = \zeta \circ \xi_1$, the first term equals $|*F_1 \circ K_1 - *F_1 \circ \xi_1|$, which is bounded by

$$\left|\frac{\partial * F_1}{\partial x_j}\right| (|\nu| \gamma m (s - \frac{s-\sigma}{4} \ell) + |\overset{1}{u}_1|) + \left|\frac{\partial * F_1}{\partial y_j}\right| |\overset{2}{u}_1| + \left|\frac{\partial * F_1}{\partial \eta_t}\right| |\overset{3}{u}_1| .$$

In view of $\xi_2 \circ \Lambda = \Lambda \circ \hat{\xi}$ the second term equals $|\Delta F \circ \Lambda^{-1} \circ K_2 \circ \Lambda - \Delta F \circ \hat{\xi}|$, which is bounded by

$$\left|\frac{\partial \Delta F}{\partial x_j}\right| (|\nu| \gamma m (s - \frac{s-\sigma}{4} \ell) + |\overset{1}{u}_2|) + \left|\frac{\partial \Delta F}{\partial y_j}\right| |\overset{2}{u}_2| + \left|\frac{\partial \Delta F}{\partial \eta_t}\right| |\overset{3}{u}_2| .$$

The third term is bounded by

$$\left|\frac{\partial F_1}{\partial x_j}\right| |\Delta \overset{1}{u}| + \left|\frac{\partial F_1}{\partial y_j}\right| |\Delta \overset{2}{u}| + \left|\frac{\partial F_1}{\partial \eta_t}\right| |\Delta \overset{3}{u}| .$$

Putting these estimates together we obtain the desired inequality (46). X

To estimate $\Delta \delta^{\tau}$ we have to estimate $\Delta(\alpha^{\tau} \circ A - \alpha^{\tau}_{\omega})$ and $\Delta(f^{\tau} \circ GA - f^{\tau}_{-\omega})$.

Derivatives of $\Delta \alpha^{\tau}$ and Δf^{τ} on $\overset{1}{D}_{\ell}, 1 \le \ell \le 4$, can be estimated by Cauchy' s formula.

Apply Δ-lemma to $F_i = \overset{\tau}{\alpha}_i$, $K_i = A_i$ $(\mu = 1,\ \nu = 1,\ \overset{\tau}{u}_i = \overset{\tau}{f}_i)$. By Cauchy's formula on domain D_1^1 $|*\overset{\tau}{\alpha}_1| < 4\gamma d|\Delta\omega|/(\tau-\rho)$. Using Cauchy's formula again, on D_2^1 one can estimate derivatives of $*\overset{\tau}{\alpha}_1$. Now in virtue of (46) we obtain on D_3^1

$$|\Delta(\overset{\tau}{\alpha}\circ A - \overset{\tau}{\alpha}_\omega)| < \frac{C_{13}\gamma|\Delta\omega|(d+d')}{(\tau-\rho)^2}\left(\frac{d}{s}+s\right).$$

Apply Δ-lemma to $F_i = \overset{\tau}{f}_i$, $K_i = G_i A_i$ $(\mu = -1,\ \nu = -1,\ \overset{1}{u}_i = -\overset{1}{f}_i + \overset{1}{\alpha}_i \circ A_i$, $\overset{2}{u}_i = \overset{2}{f}_i + \overset{2}{\alpha}_i \circ A_i$, $\overset{3}{u}_i = \overset{3}{f}_i + \overset{3}{\alpha}_i \circ A_i)$. By Cauchy's formula on domain $D_{0.5}^1$ (for its definition see the item F of § 1.3) $|*\overset{\tau}{f}_1| < 8\gamma d^1|\Delta\omega|/(\tau-\rho)$. Now, using Cauchy's formula again, on D_1^1 one can estimate derivatives of $*\overset{\tau}{f}_1$. To profit by Δ-lemma it remains to estimate $\overset{\tau}{u}_i$ on D_3^i and $\Delta\overset{\tau}{u}$ on D_3^1. It is obvious that on D_3^i $|\overset{\tau}{u}_i| < 2\gamma d$. On D_3^1 we have

$$|\Delta\overset{\tau}{u}| \leq |\Delta\overset{\tau}{f}| + |\Delta(\overset{\tau}{\alpha}\circ A)| = |\Delta\overset{\tau}{f}| + |\overset{\tau}{\alpha}_2\circ A_2\circ\Lambda - \overset{\tau}{\alpha}_1\circ A_1|$$

$$\leq |\Delta\overset{\tau}{f}| + |\overset{\tau}{\alpha}_2\circ A_2\circ\Lambda - \overset{\tau}{\alpha}_2\circ\Lambda\circ A_1| + |\overset{\tau}{\alpha}_2\circ\Lambda\circ A_1 - \overset{\tau}{\alpha}_1\circ A_1|$$

$$\leq |\Delta\omega|d' + \frac{2\gamma d}{\tau-\rho}|\Delta\omega|(1+d') + \frac{3\gamma d}{s}|\Delta\omega|d' + \frac{2\gamma d}{\tilde{\tau}-\tilde{\rho}}|\Delta\omega|d' + |\Delta\omega|d'$$

$$< C_{14}|\Delta\omega|\left(\frac{d}{\tau-\rho}+d'\right)$$

(we used $d < s/6$, $d < (\tau-\rho)/24$ and $d < (\tilde{\tau}-\tilde{\rho})/24$). Now in virtue of (46) we obtain on D_3^1

$$|\Delta(\overset{\tau}{f}\circ GA - \overset{\tau}{f}_{-\omega})| < \frac{C_{15}\gamma|\Delta\omega|(d+d')}{(\tau-\rho)^2}\left(\frac{d}{s}+s\right).$$

Thus, on D_3^1

$$|\Delta \delta^\tau| < \frac{C_{16}\, \gamma\, |\Delta\omega|(d+d')}{(\tau-\rho)^2}\left(\frac{d}{s}+s\right).$$

E'. Involutivity property of G for $\kappa>0$.

Let the function $\delta^4 = \alpha^3 + \alpha_-^3 = \alpha_-^3 - \alpha^3 \circ G$ be equipped with the lower index i. Estimate $\Delta\langle\alpha^3\rangle = \frac{1}{2}\langle\Delta\delta^4\rangle$ on D_2^1. Apply Δ-lemma to $F_i = \alpha_i^3$, $K_i = G_i$ ($\mu=-1, \nu=0, u_i^\tau = \alpha_i^\tau$). In this case $*\alpha_i^3 = 0$, and in virtue of (46) we obtain on D_2^1

$$|\Delta\langle\alpha^3\rangle| < C_{17}\,\gamma\,|\Delta\omega| d d' s^{-1}.$$

F'. Mappings U_i.

In this item we prove the inequality (12) for $|\Delta\Psi^\tau|$. On account of the estimates of the item A' we have on the domain $D_{0.25}^1$

$$|\Delta\Psi^2| < \frac{|\Delta\omega| d'}{\gamma} + \frac{2C_{12}\, d\,|\Delta\omega|}{\gamma c^2}\left(\frac{16}{\tau-\rho}\right)^{3m+3}$$

$$+\ \frac{2C_5\, d'\,|\Delta\omega|}{\gamma c}\left(\frac{16}{\tau-\rho}\right)^{2m+1}.$$

Now on the domain $D_{0.5}^1$ we can estimate $\Delta\Psi^1$ and $\Delta\Psi^3$:

$$|\Delta\Psi^1| < \frac{|\Delta\omega| d'}{2} + \frac{2C_{12}\, d\,|\Delta\omega|}{\gamma c^2}\left(\frac{16}{\tau-\rho}\right)^{3m+3}\left(1+\frac{C_5}{c}\left(\frac{16}{\tau-\rho}\right)^{2m+1}\right)$$

$$+\ \frac{2C_5\,|\Delta\omega|}{\gamma c}\left(\frac{16}{\tau-\rho}\right)^{2m+1}\left(d' + \frac{C_{12}\, d}{c^2}\left(\frac{16}{\tau-\rho}\right)^{3m+3} + \frac{C_5\, d'}{c}\left(\frac{16}{\tau-\rho}\right)^{2m+1}\right),$$

$$|\Delta\Psi^3| < \frac{2C_{12}\, d\,|\Delta\omega|}{\gamma c^2}\left(\frac{8}{\tau-\rho}\right)^{3m+3}$$

$$+\frac{2C_5 d'|\Delta\omega|}{\gamma c}\left(\frac{8}{\tau-\rho}\right)^{2m+1} .$$

Finally on the domain $D^1_{0.5}$ we obtain the desired estimate (12). For later use the following less delicate estimate of $\Delta\Psi^\tau$ will suffice: on $D^1_{0.5}$

$$|\Delta\Psi^\tau| < \frac{C_{18}|\Delta\omega|}{\gamma c^3}\,\frac{d+d'}{(\tau-\rho)^{5m+4}} .$$

H'. Estimate of $\mathcal{U}_i^{-1} A_i \mathcal{U}_i$.

In this and the next items we shall prove (without detailed calculations) the estimate (15).

Estimate Δh^τ. In view of the result of the item D' on D^1_4

$$|\Delta h^{\tau,1}| < \frac{C_{16}\gamma|\Delta\omega|(d+d')}{2(\tau-\rho)^2}\left(\frac{d}{s}+s\right).$$

To estimate $\Delta h^{\tau,2}$ we apply Δ-lemma to $F_i = f_i^\tau$, $K_i = \mathcal{U}_i$ $(\mu=1, \nu=0, u_i^\tau = \Psi_i^\tau)$. In this case $*f_i^\tau = 0$, and we obtain on D^1_4

$$|\Delta h^{\tau,2}| < \frac{C_{19}\, d(d+d')}{c^3 s}\,\frac{|\Delta\omega|}{(\tau-\rho)^{5m+4}} .$$

To estimate $\Delta h^{\tau,3}$ we apply Δ-lemma to $F_i = \Psi_i^\tau$, $K_i = \tilde{A}_i$ $(\mu=1, \nu=1, u_i^\tau = h_i^\tau)$. By Cauchy's formula one can estimate $*\Psi_i^\tau$ on

$$\left\{(x,y,\eta)\in D_0^i \;\middle|\; |\operatorname{Im} x_j| < \tau - \frac{3}{16}(\tau-\rho)\right\}$$

and, after this, derivatives of $*\Psi_1^\tau$ and $\Delta\Psi^\tau$ on D^1_1. The functions h_i^τ on D^i_4 have been already estimated (14). Realizing this programme explicitly and minding $d < 1/6 \min\{s, (\tau-\rho)/4, (\tilde{\tau}-\tilde{\rho})/4\}$

we find in virtue of (46) that on D_4^1

$$|\Delta h^{\tau,3}| < \frac{C_{20}(d+d')|\Delta\omega|}{c^5(\tau-\rho)^{9m+7}}\left(\frac{d}{s}+s\right)+2\Theta|\Delta h^1|+6\Theta|\Delta h^2|+\Theta|\Delta h^3| .$$

We obtain the system of equations

$$|\Delta h^{\tau}| = 2\Theta|\Delta h^1|+6\Theta|\Delta h^2|+\Theta|\Delta h^3|+\varepsilon'_{\tau}$$

where

$$\varepsilon'_{\tau} < \frac{C_{21}(d+d')}{c^5}\,\frac{|\Delta\omega|}{(\tau-\rho)^{9m+7}}\left(\frac{d}{s}+s\right).$$

Now the same reasoning as at the end of the item H of § 1.3 provides us with the desired estimate of Δh^{τ}.

I'. Estimate of $\mathcal{U}_i^{-1}\,\sigma_i\,\mathcal{U}_i$.

Estimate $\Delta\beta^{\tau}$. We have

$$\beta_i^{1,1} = L^i(I_i^1+I_i^2+I_i^3),$$

where

$$I_i^1=\gamma L^i(\langle\delta_i^2\rangle-\delta_i^2),\quad I_i^2=\frac{\gamma}{2}\langle\delta_i^2\rangle-\gamma\delta_i^2+\delta_i^1,\quad I_i^3=\frac{\gamma}{2}\langle\delta_i^2\rangle-\langle\delta_i^1\rangle,$$

$$\beta_i^{2,1}=-\gamma^{-1}(I_i^1+I_i^3)$$

and for $\kappa>0$

$$\beta_i^{3,1}=L^i(\delta_i^3-\langle\delta_i^3\rangle)+\langle\alpha_i^3\rangle .$$

Now using the estimates of δ_i^τ on D_3^i, $\Delta\delta^\tau$ on D_3^1, $\Delta\langle d^3\rangle$ on D_2^1 for $\varkappa > 0$, established by us before, and properties of the operator L^i we can estimate $\Delta\beta^{\tau,1}$ on D_4^1. Omitting lengthy calculations write down the result:

$$|\Delta\beta^{\tau,1}| < \frac{C_{22}(d+d')}{c^3}\frac{|\Delta\omega|}{(\tau-\rho)^{5m+5}}\left(\frac{d}{5}+5\right).$$

One can estimate $\Delta\beta^{\tau,2}$ similarly to $\Delta h^{\tau,2}$ and $\Delta\beta^{\tau,3}$ similarly to and even more simply than $\Delta h^{\tau,3}$ (since applying Δ-lemma to $F_i=\psi_i^\tau$, $K_i=\tilde{G}_i$ ($\mu=1, \nu=0, u_i^\tau=\beta_i^\tau$) we have $*\psi_i^\tau=0$). As a result one obtains for $\Delta\beta^{\tau,2}$ and $\Delta\beta^{\tau,3}$ on D_4^1 the same estimates as for $\Delta h^{\tau,2}$ and $\Delta h^{\tau,3}$ (with another constants C_{23} and C_{24} in place of C_{19} and C_{20} respectively). The concluding step of reasoning, providing the desired estimate of $\Delta\beta^\tau$, is the same as in the item H'.

Part 2

The continuous time case: Kolmogorov tori of perturbations of reversible vectorfields

§ 1.7. Preliminaries

Let $K>0$, $\varepsilon>0$. A number $\omega\in\mathbb{R}^m$ is called a number of type $\mathcal{H}_m(K,\varepsilon)$, if for all $q\in\mathbb{Z}^m\setminus\{0\}$ the following inequality holds

$$|(q,\omega)| \geqslant \frac{K}{|q|^{m-1+\varepsilon}}.$$

The following lemma is well known from the Diophantine approximations theory.

ω-LEMMA 2. Let $C>0, R>0$ and let $B_R \subset \mathbb{R}^m$ be a ball of radius R. Then for each fixed $\varepsilon>0$

$$\frac{\operatorname{mes}\{\omega\in B_R \mid \omega \text{ is of type } \mathcal{H}_m(Rc,\varepsilon)\}}{\operatorname{mes} B_R} \Rightarrow 1 \ (c\to 0)$$

uniformly with respect to $R>0$ and to all balls B_R.

We shall use the following standard abridged notations: if $Y=(Y_1,\ldots,Y_N)$ and a function F depends on $X=(X_1,\ldots,X_N)$ (and possibly on some other variables) then

$$YF_X = Y\frac{\partial F}{\partial X} = \sum_{\nu=1}^{N} Y_\nu \frac{\partial F}{\partial X_\nu} .$$

Analogously we shall write down a vectorfield:

$$Y\frac{\partial}{\partial X} = \sum_{\nu=1}^{N} Y_\nu \frac{\partial}{\partial X_\nu} .$$

Now consider a domain $D\subset \mathbb{R}^{2m+\kappa}$; a smooth diffeomorphism $G: D\to D$ and a smooth vectorfield V on D, reversible with respect to G ($G_* V = -V$) , such that D is smoothly foliated into m-dimensional tori, which are invariant under the flow of V and the action of G . Suppose that one has chosen in D a coordinate system (x, w) , where $x=(x_1,\ldots,x_m)$ are angular coordinates on T^m defined $\operatorname{mod} 2\pi$ and $w=(w_1,\ldots,w_{m+\kappa})$ are coordinates on a domain in the space $\mathbb{R}^{m+\kappa}$, such that these tori are given by equalities $w=\text{const}$ and

$$V=\omega(w)\frac{\partial}{\partial x}, \quad \sigma:(x,w)\mapsto(F(x,w),w) \tag{48}$$

(i.e. the flow induced by V on each torus is quasiperiodic).

A vectorfield V defined by the formula (48) is called slightly integrable, or integrable in a generalized sense (for $\kappa=0$ - integrable).

PROPOSITION 1.2. Assume that the rank of the mapping $w\mapsto\omega(w)$ is equal to m everywhere. Then σ is an involution and in a neighbourhood of each torus $w=\overset{\circ}{w}=const$ one can choose a coordinate system (x',y,η) (where $x'\in T^m$, $y\in\mathbb{R}^m$, $\eta\in\mathbb{R}^\kappa$) in which the tori under consideration are given by equalities $y=const, \eta=const$, and

$$V=y\frac{\partial}{\partial x'}, \quad \sigma:(x',y,\eta)\mapsto(-x',y,\eta). \tag{49}$$

The proof is quite similar to that of Proposition 1.1 (see § 1.1). We would like to remark no more than that in the vectorfield case one has the condition $(q,y)F_q(y,\eta)\equiv 0$ in place of $(e^{i(q,y)}-1)F_q(y,\eta)\equiv 0$.

The case $m=1$ of Proposition 1.2 is worthy of a special note. Firstly, if $m=1$ then it is not necessary to postulate the existence of coordinates (x,w) on the domain D in which V and σ are of the form (48) - such coordinates always exist provided there are no equilibria of V in D. Indeed, if in certain coordinates $(\tilde{x},w)$ (where $\tilde{x}=\tilde{x} \bmod 2\pi\in S^1$, $w\in\mathbb{R}^{\kappa+1}$) the invariant circles are given by equalities $w=const$ and the field V is $\omega(\tilde{x},w)\partial/\partial\tilde{x}$, then in coordinates (x,w), where

$$x=2\pi\left(\int_0^{2\pi}\frac{dt}{\omega(t,w)}\right)^{-1}\int_0^{\tilde{x}}\frac{dt}{\omega(t,w)},$$

V and G have the form (48). Secondly, for $m=1$ to guarantee the involutivity of G one need not require the nondegeneracy of the mapping $w \mapsto \omega(w)$, it is enough that $\omega(w)\neq 0$ almost everywhere. This almost trivial statement can be immediately deduced from the above calculations involving Fourier series; for its another proof see Chapter 3 (Proposition 3.1).

Our purpose is to investigate the preservation of invariant tori under small reversible (weakly reversible, if $k=0$) perturbations of the vectorfield V and the diffeomorphism G (49). All fields and mappings we shall consider will be analytic and, moreover, have been already extended into the complex space. As well as in Part 1, instead of the vectorfield V in (49) we will consider the field $\gamma y\,\partial/\partial x'$, where $\gamma \in (0,1]$, but in addition to that suppose that the real part of a domain, over which the coordinate y varies, contains a unit ball.

§ 1.8. Principal theorem

THEOREM 1.2. Let symbols Ω, D_*, r_0, $\tilde{r}_0$, $B_R(b)$, D, γ and C have the same meaning as in Theorem 1.1. Consider a vectorfield V on D and a mapping $G: D \to \mathbb{C}^{2m+k}$ of the following form:

$$V(x,y,z)=(\gamma y+\overset{1}{f}(x,y,z))\frac{\partial}{\partial x}+\overset{2}{f}(x,y,z)\frac{\partial}{\partial y}+\overset{3}{f}(x,y,z)\frac{\partial}{\partial z},$$

(50)

$$G:(x,y,z)\mapsto(-x+\overset{1}{\alpha}(x,y,z),\ y+\overset{2}{\alpha}(x,y,z),\ z+\overset{3}{\alpha}(x,y,z))$$

where $\overset{\tau}{f}$ and $\overset{\tau}{\alpha}$ are normal in D functions.

Assume that on the domain $\{(x,y,z)\in D \mid G(x,y,z)\in D\}$ the equality $TG\circ V=-V\circ G$ holds, and if $k>0$ then in addition the equality $G^2=id$ holds.

Introduce the notation $\Omega'_{\gamma,c} = \{\omega \in \gamma\Omega \mid \omega$ is of type $\mathcal{H}_m(\gamma c, 1)\}$.

Then for each $\varepsilon > 0$ there exists $\delta > 0$, depending only on ε, D and c but not on γ, such that if on D $|f^\tau| < \gamma\delta$ and $|\alpha^\tau| < \gamma\delta$ then for each $\omega \in \Omega'_{\gamma,c}$ the field V and the mapping G have a common invariant $(m+\kappa)$-dimensional manifold given by (4), where Φ^τ_ω are normal in the domain (5) functions, such that the restriction of V to the manifold (4) is $\omega\partial/\partial y$ (in coordinates (y, x)) and the diffeomorphism of (4) induced by G is $(y, x) \longmapsto (-y, x)$ (so that (4) is foliated into invariant under V and G spaces $x = \text{const}$), and inequality (6) holds. Moreover, for every two ω^1 and ω^2 in $\Omega'_{\gamma,c}$ estimate (7) holds.

The remark made right after the formulation of Theorem 1.1 remains true (of course, the words "the action of A^n are to be replaced by "the flow of V ").

Theorem 1.2 implies the same consequences on the measure of the union of the real invariant cylinders and on the involutivity of G for $\kappa = 0$ as Theorem 1.1 does.

As well as in the discrete time case, the main part of the proof of Theorem 1.2 is contained in the following main lemma. All numbers $C_1, C_2, \ldots$ in the formulation and the proof of the lemma are positive constants (depending on m and κ only), whose values, generally speaking, differ from those of denoted likewise constants in Main Lemma 1.

§ 1.9. Main lemma

MAIN LEMMA 2. Fix $\gamma, c \in (0,1]$ and $\omega^1, \omega^2 \in \mathbb{R}^m$ of type $\mathcal{H}_m(\gamma c, 1)$. Let numbers $\rho, r, \tilde{\rho}, \tilde{r}, \sigma, s, d, d'$, domains D^i_ℓ, the difference $\Delta\omega$ and the mapping $\Lambda : D^1_0 \to D^2_0$ be introduced in the same manner as in the formulation of Main Lemma 1. In addition assume that

$$\Theta = \frac{C_1}{c^2} \frac{1}{(\tau-\rho)^{4m}} \frac{d}{s} < \frac{1}{15}$$

(observe that Θ is defined here a little differently from the analogous denoted likewise magnitude in Main Lemma 1 is; the similar remark will refer to C_* and C_{**}).

Let V_i and G_i be a vectorfield and a mapping respectively defined on D_0^i by the formulas (50) in which the functions f^τ and α^τ (they, as before, are assumed to be normal) are equipped with the lower index i .

Suppose on D_0^i the inequalities (8) hold.

Assume that $TG_i \circ V_i = -V_i \circ G_i$ on D_1^i (the weak reversibility condition), and if $\kappa > 0$ then assume in addition that $G_i^2 = id$ on D_1^i .

Finally, let the inequalities (9) hold on D_0^1 .

The lemma states that by all these assumptions there exists a mapping $\mathcal{U}_i$ on D_1^i of the form (10), possessing the following properties.

a) Functions ψ_i^τ are normal in D_1^i and satisfy the inequalities similar to (11) and (12), namely,

$$|\psi_i^\tau| < \Theta s = \frac{C_1}{c^2} \frac{d}{(\tau-\rho)^{4m}} \tag{51}$$

on D_1^i and

$$|\psi_2^\tau \circ \Lambda - \psi_1^\tau| < \frac{C_2}{\gamma c^2} \frac{|\Delta\omega|}{(\tau-\rho)^{4m}} \left(d' + \frac{d}{c(\tau-\rho)^{m+1}}\right) \tag{52}$$

on $\overset{1}{D}_1$.

b) $\mathcal{U}_i \overset{i}{D}_4 \subset \overset{i}{D}_3$ and $\overset{-1}{\mathcal{U}_i} \overset{i}{D}_2 \subset \overset{i}{D}_1$ (whence $\overset{-1}{\mathcal{U}_i} \sigma_i \mathcal{U}_i \overset{i}{D}_4 \subset \overset{i}{D}_1$).

c) On $\overset{i}{D}_4$ the vectorfield $(\overset{-1}{\mathcal{U}_i})_* V_i$ and the mapping $\overset{-1}{\mathcal{U}_i} \sigma_i \mathcal{U}_i$ have the form

$$((\overset{-1}{\mathcal{U}_i})_* V_i)(x,y,\eta)$$

$$= (\gamma y + \overset{1}{h}_i(x,y,\eta))\frac{\partial}{\partial x} + \overset{2}{h}_i(x,y,\eta)\frac{\partial}{\partial y} + \overset{3}{h}_i(x,y,\eta)\frac{\partial}{\partial \eta}, \tag{53}$$

$$\overset{-1}{\mathcal{U}_i} \sigma_i \mathcal{U}_i : (x,y,\eta) \mapsto (-x + \overset{1}{\beta}_i(x,y,\eta),\ y + \overset{2}{\beta}_i(x,y,\eta),\ \eta + \overset{3}{\beta}_i(x,y,\eta))$$

where functions $\overset{\tau}{h}_i$ and $\overset{\tau}{\beta}_i$ are normal in $\overset{i}{D}_4$ and satisfy on $\overset{i}{D}_4$ and $\overset{1}{D}_4$ the inequalities

$$|\overset{\tau}{h}_i| < \gamma C_*, \quad |\overset{\tau}{\beta}_i| < \gamma C_* \tag{54}$$

and

$$|\overset{\tau}{h}_2 \circ \Lambda - \overset{\tau}{h}_1| < |\Delta\omega| C_{**}, \quad |\overset{\tau}{\beta}_2 \circ \Lambda - \overset{\tau}{\beta}_1| < |\Delta\omega| C_{**} \tag{55}$$

respectively, which differ from inequalities (14) and (15) only by values of constants C_* and C_{**} :

$$C_* = \frac{C_3}{c^2} \frac{d}{(\tau-\rho)^{4m+1}} \left(\frac{d}{s} + s\right),$$

$$C_{**} = \frac{C_4}{c^5} \frac{d+d'}{(\tau-\rho)^{9m+2}} \left(\frac{d}{s} + s\right).$$

We will carry out the proof of Main Lemma 2 in this section, as well as that of Main Lemma 1 in § 1.3, incompletely, namely, we shall not verify inequalities (52) and (55) (and, accordingly, not use inequalities (9)). We postpone the proof of estimates (52) and (55) to § 1.11. As well as in § 1.3, we will grop the index i everywhere in the present section.

We shall often refer to the items A-I of the proof of Main Lemma 1, denoting them by A.1,..., I.1.

A. OPERATOR $\mathcal{M}$.

Let symbols $W, \tau', \mathfrak{M}, \langle\ \rangle$ and $\mathfrak{M}_0$ have the same meaning as in A.1. Define the operator $\mathcal{M}: \mathfrak{M}_0 \to \mathfrak{M}_0$ by the equality

$$\omega \frac{\partial(\mathcal{M}F)}{\partial x} = F .$$

Suppose $F \in \mathfrak{M}_0$ and $|F| < C_0$ for all x and w. Let

$$F(x,w) = \sum_{q \neq 0} F_q(w) e^{i(q,x)} .$$

Then

$$(\mathcal{M}F)(x,w) = -i \sum_{q \neq 0} \frac{F_q(w)}{(q,\omega)} e^{i(q,x)} .$$

Similarly to A.1 we obtain, that for $|\operatorname{Im} x_j| < \rho' < \tau'$

$$|\mathcal{M}F| < \frac{C_5 C_0}{\gamma C} \frac{1}{(\tau' - \rho')^{2m}} .$$

B. HOMOLOGICAL EQUATIONS.

Main Lemma 2 asserts that by means of a fit change of variables

$\mathcal{U}$, close to the identity map, we can greatly diminish the difference of the perturbed field V and the perturbed mapping G from unperturbed ones

$$V_0 = \gamma y \frac{\partial}{\partial x} \quad , \; G_0 : (x,y,z) \mapsto (-x,y,z) .$$

In this item we will formulate and prove an infinitesimal analogue of this statement.

Define Z in the same manner as in B.1. Let the notations $\overset{\tau}{\zeta}$ relating to a field ζ on $T^m \times \mathbb{R}^m \times \mathbb{R}^k$ or to an element ζ of Z have the former meaning, too. G_0 acts on Z by the formula $G_0 : \zeta \mapsto (G_0)_* \zeta$, $\zeta \in Z$. Since $V_0^2 = 0$ and $V_0^3 = 0$, one can regard the operator in the space of all vectorfields on $T^m \times \mathbb{R}^m \times \mathbb{R}^k$ defined by $\zeta \mapsto [V_0 , \zeta]$ as a mapping $Z \to Z$. Here $[\;,\;]$ denotes Poisson brackets, i.e.

$$\overset{\tau}{[X,Y]} = \overset{1}{Y}\overset{\tau}{X}_x + \overset{2}{Y}\overset{\tau}{X}_y + \overset{3}{Y}\overset{\tau}{X}_z - \overset{1}{X}\overset{\tau}{Y}_x - \overset{2}{X}\overset{\tau}{Y}_y - \overset{3}{X}\overset{\tau}{Y}_z$$

(X and Y being arbitrary fields on $T^m \times \mathbb{R}^m \times \mathbb{R}^k$).

For the future all fields except V_ε ought to be considered as elements of Z .

For an arbitrary function F on T^m the symbol F_- will denote the function $F_-(x) = F(-x)$.

Assume V_0 and G_0 to be included into curves V_ε and G_ε so that $TG_\varepsilon \circ V_\varepsilon = -V_\varepsilon \circ G_\varepsilon$ for all ε . For $k>0$ assume in addition that $G_\varepsilon^2 = id$ for all ε.

Define the fields $v, g \in Z$ by

$$v = \frac{d}{d\varepsilon} V_\varepsilon \Big|_{\varepsilon=0} \quad , \; g(-x) = \frac{d}{d\varepsilon} G_\varepsilon (x, \gamma^{-1}\omega, \overset{\circ}{z}) \Big|_{\varepsilon=0} .$$

Then the equality

$$\frac{d}{d\varepsilon}(T\sigma_\varepsilon \circ V_\varepsilon)_{|\varepsilon=0} = -\frac{d}{d\varepsilon}(V_\varepsilon \circ \sigma_\varepsilon)_{|\varepsilon=0} \tag{56}$$

means that

$$[V_0, g] + v + (\sigma_0)_* v = 0, \tag{57}$$

i.e.

$$\begin{aligned} -\omega g_x^1 + \gamma g^2 + v^1 - v_-^1 &= 0, \\ -\omega g_x^2 + v^2 + v_-^2 &= 0, \\ -\omega g_x^3 + v^3 + v_-^3 &= 0. \end{aligned} \tag{58}$$

PROPOSITION. There exists a curve of diffeomorphisms $\mathcal{U}_\varepsilon$ (where $\mathcal{U}_0 = id$) such that

$$\frac{d}{d\varepsilon} V_\varepsilon \circ \mathcal{U}_{\varepsilon\,|\varepsilon=0} = \frac{d}{d\varepsilon} T\mathcal{U}_\varepsilon \circ V_{0\,|\varepsilon=0}, \quad \frac{d}{d\varepsilon} \sigma_\varepsilon \mathcal{U}_{\varepsilon\,|\varepsilon=0} = \frac{d}{d\varepsilon} \mathcal{U}_\varepsilon \sigma_{0\,|\varepsilon=0}. \tag{59}$$

PROOF. (59) may be transcribed in the form

$$\begin{cases} [V_0, u] + v = 0 & (60_1) \\ (\sigma_0)_* u + g - u = 0 & (60_2) \end{cases}$$

where

$$u = \frac{d}{d\varepsilon} \mathcal{U}_{\varepsilon\,|\varepsilon=0}.$$

The equations (60) are called the homological equations of the original problem. We will show that on condition (57) (in the case $\varkappa > 0$ - in combination with the condition $\sigma_\varepsilon^2 = id$) they are solvable.

Study the equation $[V_0, u] + \tilde{u} = 0$, where $\tilde{u}$ is a known field and u is an unknown one. Transcribe it for every component separately:

$$-\omega \overset{1}{u}_x + \gamma \overset{2}{u} + \overset{1}{\tilde{u}} = 0, \quad -\omega \overset{2}{u}_x + \overset{2}{\tilde{u}} = 0, \quad -\omega \overset{3}{u}_x + \overset{3}{\tilde{u}} = 0.$$

A solution exists if and only if $\langle \overset{2}{\tilde{u}} \rangle = 0$ and $\langle \overset{3}{\tilde{u}} \rangle = 0$. In this case all possible solutions are given by formulas

$$\overset{2}{u} = -\gamma^{-1} \langle \overset{1}{\tilde{u}} \rangle + \mathcal{M}(\overset{2}{\tilde{u}}), \quad \overset{1}{u} = \mathcal{M}(\gamma \overset{2}{u} + \overset{1}{\tilde{u}}) + K_1, \quad \overset{3}{u} = \mathcal{M}(\overset{3}{\tilde{u}}) + K_3, \tag{61}$$

$K_1 \in \mathbb{R}^m$ and $K_3 \in \mathbb{R}^\kappa$ being arbitrary constants.

(58) implies that $\langle \overset{2}{v} \rangle = 0$ and $\langle \overset{3}{v} \rangle = 0$. Therefore (60_1) is solvable.

Verify that if u is a solution of (60_1) then $(G_0)_* u + g$ is a solution of (60_1) too. We have to show that $[V_0, (G_0)_* u + g] + v = 0$. As is easy to see, $(G_0)_* V_0 = -V_0$ implies $(G_0)_* [V_0, u] = -[V_0, (G_0)_* u]$. Therefore by (57) $[V_0, (G_0)_* u + g] + v = -(G_0)_* [V_0, u] + [V_0, g] + v = -(G_0)_* ([V_0, u] + v) = 0$ (since u is a solution of (60_1)).

Thus, if u is a solution of (60_1) then $(G_0)_* u + g$ is a solution of (60_1) too. Further reasons repeat ones of B.1 word for word. Solutions of (60) are

$$\overset{2}{u} = -\gamma^{-1} \langle \overset{1}{v} \rangle + \mathcal{M} \overset{2}{v}, \quad \overset{1}{u} = \tfrac{1}{2} \langle \overset{1}{g} \rangle + \mathcal{M}(\gamma \overset{2}{u} + \overset{1}{v}), \quad \overset{3}{u} = K_3 + \mathcal{M} \overset{3}{v}, \tag{62}$$

$K_3 \in \mathbb{R}^\kappa$ being an arbitrary constant.

If $\kappa = 0$ then a solution of (60) is unique. X

The remark made at the end of B.1 remains true (A_ε and (16) are to be replaced by V_ε and (56) respectively, observe that (20_2)

and (60_2) coincide).

C. COHOMOLOGIC INTERPRETATION.

One may easily generalize cohomology of groups to algebraic systems (Ξ, Π, Z), where

a) Ξ and Z are abelian additive groups, Π is a multiplicative group;

b) there are fixed homomorphisms

$$\Pi \to \operatorname{Aut} Z, \quad \pi \mapsto [\zeta \mapsto \pi(\zeta)],$$

$$\Xi \to \operatorname{End}^+ Z, \quad \xi \mapsto [\zeta \mapsto \xi(\zeta)],$$

$$\Pi \to \operatorname{Aut} \Xi, \quad \pi \mapsto [\xi \mapsto \pi \xi]$$

and an antihomomorphism

$$\Pi \to \operatorname{Aut} \Xi, \quad \pi \mapsto [\xi \mapsto \xi \pi],$$

here $\operatorname{End}^+ Z$ denotes the additive group of the ring $\operatorname{End} Z$ (so that

$$(\pi_1 \pi_2)(\zeta) = \pi_1(\pi_2(\zeta)), \quad (\xi_1 + \xi_2)(\zeta) = \xi_1(\zeta) + \xi_2(\zeta),$$

$$(\pi_1 \pi_2)\xi = \pi_1(\pi_2 \xi), \quad \xi(\pi_1 \pi_2) = (\xi \pi_1)\pi_2);$$

c) the following conditions hold

$$\xi(\pi(\zeta)) = (\xi\pi)(\zeta), \quad \pi(\xi(\zeta)) = (\pi\xi)(\zeta). \tag{63}$$

By definition the space B^n of all n-dimensional cochains (for $n \in \mathbb{N}$) is the abelian group of functions

$$F:\Pi^n \cup \left(\bigcup_{\nu=1}^{n} \Pi^{\nu-1} \times \Xi \times \Pi^{n-\nu}\right) \to Z ,$$

which are linear in the argument belonging to Ξ (if it is present) and vanish if at least one argument belonging to Π has the value 1. By definition set $B^0 = Z$.

The coboundary homomorphism $\delta_n : B^n \to B^{n+1}$ (where $n \in \mathbb{Z}_+$) is defined in the following manner. Let $F \in B^n$. Then

a) for any $\pi_1, \ldots, \pi_{n+1} \in \Pi$

$$(\delta_n F)(\pi_1, \ldots, \pi_{n+1}) = (-1)^{n+1} \pi_1(F(\pi_2, \ldots, \pi_{n+1})) \tag{64}$$

$$+ \sum_{\nu=1}^{n} (-1)^{n+\nu+1} F(\pi_1, \ldots, \pi_{\nu-1}, \pi_\nu \pi_{\nu+1}, \pi_{\nu+2}, \ldots, \pi_{n+1}) + F(\pi_1, \ldots, \pi_n);$$

b) if the νth argument of $\delta_n F$, where $1 \leq \nu \leq n$, is $\xi \in \Xi$ then in the right hand side of (64) π_ν is to be replaced by ξ;

c) if the $(n+1)^{th}$ argument of $\delta_n F$ is $\xi \in \Xi$ then in the right hand side of (64) the term $F(\pi_1, \ldots, \pi_n)$ is to be eliminated while in preserved $n+1$ terms π_{n+1} is to be replaced by ξ.

EXAMPLES.

$$(\delta_0 \zeta)(\pi) = -\pi(\zeta) + \zeta , \quad (\delta_0 \zeta)(\xi) = -\xi(\zeta) ,$$

$$(\delta_1 F)(\pi_1, \pi_2) = \pi_1(F(\pi_2)) - F(\pi_1 \pi_2) + F(\pi_1),$$

$$(\delta_1 F)(\xi, \pi) = \xi(F(\pi)) - F(\xi \pi) + F(\xi) ,$$

$$(\delta_1 F)(\pi, \xi) = \pi(F(\xi)) - F(\pi \xi) .$$

As is easy to verify, $\delta_{n+1} \circ \delta_n = 0$ for all $n \in \mathbb{Z}_+$. By definition $H^*(\Xi, \Pi, Z)$ is the cohomology of the obtained cochain complex. For $\Xi = 0$ we get the usual cohomology $H^*(\Pi, Z)$, where Π is a multiplicative group and Z is a Π-module.

Now let Z be the described above (in B.1) factor of the space of all vectorfields on $T^m \times \mathbb{R}^m \times \mathbb{R}^k$; Z will be considered as a $\mathbb{Z}$-module in this item although it is equipped with the $\mathbb{R}$-module structure. Furthermore, let Π be the group $\mathbb{Z}_2 = \{\sigma_0 ; id\}$ and Ξ be a two-dimensional lattice $\mathbb{Z}^2$ generated by symbols V_0 and $(V_0 \sigma_0)$.

Assume the homomorphisms $\Pi \to Aut\, Z$ and $\Xi \to End^+ Z$ to be given by

$$\sigma_0(\zeta) = (\sigma_0)_* \zeta, \; V_0(\zeta) = [V_0, \zeta], \; (V_0 \sigma_0)(\zeta) = [V_0, (\sigma_0)_* \zeta]$$

for all $\zeta \in Z$.

Assume the left and right actions of Π on Ξ by automorphisms (in our case Π is abelian and, consequently, the notions of a left action of Π and a right one coincide) to be given by

$$\sigma_0 V_0 = -(V_0 \sigma_0), \; \sigma_0 (V_0 \sigma_0) = -V_0, \; V_0 \sigma_0 = (V_0 \sigma_0), \; (V_0 \sigma_0) \sigma_0 = V_0 .$$

One can easily verify the fulfillment of (63).

As is not hard to show, all one-dimensional cocycles $F: \Pi \cup \Xi \to Z$ have the form

$$F(id) = 0 \; , \; F(\sigma_0) = g \; , \qquad (65)$$
$$F(n_1 V_0 + n_2 (V_0 \sigma_0)) = (n_1 + n_2) v + n_2 [V_0, g]$$

$(n_1, n_2 \in \mathbb{Z})$, where v and g are arbitrary elements of Z satisfying relations (57) and (24). At the same time equations (60) mean that the cocycle F given by such a way is the coboundary of the element $u \in Z$. Thus the solvability of homological equations (60) on conditions (57) and (24) (for the case $\mathcal{K}=0$ (24) is a consequence of (57)) is equivalent to

$$H^1(\Xi, \Pi, Z) = 0 .$$

D. WEAK REVERSIBILITY CONDITION.

Return to the perturbed field V and the perturbed mapping G defined on D_0. The estimates of derivatives of f^τ and d^τ on D_ℓ $(1 \leq \ell \leq 4)$ obtained in D.1 remain valid.

For an arbitrary function F defined on D_0 the symbol F_- will denote the function $F_-(x, y, \eta) = F(-x, y, \eta)$.

The equality $TG \circ V = -V \circ G$ on D_1 may be written down in the following way

$$\begin{cases} \gamma y \overset{1}{d}_x + \overset{1}{f}\overset{1}{d}_x + \overset{2}{f}\overset{1}{d}_y + \overset{3}{f}\overset{1}{d}_\eta - \overset{1}{f} + \gamma \overset{2}{d} + \overset{1}{f} \circ G = 0 \\ \gamma y \overset{2}{d}_x + \overset{1}{f}\overset{2}{d}_x + \overset{2}{f}\overset{2}{d}_y + \overset{3}{f}\overset{2}{d}_\eta + \overset{2}{f} + \overset{2}{f} \circ G = 0 \\ \gamma y \overset{3}{d}_x + \overset{1}{f}\overset{3}{d}_x + \overset{2}{f}\overset{3}{d}_y + \overset{3}{f}\overset{3}{d}_\eta + \overset{3}{f} + \overset{3}{f} \circ G = 0 . \end{cases}$$

There hold the estimates

$$|\overset{\tau}{f} \circ G - \overset{\tau}{f}_-| < \gamma^2 d^2 \left(\frac{4}{\tau - \rho} + \frac{6}{s} + \frac{4}{\tilde{\tau} - \tilde{\rho}} \right) < \frac{8\gamma^2 d^2}{s},$$

$$|\gamma y \overset{\tau}{d}_x - \omega \overset{\tau}{d}_x| < \frac{\gamma^2 m (s + \sigma) d}{\tau - \rho} < \frac{4\gamma^2 m s d}{3(\tau - \rho)},$$

$$|\overset{1}{f}\overset{\tau}{d}_x| < \frac{\gamma^2 d^2}{25}, \quad |\overset{2}{f}\overset{\tau}{d}_y| < \frac{3\gamma^2 d^2}{s}, \quad |\overset{3}{f}\overset{\tau}{d}_\eta| < \frac{\gamma^2 d^2}{25}$$

on D_2. Therefore on D_2

$$\begin{cases} \omega\alpha_x^1 - f^1 + \gamma\alpha^2 + f_-^1 = \delta^1 \\ \omega\alpha_x^2 + f^2 + f_-^2 = \delta^2 \\ \omega\alpha_x^3 + f^3 + f_-^3 = \delta^3 \end{cases} \tag{66}$$

where

$$|\delta^\tau| < C_6 \gamma^2 d\left(\frac{d}{s} + \frac{s}{\tau-\rho}\right).$$

E. Using the involutivity property of G for $\kappa > 0$, one can prove the estimate $|\langle\alpha^3\rangle| < C_7 \gamma^2 d^2 s^{-1}$ on D_2 in exactly the same manner as in E.1.

F. MAPPING $\mathcal{U}$.

To define $\mathcal{U}: (x, y, \eta) \mapsto (x + \psi^1, y + \psi^2, \eta + \psi^3)$ one must substitute $\mathcal{M}$ for L in (28) (see (62)), i.e.

$$\begin{cases} \psi^2 = -\gamma^{-1}\langle f^1\rangle + \mathcal{M}(f^2 - \langle f^2\rangle) \\ \psi^1 = \tfrac{1}{2}\langle\alpha^1\rangle + \mathcal{M}(\gamma\psi^2 + f^1) \\ \psi^3 = \mathcal{M}(f^3 - \langle f^3\rangle). \end{cases} \tag{67}$$

Analogously to F.1 on the domain $D_{0.5}$ we obtain the estimate

$$|\psi^\tau| < \frac{C_1}{c^2} \frac{d}{(\tau-\rho)^{4m}} = \Theta s .$$

The estimates of derivatives of ψ^τ on D_1 written down in F.1 remain valid.

G. It is necessary to modify nothing in the reasonings of G.1 to prove that $\mathcal{U}_*^{-1}V$ and $\mathcal{U}^{-1}G\mathcal{U}$ are well defined on D_4.

H. ESTIMATE OF $\mathcal{U}_*^{-1}V$.

Let for $(x, y, \eta) \in D_4$ the field $\tilde{V} = \mathcal{U}_*^{-1}V$ be written in the form (53). Transcribe the equality $T\mathcal{U}\circ\tilde{V}=V\circ\mathcal{U}$ in a more detailed way:

$$\begin{cases} h^1=-h^1\psi^1_x-h^2\psi^1_y-h^3\psi^1_\eta+\gamma\psi^2+f^1\circ\mathcal{U}-\gamma y\psi^1_x \\ h^2=-h^1\psi^2_x-h^2\psi^2_y-h^3\psi^2_\eta+f^2\circ\mathcal{U}-\gamma y\psi^2_x \\ h^3=-h^1\psi^3_x-h^2\psi^3_y-h^3\psi^3_\eta+f^3\circ\mathcal{U}-\gamma y\psi^3_x \ . \end{cases}$$

Represent h^τ as $h^\tau=h^{\tau,1}+h^{\tau,2}+h^{\tau,3}+h^{\tau,4}$, where

$$h^{1,1}=\gamma\psi^2+f^1-\omega\psi^1_x\,,\quad h^{2,1}=f^2-\omega\psi^2_x\,,\quad h^{3,1}=f^3-\omega\psi^3_x\,,$$

$$h^{\tau,2}=f^\tau\circ\mathcal{U}-f^\tau,\ h^{\tau,3}=\omega\psi^\tau_x-\gamma y\psi^\tau_x,\ h^{\tau,4}=-h^1\psi^\tau_x-h^2\psi^\tau_y-h^3\psi^\tau_\eta.$$

By the definition of ψ^τ we have $h^{1,1}=0,\ h^{2,1}=\langle f^2\rangle, h^{3,1}=\langle f^3\rangle$. By (66) $\langle f^2\rangle=\tfrac{1}{2}\langle\delta^2\rangle$ and $\langle f^3\rangle=\tfrac{1}{2}\langle\delta^3\rangle$. Thus,

$$|h^{\tau,1}|<\frac{1}{2}C_6\gamma^2 d\left(\frac{d}{s}+\frac{s}{r-\rho}\right).$$

It is easy to obtain the estimates

$$|h^{\tau,2}|<\frac{8}{3}\gamma d\Theta\ ,$$

$$|h^{\tau,3}|<\frac{8m\gamma}{3}\,\frac{\Theta s^2}{r-\rho}\,,$$

$$|h^{\tau,4}|<2\Theta|h^1|+6\Theta|h^2|+\Theta|h^3|\ .$$

Now we get the desired estimate of h^τ similarly to H.1.

I. ESTIMATE OF $\mathcal{U}^{-1}G\,\mathcal{U}$.

Let for $(x,y,\eta)\in D_4$ the mapping $\tilde{G}=\mathcal{U}^{-1}G\,\mathcal{U}$ be written in the form (53) coinciding with (13). Define the decomposition $\beta^\tau=\beta^{\tau,1}$

$+\beta^{\tau,2}+\beta^{\tau,3}$ in the same way as in I.1.

By the definition (67) of ψ^1 we have $\langle\beta^{1,1}\rangle=0$ and $\beta^{1,1}=\mathcal{M}I$, where

$$I=\gamma\psi_-^2-\gamma\psi^2+f_-^1-f^1+\omega\alpha_x^1 .$$

Represent I in the form $I=I^1+I^2+I^3$, where

$$I^1=\gamma(\psi_-^2-\psi^2-\alpha^2+\langle\alpha^2\rangle),$$

$$I^2=f_-^1-f^1+\gamma\alpha^2+\omega\alpha_x^1,\quad I^3=-\gamma\langle\alpha^2\rangle.$$

$\langle I^1\rangle=0$, consequently the definition (67) of ψ^2 easily implies that $I^1=\gamma\mathcal{M}(\langle\delta^2\rangle-\delta^2)$. Furthermore, $I^2=\delta^1$ and $I^3=-\langle\delta^1\rangle$ (for the definition of δ^τ see (66)).

As is easy to verify, $\beta^{2,1}=-\gamma^{-1}(I^1+I^3)$. To estimate $\beta^{3,1}$ for $\varkappa>0$ we represent $\beta^{3,1}$ as $\beta^{3,1}=I^4+\langle\alpha^3\rangle$, where $I^4=-\psi_-^3+\psi^3+\alpha^3-\langle\alpha^3\rangle$. The definition (67) of ψ^3 in combination with $\langle I^4\rangle=0$ implies $I^4=\mathcal{M}(\delta^3-\langle\delta^3\rangle)$.

Now the rest of bounding β^τ is the same as in I.1.

This completes the proof of Main Lemma 2 (without (52) and (55)).

REMARK 1. Suppose that $\alpha^\tau=0$, i.e. $\sigma=\sigma_0$. Then f^2 and f^3 are odd and f^1 is even with respect to x (actually this is equivalent to $(\sigma_0)_*V=-V$ on D_1), in particular, $\delta^\tau=0$, $\langle f^2\rangle=0$, $\langle f^3\rangle=0$. The functions ψ^2 and ψ^3 defined by (67) are even and the function ψ^1 is odd with respect to x (since the operator $\mathcal{M}$ carries even (odd) functions to odd (respectively even) ones). Therefore $\mathcal{U}$ commutes with σ_0, i.e. $\beta^\tau=0$.

An infinitesimal analogue to the case $\alpha^\tau=0$ is the following one. Rewrite the equations (57) and (60) for $g=0$:

$$v+(\sigma_0)_*v=0, \tag{68}$$

$$\begin{cases} [V_0, u] + v = 0 \\ (\sigma_0)_* u - u = 0 . \end{cases} \tag{69}$$

In virtue of (68) the system of equations (69) may be transcribed in the form

$$\begin{cases} [V_0, u] + \frac{1}{2}(v - (\sigma_0)_* v) = 0 \\ (\sigma_0)_* u - u = 0 . \end{cases} \tag{70}$$

It is easy to verify that (70) has a solution (unique, if $\kappa = 0$) independently whether (68) is valid.

REMARK 2. The case $\sigma = \sigma_0$ (i.e. when the involution is not subjected to perturbing) corresponds to $g = 0$ on the infinitesimal level, which means solving (31) on condition (30) (for reversible diffeomorphisms) or (69) on condition (68) (for reversible vectorfields). But the solvability of (31) or (69) on condition (30) or (68) respectively has no as an adequate cohomological interpretation as the solvability of (20) on conditions (17) and (24) or that of (60) on conditions (57) and (24) has: setting $g = 0$ in (26) or (65) we should not have got all cocycles. It is from this point of view that it is natural to perturb not only the (slightly) integrable reversible diffeomorphism A_0 or vectorfield V_0 but the reversing involution σ_0 too.

§ 1.10. Final remarks

Now one may carry out the iteration process (the construction of an infinite sequence of changes of variables) in exactly the same manner as in § 1.4 for the discrete time case. In order to prove the invariance of the manifold (4) under the field V and to verify that the restriction of V to (4) has the desired form one has to observe that on D_∞^i

$$\frac{\partial H_i^{(n),\tau}}{\partial x_j} \longrightarrow \frac{\partial \Phi_{\omega^i}^{\tau}}{\partial x_j}, \quad \frac{\partial H_i^{(n),\tau}}{\partial \eta_t} \longrightarrow \frac{\partial \Phi_{\omega^i}^{\tau}}{\partial \eta_t} \quad (n \to \infty)$$

and

$$\left| \frac{\partial H_i^{(n),\tau}}{\partial y_j} \right| \left| f_i^{(n+1),2} \right| < P_n^2 \gamma d_{n+1} < \gamma \left(\frac{8}{5}\right)^n d_{n+1} \to 0 \quad (n \to \infty).$$

This completes the proof of Theorem 1.2.

REMARK 1. All statements of Theorem 1.2 remain true (up to obvious slight modifications of some formulas) if the field V on D has the form

$$V(x, y, \eta)$$

$$= (\theta + \gamma y + f^1(x,y,\eta))\frac{\partial}{\partial x} + f^2(x,y,\eta)\frac{\partial}{\partial y} + f^3(x,y,\eta)\frac{\partial}{\partial \eta}$$

differing from (50) by the presence of a constant $\theta \in \mathbb{R}^m$.

Replacing the coordinate y by $\tilde{y} = y + \gamma^{-1}\theta$ we reduce the field V to the form (50).

REMARK 2. The case $m=1$ of Theorem 1.2 is worthy of the separate consideration. For $m=1$ ω-lemma 2 becomes trivial and, moreover, for each $K>0$ the class of numbers $\omega \in \mathbb{R}$ of type $\mathcal{H}_1(K,\varepsilon)$ does not depend on $\varepsilon > 0$ and coincides with the set $\{\omega \in \mathbb{R} \mid |\omega| \geq K\}$. For each $c \in (0,1)$, $R > 0$ and line segment

$B_R \subset \mathbb{R}$ of length $2R$ the set $\{\omega \in B_R \,|\, |\omega| \geq Rc\}$ is either a line segment or the union of two segments, and its measure is no less than $2R(1-c)$.

Therefore if in Theorem 1.2 $m=1$ then for sufficiently small f^τ and d^τ there exists a whole subinterval $\Omega_1 \subset \Omega$ such that $S^1 \times \Omega_1 \times O(B_R(b))$ (the last factor is some neighbourhood of $B_R(b)$) is foliated into $(k+1)$-dimensional cylinders, which in turn are foliated into invariant under the field V and mapping G circles.

Thus, for $m=1$ any small reversible (and for $k=0$ even weakly reversible) perturbation of a nondegenerate slightly integrable reversible vectorfield is still slightly integrable.

If for $k=0$, as well as for $k \geq 1$, we confine ourselves to the consideration of reversible perturbations only, then the nondegeneracy condition becomes unnecessary. To be more precise, the following statement holds.

PROPOSITION. If $m=1$, any sufficiently small reversible perturbation of a slightly integrable reversible vectorfield is still slightly integrable.

We shall prove this (almost trivial) proposition in § 3.1.

In inquiring into weakly reversible perturbations of integrable reversible fields in a plane (i.e. for $m=1$, $k=0$) the nondegeneracy condition is essential.

EXAMPLE. Consider the following degenerate integrable vectorfield V on the cylinder $S^1 \times \mathbb{R}$, reversible with respect to the involution G:

$$V = \omega \frac{\partial}{\partial x}, \quad G : (x, y) \mapsto (-x, y), \quad G_* V = -V.$$

Here x is an angular $\mathrm{mod}\, 2\pi$ coordinate on S^1 and y is a coordinate on $\mathbb{R}$.

Let V'_ε and G'_ε be the following small perturbations of the field V and the diffeomorphism G respectively (ε being a small positive parameter):

$$V'_\varepsilon = \omega\frac{\partial}{\partial x} + \varepsilon e^{-\frac{1}{\varepsilon}} \sin\frac{y}{\varepsilon}\frac{\partial}{\partial y},$$

$$G'_\varepsilon : (x,y) \mapsto (-x, y+\pi\varepsilon), \ (G'_\varepsilon)_* V'_\varepsilon = -V'_\varepsilon .$$

V'_ε and G'_ε are analytic and the differences $V'_\varepsilon - V$ and $G'_\varepsilon - G$ tend to 0 as $\varepsilon \to 0$ even if extended into the complex domain $\{ |\operatorname{Im} x|<1, |\operatorname{Im} y| < 1\}$. At the same time G'_ε is not an involution and for any ε closed trajectories of the field V'_ε (circles $y = n\pi\varepsilon, n \in \mathbb{Z}$) form a set of measure zero.

REMARK 3. For $m>1, (m+k)$-dimensional cylinders in $T^m \times \Omega \times O(B_R(b))$, foliated into m-dimensional tori invariant under V and G , form a Cantor set but of a more regular structure than in the discrete time case. Namely, these cylinders are organized into one-parameter families. The ratio of the quasiperiodic motion frequencies $(\omega_1 : \ldots : \omega_m)$ is the same for all tori into which cylinders constituting a given fixed family are foliated.

Indeed, consider an arbitrary number $\omega \in \Omega'_{\gamma,c}$. For each $\lambda \in \mathbb{R}$, $1 \leq \lambda < 1 + \lambda_0$, the number $\lambda\omega$ also belongs to $\Omega'_{\gamma,c}$. The cylinders corresponding to numbers $\lambda\omega$ for all $\lambda \in (1, 1+\lambda_0)$ are organized into an analytic one-parameter family.

§ 1.11. Appendix

In this section we prove inequalities (52) and (55) of Main Lemma 2. We shall use notations of the items A, D-F, H-I of § 1.9

and refer to the items A', D'-F', H'-I' of § 1.6 denoting them by A'.1,...,I'.1. We shall also use Δ-lemma in D'.1.

A'. Operators $\mathcal{M}^i$.

Let sets $W, \mathfrak{M}, \mathfrak{M}_0$ and the operator $\mathcal{M}$, as well as the number $\omega \in \mathbb{R}^m$, be equipped with the upper index $i \in \{1; 2\}$. Let bijections Λ_0 and Λ be defined in the same manner as in A'.1. Suppose $F^i \in \mathfrak{M}_0^i$, $|F^i| < C_0$ and $|F^2 \circ \Lambda - F^1| < |\Delta\omega| C_0'$. Similarly to A'.1 we obtain that for $|Im x_j| < \rho' < \tau'$

$$|(\mathcal{M}^2 F^2) \circ \Lambda - \mathcal{M}^1 F^1|$$

$$< \frac{C_8 C_0 |\Delta\omega|}{\gamma^2 c^2} \frac{1}{(\tau' - \rho')^{3m+1}} + \frac{C_5 C_0' |\Delta\omega|}{\gamma c} \frac{1}{(\tau' - \rho')^{2m}} .$$

D'. Weak reversibility condition.

Return to the perturbed field V_i and mapping G_i defined on D_0^i. From now on, $\Lambda : D_0^1 \longrightarrow D_0^2$, $\Lambda : (x, y, \eta) \longmapsto (x, y + \gamma^{-1} \Delta\omega, \eta)$. Adopt the same agreement on the notation ΔF as in D'.1.

We equip the functions δ^τ in (66) with the lower index i. The goal of this item is to estimate $\Delta\delta^\tau$. To do it one need bound $\Delta(f^\tau \circ G - f^\tau_-)$, $\Delta(\gamma y d_x^\tau - \omega d_x^\tau)$ (i.e. $\Delta((\gamma y - \omega) d_x^\tau)$ $= (\gamma y - \omega^1) \Delta d_x^\tau)$, $\Delta(f^1 d_x^\tau)$, $\Delta(f^2 d_y^\tau)$, and $\Delta(f^3 d_\eta^\tau)$.

Apply Δ-lemma to $F_i = f_i^\tau$, $K_i = G_i$ $(\mu = -1, \nu = 0, u_i = d_i^\tau)$. In this case $* f_i^\tau = 0$, and we obtain on D_2^1

$$|\Delta(f^\tau \circ G - f^\tau_-)| < \frac{C_9 \gamma |\Delta\omega| d d'}{s} .$$

Furthermore, on D_2^1

$$|\Delta(\gamma y d_x^\tau - \omega d_x^\tau)| < \gamma m (s + \sigma) d' \frac{|\Delta\omega|}{\tau - \rho} < \frac{4m\gamma |\Delta\omega| d' s}{3(\tau - \rho)} .$$

Finally, on D_2^1

$$|\Delta(f^1 \alpha_x^\tau)|$$

$$\leq \max_j (|f_2^1 \circ \Lambda| \left|\frac{\partial \Delta \alpha^\tau}{\partial x_j}\right| + |\Delta f^1| \left|\frac{\partial \alpha_1^\tau}{\partial x_j}\right|) < \gamma |\Delta\omega| d d' s^{-1}$$

and similarly

$$|\Delta(f^2 \alpha_y^\tau)| < 6\gamma |\Delta\omega| d d' s^{-1}, \ |\Delta(f^3 \alpha_z^\tau)| < \gamma |\Delta\omega| d d' s^{-1}.$$

Thus, on D_2^1

$$|\Delta\delta^\tau| < C_{10}\gamma |\Delta\omega| d' \left(\frac{d}{s} + \frac{s}{\tau-\rho}\right).$$

E'. One can prove the estimate

$$|\Delta \langle \alpha^3 \rangle| < C_{11}\gamma |\Delta\omega| d d' s^{-1}$$

on D_2^1 for $\kappa > 0$ in exactly the same manner as in E'.1.

F'. Mappings $\mathcal{U}_i$.

Analogously to F'.1 on the domain $D_{0.5}^1$ we obtain the desired estimate (52) of $\Delta\Psi^\tau$. For later use the following less delicate estimate of $\Delta\Psi^\tau$ will suffice: on $D_{0.5}^1$

$$|\Delta\Psi^\tau| < \frac{C_{12}|\Delta\omega|}{\gamma c^3} \frac{d+d'}{(\tau-\rho)^{5m+1}}.$$

H'. Estimate of $(\mathcal{U}_i^{-1})_* V_i$.

In this and the next items we shall prove (without detailed calculations) the estimate (55).

Estimate Δh^{τ}. In view of the result of the item D' on D_4^1

$$|\Delta h^{\tau,1}| < \frac{1}{2} C_{10} \gamma |\Delta\omega| d' \left(\frac{d}{s} + \frac{s}{\tau-\rho}\right).$$

One can estimate $\Delta h^{\tau,2}$ in the same manner as in H'.1. We obtain on D_4^1

$$|\Delta h^{\tau,2}| < \frac{C_{13} d(d+d')}{c^3 s} \frac{|\Delta\omega|}{(\tau-\rho)^{5m+1}}.$$

Furthermore, $\Delta h^{\tau,3} = (\omega^1 - \gamma y)\Delta\Psi_x^{\tau}$, whence on D_4^1

$$|\Delta h^{\tau,3}| < \frac{C_{14}(d+d')s}{c^3} \frac{|\Delta\omega|}{(\tau-\rho)^{5m+2}}.$$

Finally, estimate $\Delta h^{\tau,4}$. The functions h_2^{τ} on D_4^2, i.e. $h_2^{\tau}\circ\Lambda$ on D_4^1, have been already estimated (54). One can estimate the derivatives of $\Delta\Psi^{\tau}$ on D_4^1 by Cauchy's formula. Putting all this together and minding $d<(\tau-\rho)/24$ we obtain

$$|\Delta h^{\tau,4}| \le \max_{j,t}\Big(|h_2^1\circ\Lambda| \left|\frac{\partial\Delta\Psi^{\tau}}{\partial x_j}\right| + |\Delta h^1| \left|\frac{\partial\Psi_1^{\tau}}{\partial x_j}\right|$$

$$+|h_2^2\circ\Lambda| \left|\frac{\partial\Delta\Psi^{\tau}}{\partial y_j}\right| + |\Delta h^2| \left|\frac{\partial\Psi_1^{\tau}}{\partial y_j}\right|$$

$$+|h_2^3\circ\Lambda| \left|\frac{\partial\Delta\Psi^{\tau}}{\partial \eta_t}\right| + |\Delta h^3| \left|\frac{\partial\Psi_1^{\tau}}{\partial \eta_t}\right|\Big)$$

$$< \frac{C_{15}(d+d')|\Delta\omega|}{c^5(\tau-\rho)^{9m+2}}\left(\frac{d}{s}+s\right) + 2\Theta|\Delta h^1| + 6\Theta|\Delta h^2| + \Theta|\Delta h^3|.$$

Now analogously to H'.1 we get the desired estimate of Δh^{τ}.

I'. Estimate of $\mathcal{U}_i^{-1} G_i \mathcal{U}_i$.

Estimate $\Delta\beta^{\tau}$. We have

$$\beta_i^{1,1} = \mathcal{M}^i(I_i^1 + I_i^2 + I_i^3)$$

where

$$I_i^1 = \gamma\mathcal{M}^i(\langle\delta_i^2\rangle - \delta_i^2), \quad I_i^2 = \delta_i^1, \quad I_i^3 = -\langle\delta_i^1\rangle,$$

$$\beta_i^{2,1} = -\gamma^{-1}(I_i^1 + I_i^3)$$

and for $\kappa > 0$

$$\beta_i^{3,1} = \mathcal{M}^i(\delta_i^3 - \langle\delta_i^3\rangle) + \langle\alpha_i^3\rangle .$$

Now one can carry out all estimates in the same manner as in I'.1, and we obtain

$$|\Delta\beta^{\tau,1}| < \frac{C_{16}(d+d')}{c^3} \, \frac{|\Delta\omega|}{(\tau-\rho)^{5m+2}} \left(\frac{d}{s} + s\right),$$

$$|\Delta\beta^{\tau,2}| < \frac{C_{17}\, d(d+d')}{c^3 s} \, \frac{|\Delta\omega|}{(\tau-\rho)^{5m+1}} ,$$

$$|\Delta\beta^{\tau,3}| < \frac{C_{18}(d+d')}{c^5} \, \frac{|\Delta\omega|}{(\tau-\rho)^{9m+2}} \left(\frac{d}{s} + s\right)$$

$$+ 2\Theta|\Delta\beta^1| + 6\Theta|\Delta\beta^2| + \Theta|\Delta\beta^3| .$$

The concluding step of reasoning, providing the desired estimate of $\Delta\beta^{\tau}$, is the same as in H'.1.

NOTE. In items D' and H', estimates of the sort $\leqslant \max_n (A_n + B_n + \dots)$ re to be understood as $\leqslant \max_n A_n + \max_n B_n + \dots$.

CHAPTER 2

NORMAL FORMS FOR REVERSIBLE DIFFEOMORPHISMS AND VECTORFIELDS NEAR AN EQUILIBRIUM AND THEIR KOLMOGOROV TORI

§ 2.1. Linear reversible and infinitesimally reversible operators

This chapter deals with germs of smooth or analytic diffeomorphisms $A:(\mathbb{R}^N,0)\longrightarrow(\mathbb{R}^N,0)$ and germs of smooth or analytic vectorfields V at $0\in\mathbb{R}^N$, for which 0 is an equilibrium (i.e. $V(0)=0$). Taking into account that the germ of an analytic object at 0 is a particular case of a formal object, we also consider formal diffeomorphisms $A:(\mathbb{R}^N,0)\longrightarrow(\mathbb{R}^N,0)$ and formal vectorfields V in $\mathbb{R}^N$, for which 0 is an equilibrium (i.e. which are given by formal power series without constant term, to express this we will write down $V(0)=0$ as well as in the case of genuine fields). Writing "a vectorfield at $(\mathbb{R}^N,0)$" we will have in view either the germ of a vectorfield at $0\in\mathbb{R}^N$ or a formal vectorfield in $\mathbb{R}^N$.

We shall denote by $(\ )_\ell$, where $\ell\in\mathbb{N}$, the ℓ-jet. In particular, $(\ )_1$ will denote the linearization, which will be considered as a linear operator $\mathbb{R}^N\longrightarrow\mathbb{R}^N$. Besides that, we shall denote by E_N the identity operator $\mathbb{R}^N\longrightarrow\mathbb{R}^N$ or the unit $N\times N$ matrix.

If a linear operator $g:\mathbb{R}^N\longrightarrow\mathbb{R}^N$ is an involution and the characteristic polynomial $\det(g-\lambda E_N)$ is $(-1)^N(\lambda+1)^p(\lambda-1)^q$ (where $p+q=N$) then g is said to have the type (p,q). If a diffeomorphism $G:(\mathbb{R}^N,0)\longrightarrow(\mathbb{R}^N,0)$ is an involution, so is the linear operator $(G)_1$, and we say that G has the type (p,q) if $(G)_1$ has.

Let h_1, h_2 be linear operators $\mathbb{R}^N \to \mathbb{R}^N$. If there exists a nondegenerate linear operator $g: \mathbb{R}^N \to \mathbb{R}^N$ taking h_1 into h_2 i.e. $h_2 = g h_1 g^{-1}$ then, as usual, we call h_1 and h_2 conjugate (by g). Two $N \times N$ matrices are called similar if they represent conjugate operators (i.e. if they represent the same operator in two different bases).

If a diffeomorphism $A: (\mathbb{R}^N, 0) \to (\mathbb{R}^N, 0)$ is weakly reversible with respect to another diffeomorphism $G: (\mathbb{R}^N, 0) \to (\mathbb{R}^N, 0)$ then linear operators $(A)_1$ and $(A)_1^{-1}$ are conjugate. Likewise, if a vector-field V at $(\mathbb{R}^N, 0)$ (where $V(0) = 0$) is weakly reversible with respect to a diffeomorphism $G: (\mathbb{R}^N, 0) \to (\mathbb{R}^N, 0)$ then linear operators $(V)_1$ and $-(V)_1$ are conjugate. In both cases a conjugating linear operator is $(G)_1$.

In accordance with this we introduce the following two definitions. A linear operator $a: \mathbb{R}^N \to \mathbb{R}^N$ is reversible if it is nondegenerate and conjugate to its inverse a^{-1}. A linear operator $v: \mathbb{R}^N \to \mathbb{R}^N$ is infinitesimally reversible if it is conjugate to the operator $-v$.

Establish some simple properties of reversible and infinitesimally reversible linear operators. Not all of these properties will be used in the sequel.

In an even-dimensional space, examples of reversible and infinitesimally reversible operators are those ones which in a certain basis are represented by symplectic or infinitesimally symplectic matrices, respectively. Recall that a $(2N) \times (2N)$ matrix S is symplectic if it satisfies the relation $S^* I S = I$, where

$$I = \begin{pmatrix} 0 & -E_N \\ E_N & 0 \end{pmatrix}$$

and S^* denotes the matrix transposed to S (it is the relation that matrices of symplectic linear operators satisfy in a symplectic basis). Matrices of the form $I\mathcal{U}$, where $\mathcal{U}$ is any symmetric matrix, are said to be infinitesimally symplectic (canonical equations with a quadratic Hamilton function $\frac{1}{2}\langle \mathcal{U}x, x\rangle$, $x=(p_1,\dots,p_N,q_1,\dots,q_N)$ being a vector written in a symplectic basis, have the form $\dot{x}=I\mathcal{U}x$).

PROPOSITION 2.1. A linear operator represented by a symplectic matrix is reversible.

PROOF. We will prove a more general statement, namely, if a matrix S satisfies the relation $S^*BS=B$, where B is any nondegenerate matrix, then the matrices S and S^{-1} are similar.

Indeed, $S^*BS=B$ implies $S^*=BS^{-1}B^{-1}$, i.e. the matrices S^{-1} and S^* are similar, but every matrix $\mathcal{M}$ is similar to $\mathcal{M}^*$. X

PROPOSITION 2.2. A linear operator represented by an infinitesimally symplectic matrix is infinitesimally reversible.

PROOF. If $T=I\mathcal{U}$, where $\mathcal{U}$ is symmetric, then $I^{-1}TI=\mathcal{U}I$ $=-\mathcal{U}I^*=-T^*$. Thus, the matrix T is similar to the matrix $-T^*$ and, consequently, to the matrix $-T$. X

REMARK. One can prove a more general statement, namely, if $\mathcal{U}$ is a symmetric real matrix and R is a skew symmetric one then the matrix $R\mathcal{U}$ is infinitesimally reversible. In the case when either R or $\mathcal{U}$ is nondegenerate, this statement may be verified in exactly the same manner as for $R=I$.

The spectrum and the Jordan normal form of a reversible operator possess the following properties. If a number $\lambda\in\mathbb{C}$ is an eigenvalue of a reversible operator then so is the number λ^{-1}. All eigenvalues of a reversible operator, different from 1 and -1, are divided into real pairs (s, s^{-1}), unitary pairs $(e^{i\varphi}, e^{-i\varphi})$ and quadruplets $(r^{\pm 1}e^{\pm i\varphi})$. Jordan blocks corresponding to two elements of a pair or four elements of a quadruplet always have the same structure.

It is well known that a symplectic operator always has an even number of Jordan blocks with eigenvalue 1 of odd orders and these blocks are naturally divided into pairs. The same statement is true for eigenvalue -1. On the contrary, an arbitrary reversible operator may have an odd number of Jordan blocks with eigenvalues 1 or -1 of a given odd order.

THEOREM 2.1. If $a:\mathbb{R}^N \to \mathbb{R}^N$ is a reversible operator then an operator $g:\mathbb{R}^N \to \mathbb{R}^N$ taking a into a^{-1} can be chosen to be an involution.

It is this theorem that justifies the term "reversible".

PROOF. There exists a basis in which the matrix of the operator a is the direct sum of Jordan blocks J_1 and J_{-1}, matrices of the form

$$\begin{pmatrix} J_s & 0 \\ 0 & J_s^{-1} \end{pmatrix} \quad (s\in\mathbb{R},\ |s|>1),$$

generalized Jordan blocks $J_{\exp(i\varphi)}$ $(0<\varphi<\pi)$ and matrices of the form

$$\begin{pmatrix} J_{r\exp(i\varphi)} & 0 \\ 0 & J_{r\exp(i\varphi)}^{-1} \end{pmatrix} \quad (r>1,\ 0<\varphi<\pi)$$

where J_x denotes a Jordan block with eigenvalue $x\in\mathbb{R}$ and J_{x+iy} $(x, y\in\mathbb{R},\ y>0)$ denotes a generalized Jordan block with eigenvalues $x\pm iy$, i.e. the matrix

$$\begin{pmatrix} \begin{pmatrix} x & y \\ -y & x \end{pmatrix} & \begin{pmatrix} 1 & 0 \\ 0 & 1 \end{pmatrix} & & & 0 \\ & \begin{pmatrix} x & y \\ -y & x \end{pmatrix} & \begin{pmatrix} 1 & 0 \\ 0 & 1 \end{pmatrix} & & \\ & & \ddots & \ddots & \\ & & & \ddots & \begin{pmatrix} 1 & 0 \\ 0 & 1 \end{pmatrix} \\ 0 & & & & \begin{pmatrix} x & y \\ -y & x \end{pmatrix} \end{pmatrix}$$

Now it suffices to consider matrices of each of these four types separately.

a) Every $(2\ell)\times(2\ell)$ matrix of the form

$$\begin{pmatrix} \mathcal{M} & 0 \\ 0 & \mathcal{M}^{-1} \end{pmatrix}$$

is taken into its inverse by the involutory matrix

$$L_\ell = \begin{pmatrix} 0 & E_\ell \\ E_\ell & 0 \end{pmatrix}.$$

b) The $\ell \times \ell$ Jordan block J_1 is obviously similar to the matrix

$$C_\ell = \begin{pmatrix} 1 & 2 & 2 & \dots & 2 & 2 \\ & 1 & 2 & \dots & 2 & 2 \\ & & 1 & \dots & 2 & 2 \\ & & & \dots & \dots & \\ 0 & & & & 1 & 2 \\ & & & & & 1 \end{pmatrix}.$$

Let D_ℓ be the diagonal matrix

$$diag\,(1,-1,1,-1,\dots,(-1)^{\ell},(-1)^{\ell+1})\,.$$

As is easy to verify, $D_\ell^2 = E_\ell$ and $D_\ell C_\ell D_\ell = C_\ell^{-1}$.

The $\ell \times \ell$ Jordan block J_{-1} is similar to the matrix $-C_\ell$ which satisfies the relation $D_\ell(-C_\ell)D_\ell = -C_\ell^{-1}$.

c) Let $0<\varphi<\pi$. Consider the following $(2\ell)\times(2\ell)$ matrix

$$P_\ell = \begin{pmatrix} Q & 2Q & 2Q & \dots & 2Q & 2Q \\ & Q & 2Q & \dots & 2Q & 2Q \\ & & Q & \dots & 2Q & 2Q \\ & & & \dots & \dots & \dots \\ 0 & & & & Q & 2Q \\ & & & & & Q \end{pmatrix}$$

where

$$Q = \begin{pmatrix} \cos\varphi & \sin\varphi \\ -\sin\varphi & \cos\varphi \end{pmatrix}.$$

It is easy to verify that ranks of matrices $P_\ell - e^{i\varphi}E_{2\ell}$ and $P_\ell - e^{-i\varphi}E_{2\ell}$ equal $2\ell-1$. Therefore the matrix P_ℓ is similar to the $(2\ell)\times(2\ell)$ generalized Jordan block $J_{exp(i\varphi)}$. Let T_ℓ be the diagonal matrix

$$diag(1,-1,-1,1,1,-1,-1,1,\dots,(-1)^{\ell},(-1)^{\ell+1},(-1)^{\ell+1},(-1)^{\ell})$$

(its $(2i+1)$-th diagonal element is equal to $(-1)^i$ and $(2i+2)$-th one is equal to $(-1)^{i+1}$). Then $T_\ell^2 = E_{2\ell}$ and $T_\ell P_\ell T_\ell = P_\ell^{-1}$. X

The spectrum and the Jordan normal form of an infinitesimally reversible operator possess the following properties. If a number $\lambda \in \mathbb{C}$ is an eigenvalue of an infinitesimally reversible operator then so is the number $-\lambda$. All nonzero eigenvalues of an infinitesimally reversible operator are divided into real pairs $(x,-x)$, purely imaginary pairs $(iy,-iy)$ and quadruplets $(\pm x \pm iy)$. Jordan blocks corresponding to two elements of a pair or four elements of a quadruplet always have the same structure.

It is well known that an infinitesimally symplectic operator always has an even number of nilpotent Jordan blocks of odd orders and these blocks are naturally divided into pairs. On the contrary, an arbitrary infinitesimally reversible operator may have an odd number of nilpotent Jordan blocks of a given odd order.

THEOREM 2.2. If $v: \mathbb{R}^N \to \mathbb{R}^N$ is an infinitesimally reversible operator then an operator $g: \mathbb{R}^N \to \mathbb{R}^N$ taking v into $-v$ can be chosen to be an involution.

It is this theorem that justifies the term "infinitesimally reversible".

PROOF. There exists a basis in which the matrix of the operator v is the direct sum of nilpotent Jordan blocks J_0 , matrices of the form

$$\begin{pmatrix} J_x & 0 \\ 0 & -J_x \end{pmatrix} \quad (x \in \mathbb{R},\ x > 0)\ ,$$

generalized Jordan blocks $J_{iy}\ (y \in \mathbb{R},\ y > 0)$ and matrices of the form

$$\begin{pmatrix} J_{x+iy} & 0 \\ 0 & -J_{x+iy} \end{pmatrix} \quad (x, y > 0)\ .$$

Now it suffices to consider matrices of each of these four types separately. We shall need involutory matrices L_ℓ, D_ℓ, and T_ℓ defined in the proof of the preceding theorem.

a) Every $(2\ell)\times(2\ell)$ matrix of the form

$$\begin{pmatrix} \mathcal{M} & 0 \\ 0 & -\mathcal{M} \end{pmatrix}$$

is taken into the matrix

$$\begin{pmatrix} -\mathcal{M} & 0 \\ 0 & \mathcal{M} \end{pmatrix}$$

by the matrix L_ℓ.

b) The nilpotent $\ell\times\ell$ Jordan block J_0 satisfies the relation $D_\ell J_0 D_\ell = -J_0$.

c) The $(2\ell)\times(2\ell)$ generalized Jordan block J_{iy} $(y>0)$ satisfies the relation $T_\ell J_{iy} T_\ell = -J_{iy}$. X

REMARK. One may consider reversible and infinitesimally reversible linear operators over any field and take an interest whether the statements of Theorems 2.1 and 2.2 are still valid over an arbitrary field F. If a field F is algebraically close then the statements of Theorems 2.1 and 2.2 turn out to remain true. Namely, for each reversible operator $a: F^N \to F^N$ and infinitesimally reversible operator $v: F^N \to F^N$ an operator taking a into a^{-1} and an operator taking v into $-v$ can be chosen to be involutions.

Indeed, let us consider a reversible operator a firstly. There exists a basis in which its matrix is the direct sum of matrices of the form

$$\begin{pmatrix} J_s & 0 \\ 0 & J_s^{-1} \end{pmatrix}, \quad s\in F,\ s\neq 0,\ s\neq \pm 1$$

(they can be examined in exactly the same manner as for $F=\mathbb{R}$) and Jordan blocks $J_{\pm 1}$. If $\mathrm{char}\,F \neq 2$ then Jordan blocks $J_{\pm 1}$ can be also examined similarly to the case $F=\mathbb{R}$. Let $\mathrm{char}\,F=2$ and let J_1 be the $\ell \times \ell$ Jordan block. Consider the $\ell \times \ell$ matrix W_ℓ, whose elements w_{pq} equal 0 for $p>q$ and equal

$$\binom{\ell-p}{\ell-q} \bmod 2$$

for $p \leq q$ (the binomial coefficient modulo 2). Then $W_\ell^2 = E_\ell$ which follows from the identity

$$\sum_{n=\nu}^{\mu} \binom{\mu}{n}\binom{n}{\nu} = 2^{\mu-\nu}\binom{\mu}{\nu}$$

for $\nu \leq \mu$. On the other hand, $J_1^{-1} = W_\ell J_1 W_\ell$, which follows from the identity

$$\binom{\ell-p}{\ell-q+1} = \sum_{n=p+1}^{q} \binom{\ell-n}{\ell-q}$$

for $1 \leq p < q \leq \ell$.

Now consider an infinitesimally reversible operator v . There exists a basis is which its matrix is the direct sum of matrices of the form

$$\begin{pmatrix} J_x & 0 \\ 0 & -J_x \end{pmatrix}, \quad x \in F,\ x \neq 0,$$

and nilpotent Jordan blocks J_0 . Matrices of both types can be examined in exactly the same manner as for $F=\mathbb{R}$.

We conjecture that the statements of Theorems 2.1 and 2.2 remain valid for each field F.

Return to real operators. The type of an involution $g:\mathbb{R}^N\to\mathbb{R}^N$ reversing a given reversible operator $a:\mathbb{R}^N\to\mathbb{R}^N$ or a given infinitesimally reversible one $v:\mathbb{R}^N\to\mathbb{R}^N$ imposes certain restrictions on the spectrum of operators a or v respectively.

PROPOSITION 2.3. Let $g:\mathbb{R}^{2m+\kappa}\to\mathbb{R}^{2m+\kappa}$ be an involutory operator of type $(m, m+\kappa)$ taking a reversible operator $a:\mathbb{R}^{2m+\kappa}\longrightarrow\mathbb{R}^{2m+\kappa}$ into the operator a^{-1}. Then at least κ eigenvalues of the operator a are equal to either 1 or -1 and, moreover, a has at least κ linearly independent eigenvectors with eigenvalues 1 or -1 (i.e. $\dim\operatorname{Ker}(a-E_{2m+\kappa})+\dim\operatorname{Ker}(a+E_{2m+\kappa})\geqslant\kappa$).

PROOF. Let Π be the eigensubspace of the involution g corresponding to eigenvalue 1, and let $\Xi=\Pi\cap a\Pi$. Consider an arbitrary vector $x\in\Xi$. Since $x\in a\Pi$, $\tilde{x}=a^{-1}x\in\Pi$. Now in view of $gx=x$ (since $x\in\Pi$), $g\tilde{x}=\tilde{x}$ and $ag=ga^{-1}$ we obtain that $ax=agx=ga^{-1}x=g\tilde{x}=\tilde{x}$, i.e. $\tilde{x}\in a\Pi$. Thus, $ax=\tilde{x}\in a\Pi\cap\Pi=\Xi$ and $a^2x=a\tilde{x}=x$. We have proved that Ξ is invariant under a and that the restriction of a to Ξ is an involution. This means that the subspace Ξ has a basis consisting of eigenvectors of a with eigenvalues 1 and -1. But $\dim\Pi=m+\kappa$, whence $\dim\Xi\geqslant 2(m+\kappa)-(2m+\kappa)=\kappa$. X

REMARK. Generically the other $2m$ eigenvalues of the operator a are different from 1 and -1.

PROPOSITION 2.4. Let $g:\mathbb{R}^{2m+\kappa}\longrightarrow\mathbb{R}^{2m+\kappa}$ be an involutory operator of type $(m, m+\kappa)$ taking an infinitesimally reversible operator $v:\mathbb{R}^{2m+\kappa}\longrightarrow\mathbb{R}^{2m+\kappa}$ into the operator $-v$. Then at least κ eigenvalues of the operator v are equal to 0 and, moreover, v has at least κ linearly independent 0-eigenvectors (i.e. $\dim\operatorname{Ker}v\geqslant\kappa$).

PROOF. Let Π be the eigensubspace of the involution g corresponding to eigenvalue 1, and let $\Xi=\{x\in\Pi\mid vx\in\Pi\}$. Consider an arbitrary vector $x\in\Xi$. On account of $x\in\Pi$, $vx\in\Pi$

and $vg=-gv$ we have $vx=vgx=-gvx=-vx$, whence $vx=0$. Thus $\Xi\subset \operatorname{Ker} v$. But $\dim\Pi=m+k$ which implies that $\dim\Xi\geqslant(m+k)-((2m+k)-(m+k))=k$. X

REMARK. Generically the other $2m$ eigenvalues of the operator v are different from 0.

The local (weakly reversible) KAM-theory deals with weakly reversible diffeomorphisms $A:(\mathbb{R}^{2m+k},0)\to(\mathbb{R}^{2m+k},0)$, whose linearizations $(A)_1$ have eigenvalue 1 of multiplicity k and $2m$ eigenvalues lying in $\mathcal{U}(1)\setminus\{1;-1\}$, $\mathcal{U}(1)$ being $\{\lambda\in\mathbb{C}\,|\,|\lambda|=1\}$, and with weakly reversible vectorfields V at $(\mathbb{R}^{2m+k},0)$ (where $V(0)=0$), whose linearizations $(V)_1$ have eigenvalue 0 of multiplicity k and $2m$ nonzero purely imaginary eigenvalues. We shall call such diffeomorphisms and vectorfields slightly elliptic, for $k=0$ - elliptic.

If a slightly elliptic diffeomorphism A is not only weakly reversible but genuinely reversible and the involution reversing it is of type $(m,m+k)$ then the linearization $(A)_1$ has k linearly independent eigenvectors corresponding to eigenvalue 1. If a slightly elliptic field V is not only weakly reversible but genuinely reversible and the involution reversing it is of type $(m,m+k)$ then the linearization $(V)_1$ has k linearly independent eigenvectors corresponding to eigenvalue 0.

In future for $k\geqslant 1$ we will consider only reversible slightly elliptic diffeomorphisms and vectorfields and will assume the type of an involution reversing them to be $(m,m+k)$.

§ 2.2. Normal forms for slightly elliptic reversible diffeomorphisms near a fixed point

PROPOSITION 2.5. Let A and G be smooth germs of diffeomorphisms $(\mathbb{R}^{2m+k},0)\longrightarrow(\mathbb{R}^{2m+k},0)$, where G is an involution of type $(m, m+k)$ reversing A . Then the linearization $(A)_1$ has at least k linearly independent eigenvectors with eigenvalues 1 and -1. Generically

a) the other $2m$ eigenvalues of $(A)_1$ are different from 1 and -1;

b) through 0 there exists a smooth k-dimensional surface Ξ invariant under A and consisting of points fixed by G , such that $A|_\Xi$ is an involution.

PROOF. By Proposition 2.3 the linearization $(A)_1$ of the diffeomorphism A has at least k linearly independent eigenvectors with eigenvalues 1 and -1. It is obvious that generically the other $2m$ eigenvalues of $(A)_1$ are different from 1 and -1. Now let Π be the set of fixed points of the involution G . Π is a smooth $(m+k)$-dimensional surface passing through 0. Let $\Xi = \Pi \cap A\Pi$. In exactly the same way as in the proof of Proposition 2.3 one can show that Ξ is A-invariant and $A|_\Xi$ is an involution. But generically Π and $A\Pi$ intersect at 0 transversally, and, consequently, Ξ is a smooth k-dimensional surface. X

REMARK 1. If (in the generic case) eigenvalue -1 of $(A)_1$ has multiplicity s and eigenvalue 1 has multiplicity $k-s$ (where $0 \leq s \leq k$) then $A|_\Xi$ is obviously an involution of type $(s, k-s)$.

REMARK 2. As is easy to see, if A is slightly elliptic then the surfaces Π and $A\Pi$ intersect at 0 transversally for certain, so that the surface Ξ exists and $A|_\Xi = id$.

In future we will consider pairs of analytic diffeomorphisms $A, G: (\mathbb{R}^{2m+k}, 0) \longrightarrow (\mathbb{R}^{2m+k}, 0)$, where G is an involution of type $(m, m+k)$ and A is a slightly elliptic diffeomorphism, reversible with respect to this involution. We denote unequal to 1 eigenvalues of $(A)_1$ by $\lambda_1, \ldots, \lambda_m, \bar{\lambda}_1, \ldots, \bar{\lambda}_m$, where $\operatorname{Im} \lambda_j > 0$.

We shall assume all m numbers $\lambda_1, \ldots, \lambda_m$ to be distinct. If

$\lambda_1,\dots,\lambda_m$ are resonant then, as usual, the number

$$|q| = \sum_{j=1}^{m} |q_j|$$

is called the order of a resonance $\lambda^q = 1$, where $q \in \mathbb{Z}^m \setminus \{0\}$.
It is obvious that one can choose such a coordinate system $(z_1,\dots,z_m,$ $\xi_1,\dots,\xi_\kappa)$ with origin at 0 in $\mathbb{R}^{2m+\kappa}$ where $z_j \in \mathbb{C}, \xi_t \in \mathbb{R}$ (to be more precise, such a coordinate system

$$\left(\frac{z_1+\bar{z}_1}{2},\ \frac{\bar{z}_1-z_1}{2}i,\ \dots,\ \frac{z_m+\bar{z}_m}{2},\ \frac{\bar{z}_m-z_m}{2}i\ ,\ \xi_1,\dots,\xi_\kappa\right)$$

in which the linearization $(A)_1$ of the diffeomorphism A has the form $(A)_1 : (z,\xi) \longmapsto (\lambda z, \xi)$ and Ξ is given by equations $z_j = 0$. In this coordinate system $(\sigma)_1 : (z,\xi) \mapsto (\mu\bar{z},\xi)$,where $|\mu_j| = 1$. By a rotation of the coordinate system (i.e. a transformation of the form $(z,\xi) \longmapsto (\Lambda z, \xi)$, where $\Lambda = (\Lambda_1,\dots,\Lambda_m)$ and $|\Lambda_j| = 1$) commuting with $(A)_1$ one can put $(\sigma)_1$ into $(\sigma)_1 : (z,\xi) \mapsto (\bar{z},\xi)$. By Bochner's theorem [39] there exists an analytic change of variables keeping the 1-jet at 0 unchanged and putting σ into $\sigma : (z,\xi) \mapsto (\bar{z},\xi)$. Moreover, one can require that in the new coordinate system Ξ should be still given by equations $z_j = 0$.

Henceforth fix a coordinate system in which

$$(A)_1 : (z,\xi) \longmapsto (\lambda z,\xi),\quad \sigma : (z,\xi) \longmapsto (\bar{z},\xi),\quad \Xi = \{z=0\}.$$

Introduce the notation $\rho_j = z_j \bar{z}_j$.

PROPOSITION 2.6. Suppose there are no resonances among $\lambda_1,\dots,\lambda_m$ of order $\ell+2$ and lower ($\ell\in\mathbb{N}$). Then there exists an analytic change of variables commuting with G, leaving Ξ pointwise fixed and taking $(A)_{\ell+1}$ into the form

$$(A)_{\ell+1}: \begin{matrix} z \\ \xi \end{matrix} \longmapsto \begin{matrix} \lambda z K^{(\ell)}(\xi,\rho) \\ \xi \end{matrix}$$

where $K_j^{(\ell)}$ is a complex polynomial in ξ and ρ (of degree $\leq \ell$ if considered as a polynomial in ξ, z and $\bar{z}$) with constant term 1, and

$$(K_j^{(\ell)}\overline{K_j^{(\ell)}})_\ell = 1 .$$

Suppose there are no resonances among $\lambda_1,\dots,\lambda_m$ at all. Then there exists a formal change of variables commuting with G, leaving Ξ pointwise fixed and taking A into the form

$$A: \begin{matrix} z \\ \xi \end{matrix} \longmapsto \begin{matrix} \lambda z K(\xi,\rho) \\ \xi \end{matrix}$$

where K_j is a formal complex series in powers of ξ and ρ with constant term 1, and $K_j\overline{K_j}=1$.

PROOF. We proceed by induction on the jet number. Suppose there are no resonances among $\lambda_1,\dots,\lambda_m$ of order $d+3$ and lower (where $d\in\mathbb{Z}_+$). Assume that $(A)_{d+1}$ has been normalized, i.e. in a certain coordinate system

$$G: \begin{matrix} z \\ \xi \end{matrix} \longmapsto \begin{matrix} \bar{z} \\ \xi \end{matrix}, (A)_{d+1}: \begin{matrix} z \\ \xi \end{matrix} \longmapsto \begin{matrix} \lambda z K^{(d)}(\xi,\rho) \\ \xi \end{matrix}, \quad \Xi=\{z=0\}$$

where $K_j^{(d)}$ is a complex polynomial in ξ and ρ of degree $\leq d$ (if considered as a polynomial in ξ, z and $\bar{z}$) with constant term 1 such that

$$\left(K_j^{(d)} \overline{K_j^{(d)}}\right)_d = 1 \quad .$$

We have

$$(A)_{d+2}: \begin{array}{ccc} z & & \lambda z K^{(d)}(\xi,\rho) + \sum\limits_{|a|+|b|+|c|=d+2} P_{abc}\, \xi^a z^b \bar{z}^c \\ & \longmapsto & \\ \xi & & \xi + \sum\limits_{|a|+|b|+|c|=d+2} Q_{abc}\, \xi^a z^b \bar{z}^c \end{array}$$

where $Q_{abc} = \overline{Q_{acb}}$.

Since $A|_{\Xi} = id$ it follows that $P_{j,a00} = 0$ and $Q_{t,a00} = 0$ for all $j, t, a \; (1 \leq j \leq m, \; 1 \leq t \leq \kappa, \; |a| = d+2)$.

Denote by e_j the multiindex $(0,\ldots,0,1,0,\ldots,0)$ of length m, in which the unity occupies the jth position.

In order to normalize A consider the following change of variables

$$H: \begin{array}{ccc} z & & z + \sum\limits_{|a|+|b|+|c|=d+2} P'_{abc}\, \xi^a z^b \bar{z}^c \\ & \longmapsto & \\ \xi & & \xi + \sum\limits_{|a|+|b|+|c|=d+2} Q'_{abc}\, \xi^a z^b \bar{z}^c \end{array}$$

where

$$P'_{j,abc} = \begin{cases} \dfrac{P_{j,abc}}{\lambda_j - \lambda^{b-c}}, & b \neq c + e_j \\ 0, & b = c + e_j, \end{cases} \qquad Q'_{t,abc} = \begin{cases} \dfrac{Q_{t,abc}}{1-\lambda^{b-c}}, & \text{for } b \neq c \\ 0, & \text{for } b = c. \end{cases}$$

$Q_{abc} = \overline{Q_{acb}}$ ensures that $\sum Q'_{abc} \xi^a z^b \bar{z}^c$ is real. Since $P_{a00} = 0$ for all a $(|a| = d+2)$ it follows that $H(0,\xi) = (0,\xi)$.

H commutes with G precisely when

$$\frac{Q_{abc}}{1-\lambda^{b-c}} = \frac{Q_{acb}}{1-\lambda^{c-b}}$$

for $b \neq c$ and

$$\frac{P_{j,abc}}{\lambda_j - \lambda^{b-c}} = \frac{\overline{P_{j,abc}}}{\bar{\lambda}_j - \lambda^{c-b}}$$

for $b \neq c + e_j$. These relations easily follows from $AGA = G$.

Moreover, $AGA = G$ implies that $Q_{abc} = 0$ for $b = c$ (we have already known that $Q_{abc} = 0$ for $b = c = 0$).

Therefore,

$$(HAH^{-1})_{d+2} : \begin{matrix} z \\ \xi \end{matrix} \mapsto \begin{matrix} \lambda z K^{(d)}(\xi,\rho) + z \sum_{|a|+2|b|=d+1} \tilde{P}_{ab} \xi^a \rho^b \\ \xi \end{matrix}$$

where

$$\tilde{P}_{j,a,b} = P_{j,a,b+e_j,b}\,.$$

Denote

$$K_j^{(d)}(\xi,\rho)+\bar{\lambda}_j \sum \tilde{P}_{j,ab}\xi^a \rho^b$$

by $K_j'(\xi,\rho)$. It remains to verify that $(K_j' \bar{K}_j')_{d+1}=1$. It follows from $A \sigma A = \sigma$ that

$$(\bar{K}_j' \, K_j'(\xi, \rho K' \bar{K}'))_{d+1}=1.$$

Since $(K_j' \bar{K}_j')_d = 1$,

$$(K'(\xi,\rho K' \bar{K}'))_{d+1}=(K'(\xi,\rho))_{d+1} \;,$$

and we obtain $(K_j' \bar{K}_j')_{d+1} = 1$. X

COROLLARY. If resonances are absent then a neighbourhood of 0 in $\mathbb{R}^{2m+\kappa}$ is foliated into formal $2m$-dimensional transversal to Ξ surfaces, invariant under A and σ.

REMARK. One can show that this corollary is valid not only for slightly elliptic reversible diffeomorphisms but for any generic pairs $A, \sigma : (\mathbb{R}^{2m+\kappa},0) \to (\mathbb{R}^{2m+\kappa},0)$, where σ is an involution of type $(m, m+\kappa)$ reversing A and a diffeomorphism A is nonresonant (in a suitable sense).

DEFINITION. Let $\ell \in \mathbb{N}$. We say that $A \in \Psi_\ell$ if the following two conditions hold.

a) There are no resonances among $\lambda_1, \dots, \lambda_m$ of order $4\ell+2$ and lower.

By Proposition 2.6 this condition implies the existence of such a coordinate system (z, ξ), in which

$$(A)_{4\ell+1}: \begin{matrix} z \\ \xi \end{matrix} \longmapsto \begin{matrix} \lambda z K^{(4\ell)}(\xi,\rho) \\ \xi \end{matrix}, \quad \sigma: \begin{matrix} z \\ \xi \end{matrix} \longmapsto \begin{matrix} \bar{z} \\ \xi \end{matrix}, \quad \Xi = \{z=0\} \tag{1}$$

where $K_j^{(4\ell)}$ is a complex polynomial in ξ and ρ of degree $\leqslant 4\ell$ (if considered as a polynomial in ξ, z and $\bar{z}$) with constant term 1, and

$$\left(K_j^{(4\ell)} \overline{K_j^{(4\ell)}}\right)_{4\ell} = 1 .$$

b) Polynomials $K_j^{(4\ell)}$ in (1) have the form

$$K_j^{(4\ell)}(\xi,\rho)$$

$$= 1 + \sum_{\substack{1 \leq |a|+2|b| \leq 2\ell \\ |a| \geq 1}} S_{j,ab}\,\xi^a \rho^b + i F_j(\rho) + \sum_{2\ell+1 \leq |a|+2|b| \leq 4\ell} R_{j,ab}\,\xi^a \rho^b$$

where F_j are homogeneous polynomials in ρ of degree ℓ and $F_1,\ldots,F_m$ are functionally independent:

$$\frac{\partial(F_1,\ldots,F_m)}{\partial(\rho_1,\ldots,\rho_m)} \not\equiv 0 .$$

(As is easy to see, this property of $K_j^{(4\ell)}$ is invariant under changes of variables preserving the form (1) of the jet $(A)_{4\ell+1}$ and the involution σ.)

REMARK 1. The equality

$$(K_j^{(4\ell)} \overline{K_j^{(4\ell)}})_{2\ell} = 1$$

ensures that all polynomials F_j are real.

REMARK 2. To be less formal, the condition b) means that in the vector-polynomial $(K_1^{(4\ell)}, \dots, K_m^{(4\ell)})$ the homogeneous components of degrees $2, \dots, 2\ell-1$ are dividable by ξ (i.e. belong to the ideal generated by $\xi_1, \dots, \xi_k$) and the independent of ξ part of the homogeneous component of degree 2ℓ is nondegenerate.

REMARK 3. As is easy to verify, for $m=2$ or for $\ell=1$ the functional independence of polynomials F_j follows from their linear independence (for $\ell=1$ the condition of the functional independence of $F_1, \dots, F_m$ is merely the condition of the nondegeneracy of the linear operator $F: \mathbb{R}^m \longrightarrow \mathbb{R}^m$). For $m \geqslant 3$ and $\ell \geqslant 2$ this is no longer valid. An appropriate example will be linearly independent polynomials $F_1(\rho)=\rho_1^\ell, \dots, F_{m-1}(\rho)= \rho_{m-1}^\ell$, $F_m(\rho)= \rho_1^{\ell-1}\rho_2$ depending only on $\rho_1, \dots, \rho_{m-1}$.

§ 2.3. Weakly reversible elliptic hyperbolic diffeomorphisms near a fixed point

In the preceding section we received normal forms for reversible slightly elliptic diffeomorphisms. Here we start to investigate elliptic diffeomorphisms more circumstantially, assuming them to be not reversible but only weakly reversible. In order to show the moment of ellipticity more clearly we will firstly consider not purely elliptic but elliptic hyperbolic diffeomorphisms, whose linearizations have eigenvalues lying in $(\mathcal{U}(1) \cup \mathbb{R}) \setminus \{-1, 1\}$.

In this section we allow m to equal 0, i.e. we suppose $m \in \mathbb{Z}_+$. Fix also a number $n \in \mathbb{Z}_+$. The index i will have the range from 1 to n.

For more concise notations we shall use the double numbers algebra. Recall that the real algebra $\mathbb{K}$ of double numbers is the two-dimensional algebra over $\mathbb{R}$ containing the unity 1 (double numbers of the form $a \cdot 1$, $a \in \mathbb{R}$, may be identified with corresponding real numbers) and such a vector e linearly independent with 1 that the multiplication is determined by the relation $e^2 = 1$. Thus, double numbers may be written down as $a + be$, where $a, b \in \mathbb{R}$. There exists the involution $\sim$ of double conjugation acting on $\mathbb{K}$: $\widetilde{a+be} = a - be$. It satisfies the relations $\widetilde{w_1 w_2} = \tilde{w}_1 \tilde{w}_2$ for any $w_1, w_2 \in \mathbb{K}$ and $w\tilde{w} \in \mathbb{R}$ for any $w \in \mathbb{K}$. The functional $w \mapsto w\tilde{w}$ (i.e. $a+be \mapsto a^2 - b^2$) is a (1,1)-quadratic form on $\mathbb{K}$. If $w \neq 0$ then (w is uninvertible $\Longleftrightarrow$ w is a divisor of zero $\Longleftrightarrow w\tilde{w} = 0$).

$\mathbb{C}$ and $\mathbb{K}$ may be embedded in the four-dimensional commutative algebra $\mathbb{A}$ consisting of numbers of the form $a + bi + ce + die$ (with the multiplication obviously defined). There are involutions of complex $\bar{\ }$ $(a+bi+ce+die \mapsto a-bi+ce-die)$ and double $\sim$ $(a+bi+ce+die \mapsto a+bi-ce-die)$ conjugations on $\mathbb{A}$, which commute with each other, are compatible with the embeddings $\mathbb{C} \hookrightarrow \mathbb{A}$ and $\mathbb{K} \hookrightarrow \mathbb{A}$ and are automorphisms of the algebra $\mathbb{A}$.

For any $u \in \mathbb{A}$ one has $u\bar{u} \in \mathbb{K}$, $u\tilde{u} \in \mathbb{C}$, $u\bar{u}\tilde{u}\tilde{\bar{u}} \in \mathbb{R}$. If $u = a + bi + ce + die$ then $u\bar{u}\tilde{u}\tilde{\bar{u}} = ((a-c)^2 + (b-d)^2)((a+c)^2 + (b+d)^2)$ which is equal to the determinant of the following system of linear equations with respect to $x_1, \dots, x_4$:

$$(a+bi+ce+die)(x_1 + x_2 i + x_3 e + x_4 ie) = 0.$$

Thus, for $u \neq 0$ (u is uninvertible $\Longleftrightarrow$ u is a divisor of zero $\Longleftrightarrow$ $u\tilde{u}=0 \Leftrightarrow u\bar{u}\tilde{u}\tilde{\bar{u}}=0$).

Let $A, G : (\mathbb{R}^{2(m+n)}, 0) \to (\mathbb{R}^{2(m+n)}, 0)$ be formal diffeomorphisms and let $AGA = G$. Assume all eigenvalues of $(A)_1$ to lie in $(\mathcal{U}(1) \cup \mathbb{R}) \setminus \{-1; 1\}$ and, moreover, $(A)_1$ to have $2m$ eigenvalues $\lambda_1, \ldots, \lambda_m, \bar{\lambda}_1, \ldots, \bar{\lambda}_m$ belonging to $\mathcal{U}(1)$ and $2n$ real eigenvalues $\gamma_1, \ldots, \gamma_n, \gamma_1^{-1}, \ldots, \gamma_n^{-1}$. We fix the notations so that $\operatorname{Im} \lambda_j > 0$ and $|\gamma_\tau| > 1$.

For $n=0$ the diffeomorphism A is elliptic. If $m=0$ then A is called a hyperbolic diffeomorphism.

Let $\Psi_\tau = \frac{1}{2}(\gamma_\tau + \gamma_\tau^{-1} + (\gamma_\tau - \gamma_\tau^{-1})e) \in \mathbb{K}$. Note that $\Psi_\tau \tilde{\Psi}_\tau = 1$.

We henceforth suppose all m numbers $\lambda_1, \ldots, \lambda_m$ are distinct and all n numbers $\gamma_1, \ldots, \gamma_n$ are distinct (the second assumption is equivalent to that all n numbers $\Psi_1, \ldots, \Psi_n$ are distinct). Then one can choose such a coordinate system $(z_1, \ldots, z_m, w_1, \ldots, w_n)$ with origin at 0 in $\mathbb{R}^{2(m+n)}$, where $z_j \in \mathbb{C}$, $w_\tau \in \mathbb{K}$ (to be more precise, such a coordinate system

$$\frac{z_1+\bar{z}_1}{2}, \quad \frac{\bar{z}_1 - z_1}{2} i, \ldots, \frac{z_m + \bar{z}_m}{2}, \quad \frac{\bar{z}_m - z_m}{2} i,$$

$$\frac{w_1 + \tilde{w}_1}{2}, \quad \frac{w_1 - \tilde{w}_1}{2} e, \ldots, \frac{w_n + \tilde{w}_n}{2}, \quad \frac{w_n - \tilde{w}_n}{2} e),$$

in which the linearization $(A)_1$ of the diffeomorphism A has the form

$$(A)_1 : (z, w) \longmapsto (\lambda z, \Psi w). \tag{2}$$

In this coordinate system $(G)_1 : (z, w) \longmapsto (\mu' \bar{z}, \nu' \tilde{w})$, where $\mu'_j \in \mathbb{C} \setminus \{0\}$ and $\nu'_\tau \in \mathbb{K}$, $\nu'_\tau \tilde{\nu}'_\tau \neq 0$. Via an additional linear change of variables of the form $(z,w) \mapsto (\Lambda z, \Omega w)$, where $\Lambda_j \in \mathbb{C}, |\Lambda_j| = 1$, $\Omega_\tau \in \mathbb{K}, |\Omega_\tau \tilde{\Omega}_\tau| = 1$ (such a change of variables commutes with $(A)_1$), $(G)_1$ can be specialized further, namely, be put into the form

$$(G)_1 : (z,w) \mapsto (\mu \bar{z}, \nu \tilde{w}) \tag{3}$$

where μ_j is a positive real number and ν_τ is either a positive real number or the product of such a number by e.

We henceforth consider only such coordinate systems in which $(A)_1$ and $(G)_1$ are of the form (2) and (3), respectively. Note that $\mu_1, \ldots, \mu_m, -\mu_1, \ldots, -\mu_m, \hat{\nu}_1, \ldots, \hat{\nu}_n, -\hat{\nu}_1, \ldots, -\hat{\nu}_n$ are eigenvalues of $(G)_1$ (here by definition $\hat{\nu}_\tau = \nu_\tau$, if $\nu_\tau \in \mathbb{R}$, and $\hat{\nu}_\tau = \nu_\tau^* i \in \mathbb{C}$, if $\nu_\tau = \nu_\tau^* e$, $\nu_\tau^* \in \mathbb{R}$).

The formal series giving A is of the form

$$A : (z,w) \mapsto (\lambda z + \sum X_{abcd} z^a \bar{z}^b w^c \tilde{w}^d ,$$

$$\psi w + \sum Y_{abcd} z^a \bar{z}^b w^c \tilde{w}^d)$$

where $X_{abcd} = \widetilde{X_{abdc}}$, $Y_{abcd} = \overline{Y_{bacd}}$.

The vector-monomial

$$(\underbrace{0, \ldots, 0}_{j-1}, z^a \bar{z}^b w^c \tilde{w}^d, \underbrace{0, \ldots, 0}_{m-j}, \underbrace{0, \ldots, 0}_{n})$$

is said to be resonant if $\lambda^{a-b} \psi^{c-d} = \lambda_j$, i.e. if either $(\lambda^{a-b} = \lambda_j, \psi^{c-d} = 1)$ or $(\lambda^{a-b} = -\lambda_j, \psi^{c-d} = -1)$

and antiresonant if $\lambda^{a-b}\psi^{c-d}=\bar{\lambda}_j$, i.e. if

either $(\lambda^{a-b}=\bar{\lambda}_j,\ \psi^{c-d}=1)$ or $(\lambda^{a-b}=-\bar{\lambda}_j,\ \psi^{c-d}=-1)$.

Note that this definition is invariant under interchanging the indices c and d.

The vector-monomial

$$(\underbrace{0,\ldots,0}_{m},\ \underbrace{0,\ldots,0}_{r-1},\ z^a\bar{z}^b w^c\tilde{w}^d,\ \underbrace{0,\ldots,0}_{n-r})$$

is said to be resonant if $\lambda^{a-b}\psi^{c-d}=\psi_r$, i.e. if

either $(\lambda^{a-b}=1,\ \psi^{c-d}=\psi_r)$ or $(\lambda^{a-b}=-1,\ \psi^{c-d}=-\psi_r)$

and antiresonant if $\lambda^{a-b}\psi^{c-d}=\tilde{\psi}_r$, i.e. if

either $(\lambda^{a-b}=1,\ \psi^{c-d}=\tilde{\psi}_r)$ or $(\lambda^{a-b}=-1,\ \psi^{c-d}=-\tilde{\psi}_r)$.

Note that this definition is invariant under interchanging the indices a and b.

PROPOSITION 2.7. Let $z_0\in\mathbb{C}$, $w_0\in\mathbb{K}$, $|z_0|=1$ and $w_0\tilde{w}_0=1$. Then the number $u_0=z_0w_0-1$ is uninvertible in $\mathbb{A}$ precisely when $u_0=0$, i.e. when either $z_0=w_0=1$ or $z_0=w_0=-1$.

PROOF. Let $z_0=\alpha_1+\alpha_2 i$ and $w_0=\beta_1+\beta_2 e$. The equality $u_0\bar{u}_0\tilde{u}_0\tilde{\bar{u}}_0=0$ is equivalent to

either $(\alpha_1\beta_1-1=\alpha_1\beta_2,\ \alpha_2\beta_1=\alpha_2\beta_2)$ or $(\alpha_1\beta_1-1=-\alpha_1\beta_2,\ \alpha_2\beta_1=-\alpha_2\beta_2)$.

As is easy to see, together with $\alpha_1^2+\alpha_2^2=\beta_1^2-\beta_2^2=1$ this implies $\alpha_2=\beta_2=0$, $\alpha_1=\beta_1\in\{-1;1\}$. X

PROPOSITION 2.8 (Poincaré-Dulac, cf. [19 (Chapter 5)]). One can choose a coordinate system (z, w) so that the series giving A should contain resonant terms only.

PROOF. Suppose that the ℓth jet $(A)_\ell$ of the diffeomorphism A (where $\ell\in\mathbb{N}$) is already normalized, i.e. contains only resonant terms. Consider the change of variables

$$H: \begin{matrix} z \\ w \end{matrix} \longmapsto \begin{matrix} z + \sum\limits_{|a|+|b|+|c|+|d|=\ell+1} X'_{abcd}\, z^a \bar{z}^b w^c \tilde{w}^d \\ w + \sum\limits_{|a|+|b|+|c|+|d|=\ell+1} Y'_{abcd}\, z^a \bar{z}^b w^c \tilde{w}^d \end{matrix}$$

where coefficients $X'_{j,abcd}$ and $Y'_{\tau,abcd}$ equal zero for resonant monomials and equal

$$\frac{X_{j,abcd}}{\lambda_j-\lambda^{a-b}\psi^{c-d}} \quad\text{and}\quad \frac{Y_{\tau,abcd}}{\psi_\tau-\lambda^{a-b}\psi^{c-d}},$$

respectively, for nonresonant ones (the possibility of division in these expressions is guaranteed by Proposition 2.7). Then the $(\ell+1)$-th jet $(HAH^{-1})_{\ell+1}$ contains only resonant terms. X

PROPOSITION 2.9. If the series giving A contains only resonant terms then the series giving $\mathcal{G}$ contains only antiresonant terms.

PROOF. Let the series giving A contains only resonant terms. Consider the series giving $\mathcal{G}$:

$$\mathcal{G}:(z,w)\longmapsto(\mu\bar{z}+\sum\Gamma_{abcd}\, z^a \bar{z}^b w^c \tilde{w}^d,$$

$$\nu\tilde{w} + \sum \Phi_{abcd}\, z^a \bar{z}^b w^c \tilde{w}^d)$$

where $\Gamma_{abcd} = \widetilde{\Gamma_{abdc}}$, $\Phi_{abcd} = \overline{\Phi_{bacd}}$.

Suppose that the ℓth jet $(G)_\ell$ of the diffeomorphism G (where $\ell \in \mathbb{N}$) contains only antiresonant terms. Note that substituting a resonant series into an antiresonant one or an antiresonant one into a resonant one we get an antiresonant series. Therefore $(AGA)_{\ell+1}$ is the sum of a certain antiresonant polynomial (of degree $\leq \ell+1$) diffeomorphism and the mapping

$$F : \begin{array}{ccc} z & \longmapsto & \lambda \displaystyle\sum_{|a|+|b|+|c|+|d|=\ell+1} \Gamma_{abcd}\, \lambda^{a-b} \psi^{c-d} z^a \bar{z}^b w^c \tilde{w}^d \\ w & & \psi \displaystyle\sum_{|a|+|b|+|c|+|d|=\ell+1} \Phi_{abcd}\, \lambda^{a-b} \psi^{c-d} z^a \bar{z}^b w^c \tilde{w}^d . \end{array}$$

But $AGA=G$, whence the nonantiresonant part of F coincides with the nonantiresonant part of $(G)_{\ell+1} - (G)_\ell$. Using Proposition 2.7 we obtain that $(G)_{\ell+1}$ also contains only antiresonant terms. X

Henceforth suppose resonances among λ_j and γ_τ are absent, i.e.

$$\forall q \in \mathbb{Z}^m \setminus \{0\} \quad \lambda^q \neq 1 , \quad \forall p \in \mathbb{Z}^n \setminus \{0\} \quad \gamma^p \neq 1$$

(the second part of this conjunction is equivalent to $\psi^p \neq 1$ for each $p \in \mathbb{Z}^n \setminus \{0\}$). Let $\rho_j = z_j \bar{z}_j$ and $\sigma_\tau = w_\tau \tilde{w}_\tau$.

According to Proposition 2.8 there exists such a coordinate system, in which A is of the form

$$A : (z, w) \mapsto (\lambda z K(\rho, \sigma) , \psi w R(\rho, \sigma)) \tag{4}$$

where K_j and R_τ are complex and double, respectively, power series with constant term 1.

According to Proposition 2.9 in this coordinate system G is of the form

$$G: (z,w) \mapsto (\mu \bar{z} P(\rho,\sigma), \nu \tilde{w} Q(\rho,\sigma)) \tag{5}$$

where P_j and Q_τ are also complex and double, respectively, power series with constant term 1.

We will often drop the arguments ρ and σ of series.

Let

$$\overset{\circ}{P}_j(\rho,\sigma) = P_j(\rho K\bar{K}, \sigma R\tilde{R}) \ ,$$

$$\overset{\circ}{Q}_\tau(\rho,\sigma) = Q_\tau(\rho K\bar{K}, \sigma R\tilde{R}) \ .$$

Using these notations we may write down the weak reversibility condition $AGA = G$ as follows:

$$\begin{cases} \bar{K}_j \overset{\circ}{P}_j K_j (\mu^2 \rho K\bar{K} P^\circ \overline{P^\circ}, \ \nu\tilde{\nu}\sigma R\tilde{R} Q^\circ \widetilde{Q^\circ}) = P_j \\ \tilde{R}_\tau \overset{\circ}{Q}_\tau R_\tau (\mu^2 \rho K\bar{K} P^\circ \overline{P^\circ}, \ \nu\tilde{\nu}\sigma R\tilde{R} Q^\circ \widetilde{Q^\circ}) = Q_\tau \ . \end{cases} \tag{6}$$

THEOREM 2.3. Let $A:(\mathbb{R}^{2(m+n)},0) \to (\mathbb{R}^{2(m+n)},0)$ be a formal diffeomorphism whose linearization $(A)_1$ is reversible and has an elliptic hyperbolic spectrum, resonances being absent. Then the following conditions are equivalent:

1) A is reversible.

2) In formula (4), $K_j \bar{K}_j = 1$ and $R_\tau \tilde{R}_\tau = 1$.

3) A is weakly reversible and there exists such a reversing diffeomorphism G that $\mu_j = 1$ and $\nu_\tau = 1$ in (3).

4) A is weakly reversible and there exists such a reversing

diffeomorphism σ that $\nu_\tau = 1$ in (3).

5) A is weakly reversible and there exists such a reversing diffeomorphism σ that $\nu_\tau \in \mathbb{R}$ in (3).

PROOF. We shall prove Theorem 2.3 according to the scheme 2) $\Rightarrow$ 1) $\Rightarrow$ 3) $\Rightarrow$ 4) $\Rightarrow$ 5) $\Rightarrow$ 2).

A. 2) $\Rightarrow$ 1). Let A be written in the form (4) with $K_j \overline{K}_j = 1$ and $R_\tau \widetilde{R}_\tau = 1$. Determine a diffeomorphism σ by setting $\mu_j = 1$, $P_j = 1$, $\nu_\tau = 1$, $Q_\tau = 1$ (in (5). Then σ is an involution, (6) being valid.

B. 1) $\Rightarrow$ 3). Suppose A is reversible with respect to an involution σ written in the form (5). Then

$$(\sigma^2)_1 : (z, w) \mapsto (\mu^2 z, \nu\widetilde{\nu} w).$$

Therefore $\mu_j = 1$ and $\nu_\tau = 1$.

C. 3) $\Rightarrow$ 4) $\Rightarrow$ 5). This is trivial.

D. 5) $\Rightarrow$ 2). We have to prove that (6) and $\nu_\tau \in \mathbb{R}$ imply $K_j \overline{K}_j = 1$ and $R_\tau \widetilde{R}_\tau = 1$.

Let $(\ )^{\cdot}_\ell$ denote the ℓ-th jet with respect to ρ and σ (not to $z, \overline{z}, w$ and $\widetilde{w}$). Assume $(K_j \overline{K}_j)^{\cdot}_\ell = 1$, $(R_\tau \widetilde{R}_\tau)^{\cdot}_\ell = 1$ (where $\ell \in \mathbb{Z}_+$) and show $(K_j \overline{K}_j)^{\cdot}_{\ell+1} = 1$, $(R_\tau \widetilde{R}_\tau)^{\cdot}_{\ell+1} = 1$.

The induction assumption follows that

$$(P^\circ)^{\cdot}_{\ell+1} = (P)^{\cdot}_{\ell+1}, \quad (Q^\circ)^{\cdot}_{\ell+1} = (Q)^{\cdot}_{\ell+1},$$

$$(K(\mu^2 \rho K \overline{K} P^\circ \overline{P^\circ}, \nu\widetilde{\nu}\sigma R \widetilde{R} Q^\circ \widetilde{Q^\circ}))^{\cdot}_{\ell+1}$$
$$= (K(\mu^2 \rho P \overline{P}, \nu\widetilde{\nu}\sigma Q \widetilde{Q}))^{\cdot}_{\ell+1},$$

$$(R(\mu^2 \rho K \overline{K} P^\circ \overline{P^\circ}, \nu\widetilde{\nu}\sigma R \widetilde{R} Q^\circ \widetilde{Q^\circ}))^{\cdot}_{\ell+1}$$
$$= (R(\mu^2 \rho P \overline{P}, \nu\widetilde{\nu}\sigma Q \widetilde{Q}))^{\cdot}_{\ell+1}.$$

Therefore, rewriting (6) on the level of the $(\ell+1)$ - th jet we obtain

$$\begin{cases} (\bar{K}_j K_j(\mu^2\rho P\bar{P},\ \nu\tilde{\nu}\sigma Q\tilde{Q}))^{\cdot}_{\ell+1}=1 \\ (\tilde{R}_\tau R_\tau(\mu^2\rho P\bar{P},\ \nu\tilde{\nu}\sigma Q\tilde{Q}))^{\cdot}_{\ell+1}=1\ . \end{cases}$$

For succinctness we will often drop the indices j and τ in similar expressions.

Let $H:(\mathbb{R}^{m+n},0)\longrightarrow(\mathbb{R}^{m+n},0)$ be the following formal diffeomorphism

$$H:(\rho,\sigma)\longmapsto(\mu^2\rho P\bar{P},\nu\tilde{\nu}\sigma Q\tilde{Q}).$$

We have proved that

$$(\bar{K}(K\circ H))^{\cdot}_{\ell+1}=1,\ (\tilde{R}(R\circ H))^{\cdot}_{\ell+1}=1\ . \tag{7}$$

On the one hand, this implies that

$$((\bar{K}\circ H)(K\circ H^2))^{\cdot}_{\ell+1}=1\ ,\ (\tilde{R}\circ H)(R\circ H^2))^{\cdot}_{\ell+1}=1\ .$$

On the other hand, it follows from (7) that

$$(K(\bar{K}\circ H))^{\cdot}_{\ell+1}=1\ ,\ (R(\tilde{R}\circ H))^{\cdot}_{\ell+1}=1$$

(in virtue of equalities $\bar{K}\circ H=\overline{K\circ H}$ and $\tilde{R}\circ H=\widetilde{R\circ H}$).

Thus,

$$(K)^{\cdot}_{\ell+1}=(K\circ H^2)^{\cdot}_{\ell+1}\ ,\ (R)^{\cdot}_{\ell+1}=(R\circ H^2)^{\cdot}_{\ell+1}\,.$$

Let us show that this implies

$$(K)^{\cdot}_{\ell+1}=(K\circ H)^{\cdot}_{\ell+1},\ (R)^{\cdot}_{\ell+1}=(R\circ H)^{\cdot}_{\ell+1}.$$

Indeed, suppose that for a certain j, $1\leq j\leq m$, and a certain d, $1\leq d\leq \ell+1$, we have

$$(K_j(H(\rho,\sigma)))^{\cdot}_d=(K_j(\rho,\sigma))^{\cdot}_d+\sum_{|a|+|b|=d} g_{ab}\,\rho^a\sigma^b.$$

Then

$$(K_j(H^2(\rho,\sigma)))^{\cdot}_d$$

$$=(K_j(\rho,\sigma))^{\cdot}_d+\sum_{|a|+|b|=d} g_{ab}(1+\mu^{2a}(\nu\tilde{\nu})^b)\rho^a\sigma^b.$$

Otherwise speaking,

$$g_{ab}(1+\mu^{2a}(\nu\tilde{\nu})^b)=0$$

for each a and b. But since $\nu_r\in\mathbb{R}$ it follows that $\nu_r\tilde{\nu}_r>0$ and $1+\mu^{2a}(\nu\tilde{\nu})^b>1$. Therefore $g_{ab}=0$ for each a and b. Thus, $(K\circ H)^{\cdot}_{\ell+1}=(K)^{\cdot}_{\ell+1}$. Analogously, $(R\circ H)^{\cdot}_{\ell+1}=(R)^{\cdot}_{\ell+1}$.

Now (7) gives

$$(\bar{K}K)^{\cdot}_{\ell+1}=1,\ (\tilde{R}R)^{\cdot}_{\ell+1}=1.$$

This completes the proof of Theorem 2.3. X

As a corollary we obtain that the relation

$$K_j \bar{K}_j = 1 \; \& \; R_\tau \tilde{R}_\tau = 1$$

is invariant under changes of variables preserving the form (4) of the diffeomorphism A .

REMARK. Abandon the nonresonantness condition imposed on A and suppose only that all resonant monomials have degree $2\ell+2$ and higher (where ℓ is a fixed natural number). Then by Proposition 2.8 there exists a coordinate system in which $(A)_{2\ell+1}$ is of the form

$$(A)_{2\ell+1} : (z, w) \longmapsto (\lambda z K^{(2\ell)}(\rho, \sigma), \; \Psi w R^{(2\ell)}(\rho, \sigma))$$

where $K_j^{(2\ell)}$ and $R_\tau^{(2\ell)}$ are complex and double (respectively) polynomials in ρ and σ of degree $\leq \ell$ with constant term 1. Similarly to the proof of Theorem 2.3 one can show that if there exists such a diffeomorphism G reversing A that all $\nu_\tau \in \mathbb{R}$ in (3), then

$$(K_j^{(2\ell)} \overline{K_j^{(2\ell)}})^{\cdot}_{\ell} = 1 \quad \text{and} \quad (R_\tau^{(2\ell)} \widetilde{R_\tau^{(2\ell)}})^{\cdot}_{\ell} = 1 \, .$$

If $n = 0$, the condition 5) of Theorem 2.3 is fulfilled automatically, and we receive the following remarkable

THEOREM 2.4. Every nonresonant elliptic weakly reversible formal diffeomorphism $(\mathbb{R}^{2m}, 0) \to (\mathbb{R}^{2m}, 0)$ is reversible.

I don't know whether this statement is valid without the nonresonantness condition.

For $n \geq 1$ there exist nonresonant elliptic hyperbolic weakly reversible formal diffeomorphisms $A : (\mathbb{R}^{2(m+n)}, 0) \to (\mathbb{R}^{2(m+n)}, 0)$ which are not reversible. It is easy to construct appropriate examples even in the case of dimension two $(m = 0, \; n = 1)$, when resonances are absent automatically. Moreover, diffeomorphisms involved in these examples are generic.

Thus, let us start seeking an irreversible weakly reversible hyperbolic diffeomorphism of a plane, $(\mathbb{R}^2,0)\to(\mathbb{R}^2,0)$. We shall assume it to have the form (4). Set $\nu=e$ and $Q=1$ in (5), then the condition (6) will be reduced to $\tilde{R}R(-\sigma R\tilde{R})=1$. Pass from the double coordinate w to real coordinates

$$x=\frac{1}{2}(w(1+e)+\tilde{w}(1-e)),\quad y=\frac{1}{2}(w(1-e)+\tilde{w}(1+e)).$$

Then $w=(x+y)/2+e(x-y)/2$ and $\sigma=w\tilde{w}=xy$. In the coordinates (x,y) the diffeomorphisms G and A have the form

$$G:(x,y)\mapsto(y,-x)$$

and

$$A:(x,y)\mapsto(\gamma x B(\sigma),\gamma^{-1}yC(\sigma)),$$

respectively, where

$$B=\frac{1}{2}((1+e)R+(1-e)\tilde{R}),\quad C=\frac{1}{2}((1+e)\tilde{R}+(1-e)R).$$

B and C are real formal series in powers of σ with constant term 1. One sees $R\tilde{R}=BC$, so that

$$R\tilde{R}=1\Leftrightarrow BC=1$$

and

$$\tilde{R}R(-\sigma R\tilde{R})=1\Leftrightarrow CB(-\sigma BC)=BC(-\sigma BC)=1.$$

LEMMA. Let $B = B(\sigma)$ be a power series with constant term 1. Then

a) the condition $CB(-\sigma BC) = 1$ determines uniquely a series $C = C(\sigma)$ with constant term 1;

b) this series C satisfies the relation $BC(-\sigma BC)=1$.

PROOF. The statement a) is trivial. We have to prove b). Let $BC(-\sigma BC) = \Xi(\sigma)$. Substituting the series $-\sigma BC$ for σ into $CB(-\sigma BC)=1$ we obtain $B(\sigma\Xi)\Xi = B$. If $(\Xi)^{\cdot}_{\ell} = 1$ (where $\ell \in Z_+$) then $(B(\sigma\Xi))^{\cdot}_{\ell+1} = (B)^{\cdot}_{\ell+1}$, whence $(\Xi)^{\cdot}_{\ell+1} = 1$. Since $\Xi(0) = 1$ it follows that by induction $\Xi = 1$.

Thus, the statement b) is proved. One can receive another proof of this statement considering the series $L(\sigma) = \sigma B(\sigma)$ and $\mathcal{M}(\sigma) = \sigma C(\sigma)$. The relation $CB(-\sigma BC)=1$ is equivalent to

$$L\left(-\frac{L\mathcal{M}}{\sigma}\right) = -L$$

which implies that

$$-\frac{L\mathcal{M}}{\sigma} = L^{-1}(-L(\sigma)) \quad \text{and} \quad \mathcal{M}(\sigma) = -\frac{L^{-1}(-L(\sigma))}{L(\sigma)}\sigma$$

(here L^{-1} denotes the inverse function, i.e. $L^{-1}(L(\sigma)) \equiv \sigma$). Consequently

$$\mathcal{M}\left(-\frac{L\mathcal{M}}{\sigma}\right) = \mathcal{M}(L^{-1}(-L(\sigma))) = \frac{L^{-1}(-L(\sigma))}{L(\sigma)}\sigma = -\mathcal{M}$$

but the equality

$$\mathcal{M}\left(-\frac{L\mathcal{M}}{\sigma}\right)=-\mathcal{M}$$

is equivalent to $BC(-\sigma BC)=1$. X

The statement a) of the Lemma defines the operator $\mathcal{R}: B\mapsto C$ in the space of all real formal power series with constant term 1. The statement b) of the Lemma means that $\mathcal{R}$ is an involution.

This Lemma provides a regular method of constructing irreversible weakly reversible hyperbolic diffeomorphisms of a plane. Indeed, if an original series B is not even then the series $C=\mathcal{R}(B)$ is not equal to $1/B$. The diffeomorphism A given by such series B and C is weakly reversible (with respect to the diffeomorphism $G:(x,y)\mapsto(y,-x)$) but, since $BC\neq 1$, it is not reversible by virtue of Theorem 2.3.

Let us compute the 3-jet of the series $C=\mathcal{R}(B)$ in dependence on the 3-jet of a series B. If $(B)^{\bullet}_3(\sigma)=1+a_1\sigma+a_2\sigma^2+a_3\sigma^3$ then $(C)^{\bullet}_3(\sigma)=1+a_1\sigma+(3a_1^2-a_2)\sigma^2+(9a_1^3-6a_1a_2+a_3)\sigma^3$.

REMARK 1. The Implicit Function Theorem follows that if a series B converges (in some neighbourhood of 0) then so does the series $C=\mathcal{R}(B)$. Thus, irreversible weakly reversible hyperbolic diffeomorphisms $A:(\mathbb{R}^2,0)\longrightarrow(\mathbb{R}^2,0)$ exist in the analytic realm, too.

REMARK 2. Let $A:(\mathbb{R}^{2m},0)\longrightarrow(\mathbb{R}^{2m},0)$ be an arbitrary nonresonant elliptic symplectic formal diffeomorphism. It is well known (see, e.g., [19 (Appendix 7)]) that one can choose a canonical coordinate system z (in which the symplectic structure is

$$\frac{i}{2}\,dz\wedge d\bar{z}=\sum_{j=1}^{m}\left(d\,\frac{z_j+\bar{z}_j}{2}\wedge d\,\frac{\bar{z}_j-z_j}{2}i\right))$$

so as to have

$$A : z \longmapsto \lambda z e^{i\partial S/\partial \rho}$$

where $S = S(\rho)$ is a real formal series in powers of ρ without constant and linear terms (the Birkhoff normal form). Consequently, every nonresonant elliptic symplectic formal diffeomorphism is re-vesrible. For $m=1$ the converse statement is also true, i.e. every nonresonant elliptic reversible formal diffeomorphism of a plane can be made into a symplectic one by a suitable choice of the symplectic structure. For $m>1$ this is no longer valid. For instance, there is no symplectic structure, with respect to which the reversible dif-feomorphism

$$(z_1, z_2) \longmapsto (\lambda_1 z_1 e^{i\rho_2}, \lambda_2 z_2)$$

(here $m=2$) is symplectic.

REMARK 3. Formal normal forms for reversible diffeomorphisms were studied in [29] . To be more precise, [29] presents normal forms for a pair of involutions $(\mathbb{C}^\ell, 0) \longrightarrow (\mathbb{C}^\ell, 0)$ $(\ell \geqslant 2)$ of type $(1, \ell-1)$ which are in the generic position. One can easily transfer the results of [29] to the real case, i.e. to a generic pair of involutions $(\mathbb{R}^\ell, 0) \longrightarrow (\mathbb{R}^\ell, 0)$ $(\ell \geqslant 2)$ of type $(1, \ell-1)$ such that all eigenvalues of the product of their linearizations are real. In particular, we derive normal forms for a triplet (G, AG, A) , where $A : (\mathbb{R}^2, 0) \longrightarrow (\mathbb{R}^2, 0)$ is a hyperbolic reversible diffeomorphism and (G, AG) is a pair of involutions reversing it. These normal forms for A and G will coincide with (4) and (5) respectively (for $m = 0$, $n = 1$, $\nu=1$, $R\tilde{R} = Q\tilde{Q} = 1$) provided one passes from two real coordinates x and y to the single double coordinate in these forms via the formula $w = (x+y)/2 + e(x-y)/2$. Moreover, [29] guarantees that if A and G are analytic then one can put them into normal forms by an analytic change of variables.

§ 2.4. Weakly reversible elliptic diffeomorphisms near a fixed point

Return to elliptic weakly reversible diffeomorphisms. We shall not suppose the total absence of resonances. Let $A:(\mathbb{R}^{2m},0)\to(\mathbb{R}^{2m},0)$ be a formal weakly reversible (with respect to a diffeomorphism G) elliptic diffeomorphism. Eigenvalues of its linearization are $\lambda_1,\dots,\lambda_m,\bar\lambda_1,\dots,\bar\lambda_m$ $(\mathrm{Im}\lambda_j>0)$. We will assume all m numbers $\lambda_1,\dots,\lambda_m$ to be distinct. Recall that the order of a resonance $\lambda^q=1$ is the number

$$|q|=\sum_{j=1}^{m}|q_j|.$$

DEFINITION. Let $\ell\in\mathbb{N}$. We say that $A\in\Psi_\ell^*$ if the following two conditions hold.

a) There are no resonances among $\lambda_1,\dots,\lambda_m$ of order $2\ell+2$ and lower.

By the remark made right after the proof of Theorem 2.3 this condition implies the existence of such a coordinate system z , in which

$$(A)_{2\ell+1}: z\mapsto \lambda z K^{(2\ell)}(\rho) \tag{8}$$

where $K_j^{(2\ell)}$ is a complex polynomial in ρ of degree $\le\ell$ with constant term 1, and

$$\left(K_j^{(2\ell)}\,\overline{K_j^{(2\ell)}}\right)_\ell = 1 \ . \qquad (9)$$

b) Polynomials $K_j^{(2\ell)}$ in (8) have the form

$$K_j^{(2\ell)}(\rho) = 1 + iF_j(\rho)$$

where F_j are homogeneous polynomials in ρ of degree ℓ and $F_1, \dots, F_m$ are functionally independent.

(As is easy to see, this property of $K_j^{(2\ell)}$ is invariant under changes of variables preserving the form (8) of the jet $(A)_{2\ell+1}$.)

REMARK 1. The equality (9) ensures that all polynomials F_j are real.

REMARK 2. By Proposition 2.9 $(G)_{2\ell+1}$ has the form

$$(G)_{2\ell+1} : z \mapsto \mu \bar{z}\, P^{(2\ell)}(\rho) \quad , \qquad (10)$$

where $\mu_j \in \mathbb{R}$, $\mu_j > 0$ and $P_j^{(2\ell)}$ is a complex polynomial in ρ of degree $\leq \ell$ with constant term 1, in every coordinate system z, in which $(A)_{2\ell+1}$ has the form (8).

REMARK 3. The class Ψ_ℓ of slightly elliptic reversible diffeomorphisms introduced in § 2.2 does not coincide (for $\kappa = 0$) with Ψ_ℓ^* . Firstly, Ψ_ℓ consists of reversible diffeomorphisms whereas Ψ_ℓ^* consists of weakly reversible ones. Secondly, diffeomorphisms belonging to Ψ_ℓ are nonresonant up to order $4\ell+2$ whereas ones belonging to Ψ_ℓ^* are to be nonresonant only up to order $2\ell+2$.

THEOREM 2.5. Let $A, G : (\mathbb{R}^{2m}, 0) \to (\mathbb{R}^{2m}, 0)$ be formal diffeomorphisms and A is weakly reversible with respect to G . Let A be elliptic and let $A \in \Psi_\ell^*$ for a certain $\ell \in \mathbb{N}$. Suppose that for a certain $N \geq \ell$ there are no resonances among $\lambda_1, \dots, \lambda_m$ of order $2N+2$ and lower, where $\lambda_1, \dots, \lambda_m$ are eigenvalues of $(A)_1$

with positive imaginary parts. Then $(G^2)_{2N+1} = id$.

PROOF. Denote by Φ^+ (respectively Φ^-) the space of vector-polynomials $\varphi(z,\bar{z}) = (\varphi_1(z,\bar{z}),\dots,\varphi_m(z,\bar{z}))$ possessing the following two properties.

a) The degrees of all terms of $\varphi_j(z,\bar{z})$ lie in the interval $2N+2 \leq \deg \leq 4N+1$.

b) All terms of $\varphi_j(z,\bar{z})$ are resonant (respectively antiresonant), but $\varphi_j(z,\bar{z})$ does not contain the terms of the form $az_j\rho^q$ (respectively of the form $a\bar{z}_j\rho^q$).

By Proposition 2.8 there exists a coordinate system z in which

$$(A)_{4N+1} : z \longmapsto \lambda z K^{(4N)}(\rho) + \tilde{\varphi}(z,\bar{z}) ,$$

where $K_j^{(4N)}$ is a polynomial in ρ of degree $\leq 2N$ with constant term 1 and $\tilde{\varphi} \in \Phi^+$.

By Proposition 2.9 in this coordinate system

$$(G)_{4N+1} : z \longmapsto \mu \bar{z} P^{(4N)}(\rho) + \varphi(z,\bar{z}) ,$$

where $P_j^{(4N)}$ is a polynomial in ρ of degree $\leq 2N$ with constant term 1 and $\varphi \in \Phi^-$.

For succinctness let $K^{(4N)} = K$, $P^{(4N)} = P$. We will denote series beginning with terms of degree $\geq d$ (where $d \in \mathbb{N}$) by O_d.

It is easy to verify that

$$GA : z \longmapsto \mu\bar{\lambda}\bar{z}\bar{K}\, P(\rho K\bar{K}) + \varphi'(z,\bar{z}) + O_{4N+2} ,$$

where $\varphi' \in \Phi^-$ and, likewise,

$$A G A = z \mapsto \mu \bar{z} \bar{K} P(\rho K\bar{K}) K(\mu^2 \rho K\bar{K} P(\rho K\bar{K}) \bar{P}(\rho K\bar{K})) + \varphi''(z,\bar{z}) + O_{4N+2} ,$$

where $\varphi'' \in \Phi^-$.

This follows that

$$\bar{K} P(\rho K\bar{K}) K(\mu^2 \rho K\bar{K} P(\rho K\bar{K}) \bar{P}(\rho K\bar{K})) = P + O_{4N+1} .$$

By means of arguments similar to those in the proof of Theorem 2.3 we obtain from this that $(K\bar{K})^{\bullet}_{2N} = 1$ and $(K)^{\bullet}_{2N} = (K(\mu^2\rho P\bar{P}))^{\bullet}_{2N}$. We shall deduce, from the second of these equalities, that $\mu_j = 1$ and $(P_j \bar{P}_j)^{\bullet}_N = 1$, which will immediately imply $(G^2)_{2N+1} = id.$

Let $P_j \bar{P}_j = u_j$. Recalling that $(K_j)^{\bullet}_{\ell} = 1 + iF_j$, we get

$$(K_j(\mu^2\rho\, u(\rho)))^{\bullet}_{\ell} = 1 + iF_j(\mu^2\rho) , \quad (K_j(\rho))^{\bullet}_{\ell} = 1 + iF_j(\rho)$$

i.e. $F_j(\mu^2\rho) = F_j(\rho)$. This follows $\mu_j = 1$. Indeed, if not all $\mu_1, \dots, \mu_m$ are equal to 1 then the rank of the lattice

$$Lat = \{ q \in \mathbb{Z}^m \mid \sum_{j=1}^{m} q_j \ln \mu_j = 0 \}$$

is equal to $s < m$. Let $(q^1, \dots, q^s)$ be a basis of Lat. Since $F_j(\mu^2\rho) = F_j(\rho)$, F_j contain only terms of the form $a\rho^q$ with $q \in Lat$.

Introduce the notation

$$\mathbb{R}^d_0 = \{ (x_1, \dots, x_d) \in \mathbb{R}^d \mid \prod_{i=1}^{d} x_i \neq 0 \} .$$

Consider the mapping $F': \mathbb{R}_0^m \longrightarrow \mathbb{R}_0^s$ given by

$$F' : (\rho_1, \ldots, \rho_m) \longmapsto (\rho^{q^1}, \ldots, \rho^{q^s}).$$

The mapping

$$F\big|_{\mathbb{R}_0^m} ,$$

where $F : (\rho_1, \ldots, \rho_m) \longmapsto (F_1(\rho), \ldots, F_m(\rho))$, may be decomposed into

$$\mathbb{R}_0^m \xrightarrow{F'} \mathbb{R}_0^s \longrightarrow \mathbb{R}^m .$$

Therefore F_j can not be functionally independent.

Thus, $\mu_j = 1$. Now we have

$$(K_j(\rho \mathcal{U}))^{\cdot}_{\ell+N} = (K_j(\rho))^{\cdot}_{\ell+N} .$$

Let us deduce from this that $(\mathcal{U}_j)^{\cdot}_N = 1$. Assume $(\mathcal{U}_j)^{\cdot}_d = 1$, where $0 \leq d < N$, and prove $(\mathcal{U}_j)^{\cdot}_{d+1} = 1$. Let $(\mathcal{U}_j)^{\cdot}_{d+1} = 1 + W_j$, where W_j are homogeneous polynomials in ρ of degree $d+1$. We have

$$(K_j(\rho \mathcal{U}))^{\cdot}_{\ell+d+1} = (K_j(\rho))^{\cdot}_{\ell+d+1} + i \sum_{s=1}^{m} \frac{\partial F_j}{\partial \rho_s} \rho_s W_s(\rho) .$$

Since $F_1, \ldots, F_m$ are functionally independent it follows that $W_j \equiv 0$.

Thus, $(\mathcal{U}_j)^{\cdot}_N = 1$. X

COROLLARY. If A is nonresonant and $A \in \Psi_\ell^*$ for a certain $\ell \in N$ then G is an involution.

Thus, formal nonresonant elliptic weakly reversible diffeomorphisms A are always reversible (Theorem 2.4) and on the additional condition of nondegeneracy (there exists $\ell \in N$ such that $A \in \Psi_\ell^*$)

every diffeomorphism reversing them is an involution.

REMARK. If $m = 1$ then the absence of resonances of order $2N+2$ and lower means that λ is not a root of unity of degree $2N+2$ or lower, and the existence of $\ell \leq N$ such that $A \in \Psi_\ell^*$ means that no change of variables reduces $(A)_{2N+1}$ into $(A)_1$. Therefore, if λ is not a root of unity (the nonresonant case) and the diffeomorphism A can not be reduced to its linearization $(A)_1$ then, according to the corollary of Theorem 2.5, every diffeomorphism G reversing A is an involution.

PROPOSITION 2.10. Under the assumptions of Theorem 2.5 there exists a coordinate system z in which

$$(A)_{2N+1} : z \longmapsto \lambda z K^{(2N)}(\rho), \ (G)_{2N+1} : z \longmapsto \bar{z}$$

where $K_j^{(2N)}$ is a complex polynomial in ρ of degree $\leq N$ with constant term 1, and

$$(K_j^{(2N)} \overline{K_j^{(2N)}})_N^{\cdot} = 1 \ . \qquad (11)$$

PROOF. By the remark made right after the proof of Theorem 2.3 and by Proposition 2.9 there exists a coordinate system z in which

$$(A)_{2N+1} : z \mapsto \lambda z K^{(2N)}(\rho), \ (G)_{2N+1} : z \mapsto \mu \bar{z} P^{(2N)}(\rho)$$

where $K_j^{(2N)}$ and $P_j^{(2N)}$ are complex polynomials in ρ of degree $\leq N$ with constant term 1, and (11) holds.

For succinctness let $K^{(2N)} = K$, $P^{(2N)} = P$. Proving Theorem 2.5 we established that $\mu_j = 1$ and $(P_j \bar{P}_j)_N^{\cdot} = 1$.

Consider the series

$$Z_j = (\rho_j)^{-1/2}$$

(with constant term 1). Denote by H the following change of variables

$$H : z \longmapsto z Z(\rho) .$$

Since $(\rho_j \bar{\rho}_j)^{\cdot}_N = 1$ it follows that $(Z_j \bar{Z}_j)^{\cdot}_N = 1$ and $(Z_j \rho_j)^{\cdot}_N = (\bar{Z}_j)^{\cdot}_N$. These relations imply that

$$(H G H^{-1})_{2N+1} : z \longmapsto \bar{z}$$

and

$$(H A H^{-1})_{2N+1} = (A)_{2N+1} : z \longmapsto \lambda z K(\rho).$$

X

§ 2.5. Normal forms for slightly elliptic reversible vectorfields near an equilibrium

The theory of reversible and weakly reversible vectorfields parallels that of diffeomorphisms.

PROPOSITION 2.11. Let V be the smooth germ of a vectorfield at $(\mathbb{R}^{2m+k}, 0)$, $V(0) = 0$, which is reversible with respect to a smooth involution $G : (\mathbb{R}^{2m+k}, 0) \to (\mathbb{R}^{2m+k}, 0)$ of type $(m, m+k)$. Then the linearization $(V)_1$ has at least k linearly independent eigenvectors with eigenvalue 0. Generically

a) the other $2m$ eigenvalues of $(V)_1$ are different from 0;

b) through 0 there exists a smooth k-dimensional surface Ξ

consisting of points fixed by σ such that the vector of the field V vanishes at every point of Ξ.

PROOF. By Proposition 2.4 the linearization $(V)_1$ of the field V has at least k linearly independent eigenvectors with eigenvalue 0. It is obvious that generically the other $2m$ eigenvalues of $(V)_1$ are different from 0. Now let Π be the set of fixed points of the involution σ. Π is a smooth $(m+k)$-dimensional surface passing through 0. Let Ξ be the locus of those points of Π at which the vector of the field V is tangent to Π. Since $\sigma_* V = -V$, at every point of Ξ the vector of the field V is zero. But standard dimension arguments show that generically Ξ is a smooth k-dimensional surface. X

REMARK. As is easy to see, if V is slightly elliptic then the surface Ξ exists always.

In future we will consider pairs (V, σ), where σ is an analytic involution $(\mathbb{R}^{2m+k}, 0) \to (\mathbb{R}^{2m+k}, 0)$ of type $(m, m+k)$ and V is an analytic slightly elliptic vectorfield at $(\mathbb{R}^{2m+k}, 0)$ $(V(0) = 0)$, reversible with respect to this involution. We denote nonzero eigenvalues of $(V)_1$ by $i\varkappa_1, \dots, i\varkappa_m, -i\varkappa_1, \dots, -i\varkappa_m$, where $\varkappa_j > 0$. We shall assume all m numbers $\varkappa_1, \dots, \varkappa_m$ to be distinct. If $\varkappa_1, \dots, \varkappa_m$ are resonant then, as usual, the number

$$|q| = \sum_{j=1}^{m} |q_j|$$

is called the order of a resonance $(q, \varkappa) = 0$, where $q \in \mathbb{Z}^m \setminus \{0\}$.

Analogously to the diffeomorphisms case, it is easy to prove that, using an analytic change of variables, one can choose such a coordinate system $(z_1, \dots, z_m, \xi_1, \dots, \xi_k)$ with origin at 0 in $\mathbb{R}^{2m+k}$, where $z_j \in \mathbb{C}$, $\xi_t \in \mathbb{R}$, in which

$$(V)_1 = i\varkappa z\frac{\partial}{\partial z}, \quad \sigma:(z,\xi)\mapsto(\bar z,\xi), \quad \Xi=\{z=0\}.$$

Fix such a coordinate system. Keep the notation $\rho_j = z_j\bar z_j$. Recall that if $z_j = x_j + iy_j$ then $(u+iv)\,\partial/\partial z_j$ is to be understood as the vectorfield $u\,\partial/\partial x_j + v\,\partial/\partial y_j$.

PROPOSITION 2.12. Suppose there are no resonances among $\varkappa_1,\dots,\varkappa_m$ of order $\ell+2$ and lower $(\ell\in\mathbb{N})$. Then there exists an analytic change of variables commuting with σ, leaving Ξ pointwise fixed and taking $(V)_{\ell+1}$ into the form

$$(V)_{\ell+1} = i\varkappa z T^{(\ell)}(\xi,\rho)\frac{\partial}{\partial z}$$

where $T_j^{(\ell)}$ is a real polynomial in ξ and ρ (of degree $\leq \ell$ if considered as a polynomial in ξ, z and $\bar z$) with constant term 1.

Suppose there are no resonances among $\varkappa_1,\dots,\varkappa_m$ at all. Then there exists a formal change of variables commuting with σ, leaving Ξ pointwise fixed and taking V into the form

$$V = i\varkappa z T(\xi,\rho)\frac{\partial}{\partial z}$$

where T_j is a formal real series in powers of ξ and ρ with constant term 1.

REMARK. The reality of $T_j^{(\ell)}$ or T_j is an analogue to the relations

$$(K_j^{\ell}\,\overline{K_j^{(\ell)}})_\ell = 1$$

or

$$K_j\overline{K}_j = 1$$

respectively, from the formulation of Proposition 2.6 concerning slightly elliptic reversible diffeomorphisms.

The proof is similar to that of Proposition 2.6.

COROLLARY. If resonances are absent then a neighbourhood of 0 in $\mathbb{R}^{2m+\kappa}$ is foliated into formal $2m$-dimensional transversal to Ξ surfaces, invariant under V and σ.

REMARK. One can show that this corollary is valid not only for slightly elliptic reversible fields but for any generic pairs (V,σ), where V is a nonresonant (in a suitable sense) vectorfield at $(\mathbb{R}^{2m+\kappa},0)$ $(V(0)=0)$ reversible with respect to an involution $\sigma:(\mathbb{R}^{2m+\kappa},0)\to(\mathbb{R}^{2m+\kappa},0)$ of type $(m, m+\kappa)$.

DEFINITION. Let $\ell\in\mathbb{N}$. We say that $V\in\Psi_\ell$ if the following two conditions hold.

a) There are no resonances among $\varkappa_1,\dots,\varkappa_m$ of order $4\ell+2$ and lower.

By Proposition 2.12 this condition implies the existence of such a coordinate system (z,ξ) in which

$$(V)_{4\ell+1}=i\varkappa z T^{(4\ell)}(\xi,\rho)\frac{\partial}{\partial z},\quad \sigma:\begin{matrix} z \\ \xi\end{matrix}\mapsto\begin{matrix}\bar z\\ \xi\end{matrix},\quad \Xi=\{z=0\} \tag{12}$$

where $T_j^{(4\ell)}$ is a real polynomial in ξ and ρ of degree $\leqslant 4\ell$ (if considered as a polynomial in ξ, z and $\bar z$) with constant term 1.

b) Polynomials $T_j^{(4\ell)}$ in (12) have the form

$$T_j^{(4\ell)}(\xi,\rho)$$

$$= 1 + \sum_{\substack{1 \leq |a| + 2|b| \leq 2\ell \\ |a| \geq 1}} S_{j,ab} \xi^a \rho^b + F_j(\rho) + \sum_{\substack{2\ell+1 \leq |a|+2|b| \\ \leq 4\ell}} R_{j,ab} \xi^a \rho^b$$

where F_j are homogeneous (obviously real) polynomials in ρ of degree ℓ and $F_1, \dots, F_m$ are functionally independent.

(As is easy to see, this property of $T_j^{(4\ell)}$ is invariant under changes of variables preserving the form (12) of the jet $(V)_{4\ell+1}$ and the involution G .)

§ 2.6. Weakly reversible elliptic hyperbolic vectorfields near an equilibrium

In the preceding section we received normal forms for reversible slightly elliptic fields. Here we start to investigate elliptic fields more circumstantially, assuming them to be not reversible, but only weakly reversible. As well as in § 2.3 (in which the diffeomorphisms case is studied), we will firstly consider not purely elliptic but elliptic hyperbolic fields, whose linearizations have eigenvalues lying in $(\mathbb{R} \cup \mathbb{R}i) \setminus \{0\}$, where $\mathbb{R}i$ denotes the axis of purely imaginary numbers. As well as in § 2.3, for more concise notations we shall use the double numbers algebra. Adopt the same agreements on the numbers m and n and the index τ as at the beginning of § 2.3.

If $w_\tau = x_\tau + e y_\tau$ is one of the double coordinates then $(u + ev)\partial/\partial w_\tau$ will be understood as the vectorfield $u\,\partial/\partial x_\tau + v\,\partial/\partial y_\tau$.

Let V be a formal vectorfield at $(\mathbb{R}^{2(m+n)}, 0)$, $V(0) = 0$, and $G: (\mathbb{R}^{2(m+n)}, 0) \longrightarrow (\mathbb{R}^{2(m+n)}, 0)$ be a formal diffeomorphism. Let $G_* V = -V$. Assume all eigenvalues of $(V)_1$ to lie in

$(\mathbb{R}\cup\mathbb{R}i)\setminus\{0\}$ and, moreover, $(V)_1$ to have $2m$ purely imaginary eigenvalues $i\varkappa_1,\dots,i\varkappa_m,-i\varkappa_1,\dots,-i\varkappa_m$ and $2n$ real eigenvalues $\zeta_1,\dots,\zeta_n,\ -\zeta_1,\dots,-\zeta_n$. We fix the notations so that $\varkappa_j>0$ and $\zeta_r>0$.

For $n=0$ the field V is elliptic. If $m=0$ then V is called a hyperbolic field.

We henceforth suppose all m numbers $\varkappa_1,\dots,\varkappa_m$ are distinct and all n numbers $\zeta_1,\dots,\zeta_n$ are distinct.

Analogously to the diffeomorphisms case it is easy to prove that one can choose such a coordinate system $(z_1,\dots,z_m,\ w_1,\dots,w_n)$ with origin at 0 in $\mathbb{R}^{2(m+n)}$, where $z_j\in\mathbb{C}$, $w_r\in\mathbb{K}$, in which $(V)_1$ has the form

$$(V)_1 = i\varkappa z\frac{\partial}{\partial z}+e\zeta w\frac{\partial}{\partial w} \tag{13}$$

and $(G)_1$ has the form (3).

We henceforth consider only such coordinate systems in which $(V)_1$ and $(G)_1$ are of the form (13) and (3), respectively.

The vector-monomial

$$(\underbrace{0,\dots,0}_{j-1},\ z^a\bar{z}^b w^c\tilde{w}^d,\ \underbrace{0,\dots,0}_{m-j},\ \underbrace{0,\dots,0}_{n})$$

is said to be resonant if

$$(a-b)\varkappa=\varkappa_j \quad\text{and}\quad (c-d)\zeta=0$$

and antiresonant if

$$(a-b)\varkappa=-\varkappa_j \quad\text{and}\quad (c-d)\zeta=0\ .$$

Note that this definition is invariant under interchanging the indices c and d.

The vector-monomial

$$(\underbrace{0,\ldots,0}_{m},\ \underbrace{0,\ldots,0}_{\tau-1},\ z^a\bar{z}^b w^c \tilde{w}^d,\ \underbrace{0,\ldots,0}_{n-\tau})$$

is said to be resonant if

$$(a-b)\varkappa=0 \text{ and } (c-d)\zeta=\zeta_\tau$$

and antiresonant if

$$(a-b)\varkappa=0 \text{ and } (c-d)\zeta=-\zeta_\tau\ .$$

Note that this definition is invariant under interchanging the indices a and b.

PROPOSITION 2.13. Let $\alpha, \beta \in \mathbb{R}$. Then the number $u_0 = i\alpha + e\beta$ is uninvertible in $\mathbb{A}$ precisely when $u_0 = 0$, i.e. when $\alpha=\beta=0$.

PROOF. $u_0\bar{u}_0\tilde{u}_0\tilde{\bar{u}}_0 = (\alpha^2+\beta^2)^2$. X

PROPOSITION 2.14 (Poincaré-Dulac). One can choose a coordinate system (z, w) so that the series giving V should contain resonant terms only.

The proof is similar to that of Proposition 2.8 (one would use Proposition 2.13 instead of Proposition 2.7).

PROPOSITION 2.15. If the series giving V contants only resonant terms then the series giving G contains only antiresonant terms.

The proof is similar to that of Proposition 2.9 (one would use Proposition 2.13 instead of Proposition 2.7).

Henceforth suppose resonances among $\varkappa_j$ and ζ_τ are absent, i.e. $\varkappa_1, \ldots, \varkappa_m$ are rationally independent and so are $\zeta_1, \ldots, \zeta_n$. Keep the notations $\rho_j = z_j\bar{z}_j$ and $\sigma_\tau = w_\tau \tilde{w}_\tau$ of § 2.3.

According to Proposition 2.14, there exists such a coordinate system, in which V is of the form

$$V = i\varkappa z T(\rho,\sigma)\frac{\partial}{\partial z} + e\zeta w S(\rho,\sigma)\frac{\partial}{\partial w} \qquad (14)$$

where T_j and S_τ are complex and double, respectively, power series with constant term 1.

According to Proposition 2.15, in this coordinate system G is of the form (5).

We will often drop the arguments ρ and σ of series.

The weak reversibility condition $G_* V = -V$ may be written down as follows

$$\left\{\begin{aligned} &\varkappa \bar{T} P + \sum_{j=1}^{m} \frac{\partial P}{\partial \rho_j} \varkappa_j \rho_j (\bar{T}_j - T_j) + ie \sum_{\tau=1}^{n} \frac{\partial P}{\partial \sigma_\tau} \zeta_\tau \sigma_\tau (S_\tau - \tilde{S}_\tau) \\ &\qquad = \varkappa P T(\mu^2 \rho P \bar{P}, \nu\tilde{\nu}\sigma Q \tilde{Q}) \\ &\zeta \tilde{S} Q + \sum_{\tau=1}^{n} \frac{\partial Q}{\partial \sigma_\tau} \zeta_\tau \sigma_\tau (\tilde{S}_\tau - S_\tau) + ie \sum_{j=1}^{m} \frac{\partial Q}{\partial \rho_j} \varkappa_j \rho_j (\bar{T}_j - T_j) \\ &\qquad = \zeta Q S(\mu^2 \rho P \bar{P}, \nu\tilde{\nu}\sigma Q \tilde{Q}) \end{aligned}\right. \qquad (15)$$

(this is not contradictory, since $e(S_\tau - \tilde{S}_\tau) \in \mathbb{R}$ and $i(\bar{T}_j - T_j) \in \mathbb{R}$) .

THEOREM 2.6. Let V be a formal vectorfield at $(\mathbb{R}^{2(m+n)}, 0)$ $(V(0)=0)$ whose linearization $(V)_1$ is infinitesimally reversible and has an elliptic hyperbolic spectrum, resonances being absent. Then the following conditions are equivalent.

1) V is reversible.

2) In formula (14), the series T_j and S_τ are real.

3) V is weakly reversible and there exists such a reversing diffeomorphism G that $\mu_j = 1$ and $\nu_\tau = 1$ in (3).

4) V is weakly reversible and there exists such a reversing diffeomorphism G that $\nu_\tau = 1$ in (3).

5) V is weakly reversible and there exists such a reversing diffeomorphism G that $\nu_\tau \in \mathbb{R}$ in (3).

PROOF. One may prove Theorem 2.6 similarly to Theorem 2.3, but it is simpler to deduce Theorem 2.6 from Theorem 2.3. In order to do it one has to observe that the proof of Theorem 2.3 can be word for word transferred to that situation when coefficients of series K_j and R_τ are not complex and double numbers respectively but germs of analytic (in the real sense) functions $(\mathbb{R},0)\to\mathbb{C}$ and $(\mathbb{R},0)\longrightarrow\mathbb{K}$ respectively. Denote the spaces of these functions by $\mathcal{E}(\mathbb{C})$ and $\mathcal{E}(\mathbb{K})$ respectively.

Define the exponent of a double number analogously to the definition of the exponent of complex numbers:

$$\exp w = \sum_{d=0}^{\infty} \frac{w^d}{d!} .$$

If $w = a + be$, where $a, b \in \mathbb{R}$, then $\exp w = (\exp a)(\cosh b + e \sinh b)$.

Now consider the phase flow F_t $(t \in \mathbb{R})$ of the field V instead of V itself. If V is of the form (14) then

$$F_t : (z,w) \mapsto (\exp(i\varkappa t) z K_t(\rho,\sigma) \ , \ \exp(e\tau t) w R_t(\rho,\sigma))$$

where

$$K_{t,j} \in \mathcal{E}(\mathbb{C})[[\rho,\sigma]], \quad R_{t,\tau} \in \mathcal{E}(\mathbb{K})[[\rho,\sigma]].$$

(K_t, R_t) is the formal solution of the formal Cauchy problem

$$\begin{cases} K_{0,j} = 1 \\ R_{0,\tau} = 1 \\ \dot{K}_{t,j} = i\varkappa_j K_{t,j}(-1 + T_j(\rho K_t \bar{K}_t, \sigma R_t \tilde{R}_t)) \\ \dot{R}_{t,\tau} = e\tau_\tau R_{t,\tau}(-1 + S_\tau(\rho K_t \bar{K}_t, \sigma R_t \tilde{R}_t)) \end{cases} .$$

Then $F_t G F_t = G$ for each t.

Note that

$$K_{t,j}(0,0) = 1 , \quad R_{t,\tau}(0,0) = 1 ,$$

$$\frac{\partial}{\partial t}(K_t \bar{K}_t) = i\varkappa K_t \bar{K}_t (T(\rho K_t \bar{K}_t, \sigma R_t \tilde{R}_t) - \bar{T}(\rho K_t \bar{K}_t, \sigma R_t \tilde{R}_t)),$$

$$\frac{\partial}{\partial t}(R_t \tilde{R}_t) = e\tau R_t \tilde{R}_t (S(\rho K_t \bar{K}_t, \sigma R_t \tilde{R}_t) - \tilde{S}(\rho K_t \bar{K}_t, \sigma R_t \tilde{R}_t)).$$

Therefore the condition

$$K_{t,j} \overline{K_{t,j}} = 1 \ \& \ R_{t,\tau} \widetilde{R_{t,\tau}} = 1$$

is equivalent to the reality of T_j and S_τ.

Proving the analogue to Theorem 2.3 concerning F_t we receive Theorem 2.6. X

As a corollary we obtain that the reality property of T_j and S_τ is invariant under changes of variables preserving the form (14) of the field V.

REMARK. Abandon the nonresonantness condition imposed on V and suppose only that all resonant monomials have degree $2l + 2$ and higher (where l is a fixed natural number). Then by Proposition

2.14 there exists a coordinate system in which $(V)_{2\ell+1}$ is of the form

$$(V)_{2\ell+1} = i\varkappa z\, T^{(2\ell)}(\rho,\sigma)\frac{\partial}{\partial z} + e\zeta w\, S^{(2\ell)}(\rho,\sigma)\frac{\partial}{\partial w}$$

where $T_j^{(2\ell)}$ and $S_\tau^{(2\ell)}$ are complex and double (respectively) polynomials in ρ and σ of degree $\leq \ell$ with constant term 1. Similarly to the nonresonant case one can show that if there exists such a diffeomorphism G reversing V that all $\nu_\tau \in \mathbb{R}$ in (3) then $T_j^{(2\ell)}$ and $S_\tau^{(2\ell)}$ are real.

If $n = 0$, the condition 5) of Theorem 2.6 is fulfilled automatically, and we receive the following remarkable

THEOREM 2.7. Every nonresonant elliptic weakly reversible formal vectorfield at $(\mathbb{R}^{2m}, 0)$, for which 0 is an equilibrium, is reversible.

I don't know whether this statement is valid without the nonresonantness condition.

For $n \geqslant 1$ there exist nonresonant elliptic hyperbolic weakly reversible formal vectorfields V at $(\mathbb{R}^{2(m+n)}, 0)$ (where $V(0)=0$) which are not reversible. It is easy to construct appropriate examples even in the case of dimension two $(m = 0\ ,\ n=1)$ when resonances are absent automatically. Moreover, fields and reversing diffeomorphisms involved in these examples are generic.

Thus, construct an irreversible weakly reversible hyperbolic vectorfield on a plane $\mathbb{R}^2$. We shall assume it to have the form (14). Set $\nu = e$ and $Q = 1$ in (5), then the condition (15) will be reduced to $\tilde{S}(\sigma) = S(-\sigma)$, which means that coefficients of the even part of S are real and ones of the odd part of S are the products of real numbers by e. There corresponds a weakly reversible field V to each such series S (a reversing diffeomorphism is

$\sigma : w \mapsto e\tilde{w}$). If a series S is not even then it is not real, and the field V given by this series is not reversible by virtue of Theorem 2.6.

REMARK 1. Pass from the double coordinate w to real coordinates

$$x=\frac{1}{2}(w(1+e)+\tilde{w}(1-e)), \quad y=\frac{1}{2}(w(1-e)+\tilde{w}(1+e)).$$

Then $w=(x+y)/2+e(x-y)/2$ and $\sigma=w\tilde{w}=xy$. In the coordinates (x,y) the diffeomorphism σ and the field V have the form

$$\sigma:(x,y)\mapsto(y,-x)$$

and

$$V=\tau x B(\sigma)\frac{\partial}{\partial x}-\tau y C(\sigma)\frac{\partial}{\partial y}$$

respectively, where

$$B=\frac{1}{2}((1+e)S+(1-e)\tilde{S}), \quad C=\frac{1}{2}((1+e)\tilde{S}+(1-e)S).$$

B and C are real formal series in powers of σ with constant term 1. One sees that

$$S \text{ is real} \Longleftrightarrow B = C$$

and

$$\tilde{S}(\sigma)=S(-\sigma) \Longleftrightarrow B(\sigma)=C(-\sigma).$$

Taking any series B with constant term 1 and setting $C(\sigma)=B(-\sigma)$ we obtain a weakly reversible field V. If an original series B is not even then this field V is not reversible.

REMARK 2. Choosing a series B to be convergent (in some neighbourhood of 0) we arrive at the conclusion that irreversible weakly reversible hyperbolic fields V at $(\mathbb{R}^2,0)\,(V(0)=0)$ exist in the analytic realm, too.

REMARK 3. Let V be an arbitrary nonresonant elliptic Hamiltonian formal vectorfield at $(\mathbb{R}^{2m},0)(V(0)=0)$. It is well known (see, e.g., [19 (Appendix 7), 21 (Lecture 1)])that one can choose a canonical coordinate system z (in which the symplectic structure is $i/2\, dz \wedge d\bar{z}$) so as to have

$$V = iz\left(\varkappa + \frac{\partial H'}{\partial \rho}\right)\frac{\partial}{\partial z}$$

where $H' = H'(\rho)$ is a real formal series in powers of ρ without constant and linear terms (the Birkhoff normal form), the formal Hamilton function of this field is equal to $H = H(\rho) = \frac{1}{2}(\varkappa\rho + H'(\rho))$. Consequently, every nonresonant elliptic Hamiltonian formal vectorfield is reversible. For $m=1$ the converse statement is also true,i.e. every (necessarily nonresonant) elliptic reversible formal vectorfield on a plane can be made into a Hamiltonian one by a suitable choice of the symplectic structure. For $m>1$ this is no longer valid. For instance, there is no symplectic structure, with respect to which the reversible field

$$V = iz_1(\varkappa_1 + \rho_2)\frac{\partial}{\partial z_1} + i\varkappa_2 z_2 \frac{\partial}{\partial z_2}$$

(here $m=2$) is Hamiltonian.

§ 2.7. Weakly reversible elliptic vectorfields near an equilibrium

Return to elliptic weakly reversible fields. We shall not suppose the total absence of resonances. Let V be a formal weakly reversible (with respect to a diffeomorphism G) elliptic vectorfield at $(\mathbb{R}^{2m},0)$ $(V(0)=0)$. Eigenvalues of its linearization are $i\varkappa_1,\dots,i\varkappa_m,-i\varkappa_1,\dots,-i\varkappa_m$ $(\varkappa_j>0)$. We will assume all m numbers $\varkappa_1,\dots,\varkappa_m$ to be distinct. Recall that the order of a resonance $(q,\varkappa)=0$ is the number

$$|q| = \sum_{j=1}^{m} |q_j| .$$

DEFINITION. Let $\ell\in\mathbb{N}$. We say that $V\in\Psi_\ell^*$ if the following two conditions hold.

a) There are no resonances among $\varkappa_1,\dots,\varkappa_m$ of order $2\ell+2$ and lower.

By the remark made right after the proof of Theorem 2.6 this condition implies the existence of such a coordinate system z in which

$$(V)_{2\ell+1} = i\varkappa z\, T^{(2\ell)}(\rho)\frac{\partial}{\partial z} \tag{16}$$

where $T_j^{(2\ell)}$ is a real polynomial in ρ of degree $\leq \ell$ with constant term 1.

b) Polynomials $T_j^{(2\ell)}$ in (16) have the form

$$T_j^{(2\ell)}(\rho) = 1 + F_j(\rho)$$

where F_j are homogeneous (obviously real) polynomials in ρ of degree ℓ and $F_1, \dots, F_m$ are functionally independent.

(As is easy to see, this property of $T_j^{(2\ell)}$ is invariant under changes of variables preserving the form (16) of the jet $(V)_{2\ell+1}$.)

REMARK 1. By Proposition 2.15 $(\sigma)_{2\ell+1}$ has the form (10) in every coordinate system z in which $(V)_{2\ell+1}$ has the form (16).

REMARK 2. The class Ψ_ℓ of slightly elliptic reversible vectorfields introduced in § 2.5 does not coincide (for $\kappa = 0$) with Ψ_ℓ^* for the same reasons as in the diffeomorphisms case (see § 2.4).

THEOREM 2.8. Let V be a formal vectorfield at $(\mathbb{R}^{2m}, 0)$ $(V(0)=0)$ weakly reversible with respect to a diffeomorphism $\sigma : (\mathbb{R}^{2m}, 0) \to (\mathbb{R}^{2m}, 0)$. Let V be elliptic and let $V \in \Psi_\ell^*$ for a certain $\ell \in \mathbb{N}$. Suppose that for a certain $N \geqslant \ell$ there are no resonances among $\varkappa_1, \dots, \varkappa_m$ of order $2N+2$ and lower, where $i\varkappa_1, \dots, i\varkappa_m$ are eigenvalues of $(V)_1$ with positive imaginary parts. Then $(\sigma^2)_{2N+1} = id$.

PROOF. One may either prove this theorem analogously to Theorem 2.5 or deduce it from Theorem 2.5 (passing from the field V to its phase flow F_t).

COROLLARY. If V is nonresonant and $V \in \Psi_\ell^*$ for a certain $\ell \in \mathbb{N}$ then σ is an involution.

Thus, formal nonresonant elliptic weakly reversible vectorfields V are always reversible (Theorem 2.7) and on the additional condition of nondegeneracy (there exists $\ell \in \mathbb{N}$ such that $V \in \Psi_\ell^*$) every diffeomorphism reversing them is an involution.

REMARK. If $m=1$ then resonances are absent automatically, and the existence of $\ell \leqslant N$ such that $V \in \Psi_\ell^*$ means that no change of variables reduces $(V)_{2N+1}$ into $(V)_1$. Therefore, if the vectorfield V can not be reduced to its linearization $(V)_1$ then, according to the corollary of Theorem 2.8, every diffeomorphism σ reversing V is an involution.

PROPOSITION 2.16. Under the assumptions of Theorem 2.8 there exists a coordinate system z in which

$$(V)_{2N+1} = i\varkappa z T^{(2N)}(\rho)\frac{\partial}{\partial z}, \quad (G)_{2N+1} : z \mapsto \bar{z}$$

where $T_j^{(2N)}$ is a real polynomial in ρ of degree $\leqslant N$ with constant term 1.

The proof is similar to that of Proposition 2.10.

§ 2.8. Invariant tori near a fixed point of a reversible diffeomorphism

Let us proceed to theorems on invariant tori near equilibria of reversible and weakly reversible analytic diffeomorphisms and vectorfields. We shall prove these local statements by reducing them to "global" Theorems 1.1 and 1.2. The reduction technique bases upon using normal forms for jets of reversible and weakly reversible diffeomorphisms and vectorfields described in Propositions 2.6, 2.10, 2.12 and 2.16. For the case of plane diffeomorphisms, this technique was applied in [22 (§§ 32, 34)] . In the local theory, the nearness to an equilibrium plays the same role as the closeness to a (slightly) integrable object does in the global one.

At first, consider the diffeomorphisms case.

THEOREM 2.9. Let $A, G : (\mathbb{R}^{2m+\kappa}, 0) \longrightarrow (\mathbb{R}^{2m+\kappa}, 0)$ be the germs of analytic diffeomorphisms, and let $AGA = G$. Assume the weakly reversible diffeomorphism A to be slightly elliptic, i.e. its linearization $(A)_1$ to have κ eigenvalues equaling 1 and $2m$

eigenvalues $\lambda_1, \dots, \lambda_m, \bar{\lambda}_1, \dots, \bar{\lambda}_m$ lying in $\mathcal{U}(1) \setminus \{-1; 1\}$ $(\operatorname{Im} \lambda_j > 0)$. Suppose all m numbers $\lambda_1, \dots, \lambda_m$ are distinct.

If $\varkappa > 0$ then in addition assume G to be an involution of type $(m, m+\varkappa)$.

Let the diffeomorphism A be nondegenerate, i.e. there exists $\ell \in \mathbb{N}$ such that either $A \in \Psi_\ell$ (for $\varkappa > 0$) or $A \in \Psi_\ell^*$ (for $\varkappa = 0$) (for definitions of Ψ_ℓ and Ψ_ℓ^* see § 2.2 and § 2.4 respectively).

Then the following holds.

a) In any neighbourhood of $0 \in \mathbb{R}^{2m+\varkappa}$, there exist $(m+\varkappa)$-dimensional manifolds invariant under A and G and foliated into m-dimensional tori also invariant under A and G. The action of A on these tori is quasiperiodic, and the frequencies of this action are constants on every $(m+\varkappa)$-dimensional manifold (i.e. the frequencies are the same on all tori constituting a given $(m+\varkappa)$-dimensional manifold).

b) Moreover, one can choose neighbourhoods O_ε of $0 \in \mathbb{R}^{2m+\varkappa}$ ($\operatorname{diam}(O_\varepsilon)$ tends to zero as $\varepsilon \to 0$, $O_{\varepsilon_1} \subset O_{\varepsilon_2}$ if $\varepsilon_1 < \varepsilon_2$) in such a manner that

$$\lim_{\varepsilon \to 0} \frac{\operatorname{mes} g_\varepsilon}{\operatorname{mes} O_\varepsilon} = 1 \tag{17}$$

where g_ε denotes the union of invariant $(m+\varkappa)$-dimensional manifolds lying in O_ε.

c) For $\varkappa = 0$, G is an involution of type (m, m).

PROOF. By virtue of Proposition 2.6 (for $\varkappa > 0$) and Proposition 2.10 (for $\varkappa = 0$) together with definitions of classes Ψ_ℓ and Ψ_ℓ^*, there exists a coordinate system $(z_1, \dots, z_m, \xi_1, \dots, \xi_\varkappa)$ in $\mathbb{R}^{2m+\varkappa}$ with origin at 0 $(z_j \in \mathbb{C}, \xi_t \in \mathbb{R})$, in which

1) if $\varkappa > 0$:

$$(A)_{4\ell+1} : \begin{array}{ccc} z & \longmapsto & \lambda z\Big(1 + \sum\limits_{\substack{1\le|a|+2|b|\le 2\ell \\ |a|\ge 1}} S_{ab}\xi^a\rho^b + iF(\rho) + \sum\limits_{\substack{2\ell+1\le|a|+2|b| \\ \le 4\ell}} R_{ab}\xi^a\rho^b\Big) \\ \xi & & \xi \end{array},$$

$$\sigma : \begin{array}{ccc} z & \longmapsto & \bar{z} \\ \xi & & \xi \end{array};$$

2) if $\varkappa = 0$:

$$(A)_{2\ell+1} : z \longmapsto \lambda z(1 + iF(\rho)),$$

$$(\sigma)_{2\ell+1} : z \longmapsto \bar{z}.$$

Here $\rho_j = z_j\bar{z}_j$, $F_1, \ldots, F_m$ are functionally independent real homogeneous polynomials in ρ of degree ℓ. For $\varkappa > 0$ $S_{j,ab}$ and $R_{j,ab}$ are complex numbers.

Let $\mathbb{R}^m_+ = \{\rho \in \mathbb{R}^m \mid \rho_j > 0\}$. Choose such a point $\overset{\circ}{\rho} \in \mathbb{R}^m_+$ that

$$\frac{\partial(F_1,\ldots,F_m)}{\partial(\rho_1,\ldots,\rho_m)}\Big|_{\overset{\circ}{\rho}} \neq 0.$$

Then the mapping $F:(\rho_1,\ldots,\rho_m)\longmapsto(F_1(\rho),\ldots,F_m(\rho))$ realizes a local diffeomorphism $F: \mathcal{O}_1 \to \mathcal{O}_2$, where $\mathcal{O}_1 = \mathcal{O}(\overset{\circ}{\rho})$ is a neighbourhood of $\overset{\circ}{\rho}$ assumed to be situated in $\mathbb{R}^m_+$ and

$O_2 = O(F(\rho^\circ))$ is a neighbourhood of $F(\rho^\circ)$. By multiplying, if needed, ρ° by a suitable positive constant we may achieve O_2 to contain a close ball Ω of radius 1.

Let $\lambda_j = e^{i\theta_j}$, where $0 < \theta_j < \pi$.

Consider the "polycylindrical" coordinate system (x, y, η) on a neighbourhood O_ε of the origin in $\mathbb{R}^{2m+\kappa}$ (where $x \in T^m (x \bmod 2\pi)$, $y \in O_2 \subset \mathbb{R}^m$, $\eta \in \mathbb{R}^\kappa$ $(|\eta_t| < 2)$) that is given by the formulas

$$z_j = \varepsilon \sqrt{(F^{-1})_j(y)}\, e^{ix_j}$$

$$\xi_t = \varepsilon^{2l+1} \eta_t$$

where $\varepsilon > 0$ is sufficiently small, $\varepsilon < \varepsilon_0$, say.

In this coordinate system, we have:

1) if $\kappa > 0$

$$A: \begin{matrix} \varepsilon\sqrt{F^{-1}(y)}\, e^{ix} \\ \varepsilon^{2l+1}\eta \end{matrix} \longmapsto \begin{matrix} \varepsilon e^{i\theta}\sqrt{F^{-1}(y)}\, e^{ix}(1 + i\varepsilon^{2l} y + O(\varepsilon^{2l+1})) + O(\varepsilon^{2l+2}) \\ \varepsilon^{2l+1}\eta + O(\varepsilon^{4l+2}) \end{matrix},$$

$$G: \begin{matrix} \varepsilon\sqrt{F^{-1}(y)}\, e^{ix} \\ \varepsilon^{2l+1}\eta \end{matrix} \longmapsto \begin{matrix} \varepsilon\sqrt{F^{-1}(y)}\, e^{-ix} \\ \varepsilon^{2l+1}\eta \end{matrix};$$

2) if $\kappa = 0$

$$A: \varepsilon\sqrt{F^{-1}(y)}\, e^{ix} \longmapsto \varepsilon e^{i\theta}\sqrt{F^{-1}(y)}\, e^{ix}(1 + i\varepsilon^{2l} y) + O(\varepsilon^{2l+2}),$$

$$G: \varepsilon\sqrt{F^{-1}(y)}\, e^{ix} \mapsto \varepsilon\sqrt{F^{-1}(y)}\, e^{-ix} + O(\varepsilon^{2l+2}).$$

Therefore,

$$A: \begin{array}{l} x \\ y \\ \eta \end{array} \longmapsto \begin{array}{l} x+\theta+\varepsilon^{2l}y+f^1(x,y,\eta,\varepsilon) \\ y+f^2(x,y,\eta,\varepsilon) \\ \eta+f^3(x,y,\eta,\varepsilon) \end{array} \tag{18}$$

and

$$\sigma: \begin{array}{l} x \\ y \\ \eta \end{array} \longmapsto \begin{array}{l} -x+d^1(x,y,\eta,\varepsilon) \\ y+d^2(x,y,\eta,\varepsilon) \\ \eta+d^3(x,y,\eta,\varepsilon) \end{array} \tag{19}$$

where f^τ and d^τ are analytic on $T^m \times O_2 \times \{\eta \in \mathbb{R}^K \mid |\eta_t| < 2\} \times [0,\varepsilon_0)$ functions, and each of them is $O(\varepsilon^{2l+1})$ as $\varepsilon \to 0$. $d^\tau = 0$ for $K>0$ but we shall not need it.

There exist numbers $\tau_0 \in (0,1]$, $\tilde{\tau}_0 \in (0,1)$, $\delta_* > 0$ and a complex neighbourhood $D_* \subset \mathbb{C}^m$ of the ball Ω (with $D_* \cap \mathbb{R}^m \subset O_2$), not depending on ε and such that for each sufficiently small fixed ε the functions f^τ and d^τ can be extended into the domain

$$D = \{x \in (\mathbb{C}/2\pi\mathbb{Z})^m \mid |\mathrm{Im}\, x_j| < \tau_0\} \times \{y \in \mathbb{C}^m \mid y \in D_*\} \times \{\eta \in \mathbb{C}^K \mid |\eta_t| < 1+\tilde{\tau}_0\}$$

holomorphically in x, y and η so that $|f^\tau| < \delta_* \varepsilon^{2l+1}$ and $|d^\tau| < \delta_* \varepsilon^{2l+1}$ on D.

By introducing the new coordinate $\tilde{y} = y + \varepsilon^{-2l}\theta$ we may remove θ in (18) (confer the remark at the end of § 1.4).

Now Theorem 1.1 guarantees that for each $C \in (0,1]$, each sufficiently small $\varepsilon > 0$ ($\varepsilon < \varepsilon_*(C)$) and each ω of type $\mathcal{M}_m(\varepsilon^{2l}C, 1)$ belonging to the ball $\varepsilon^{2l}\Omega + \theta$, there exists an invariant under both

A and σ analytic manifold in O_ε that is given parametrically as follows:

$$\begin{cases} z=\varepsilon\sqrt{F^{-1}((\omega-\theta)\varepsilon^{-2\ell}+\Phi^2_\omega(\varphi,\varkappa))}\ \exp(i(\varphi+\Phi^1_\omega(\varphi,\varkappa))) \\ \xi=\varepsilon^{2\ell+1}(\varkappa+\Phi^3_\omega(\varphi,\varkappa)) \end{cases} \tag{20}$$

where $\varphi\in T^m(\varphi \bmod 2\pi)$, $\varkappa\in\mathbb{R}^\kappa(|\varkappa_t|<1+\tilde{\tau}_0/2)$. Moreover, this manifold is foliated into invariant under A and σ tori $\varkappa=\mathrm{const}$, on which the mappings A and σ induce diffeomorphisms $\varphi\mapsto\varphi+\omega$ and $\varphi\mapsto-\varphi$, respectively. Furthermore,

$$\lim_{\varepsilon\to 0}\ \sup_{\omega}\ \sup_{\varphi,\varkappa}|\Phi^\tau_\omega(\varphi,\varkappa)|=0 .$$

By Corollary 1 of Theorem 1.1 the relation (17) holds, in which g_ε denotes the union of manifolds (20) corresponding to all possible ω. For $\kappa=0$ this implies that σ is an involution, because σ is analytic and the restriction of σ to every manifold (20) is an involution. X

REMARK. It seems very likely that if A and σ are formal (possible not analytic) diffeomorphisms $(\mathbb{R}^{2m},0)\to(\mathbb{R}^{2m},0)$ such that $A\sigma A=\sigma$, A is elliptic, all eigenvalues $\lambda_1,\dots,\lambda_m$ of the linearization $(A)_1$ with positive imaginary parts are distinct and $A\in\Psi^*_\ell$ for a certain $\ell\in\mathbb{N}$, then σ is an involution, but I have no proof of this conjecture. If A is not resonant, it is known to be true (Corollary of Theorem 2.5).

§ 2.9. Weakly reversible diffeomorphisms of a plane

For $m = 1$ and $k = 0$, Theorem 2.9 asserts the existence of an invariant under A and G circle, rounding once the origin, in every neighbourhood of 0. Consequently, the fixed point 0 of the diffeomorphism A is stable. We arrive at the following result (similar to the theorem on the stability of a nondegenerate elliptic fixed point of a symplectic diffeomorphism of a plane).

THEOREM 2.10. Let $A:(\mathbb{R}^2,0)\to(\mathbb{R}^2,0)$ be an elliptic weakly reversible analytic diffeomorphism. Assume that there exists such a number $\ell\in\mathbb{N}$ that no change of variables reduces the jet $(A)_{2\ell+1}$ to $(A)_1$. Suppose the eigenvalue λ of $(A)_1$ is not a root of unity of degree $2\ell+2$ and lower. Then A is reversible and the fixed point 0 of the diffeomorphism A is stable.

The nondegeneracy condition imposed on $(A)_{2\ell+1}$ in Theorem 2.10 is essential. For an arbitrary root $\lambda\in\mathcal{U}(1)$ of unity of degree $N>2$ $(\lambda\notin\{-1;1\})$, there exist analytic reversible unstable diffeomorphisms $A:(\mathbb{R}^2,0)\to(\mathbb{R}^2,0)$, whose linearizations have eigenvalues λ and $\bar\lambda$.

EXAMPLE. Let $\lambda=e^{i\theta}$, where $\theta\in\mathbb{R}$ (one may assume $0<\theta<\pi$) and $N\theta\in 2\pi\mathbb{Z}$. Consider the following function $u:\mathbb{C}\to\mathbb{C}$:

$$u(z)=e^{i\theta/2}\left(z+\frac{i}{2}z\bar z^{N}\right).$$

The relation $u\left(\overline{A(z)}\right)=\overline{u(z)}$ defines a reversible diffeomorphism $A:(\mathbb{C},0)\to(\mathbb{C},0)$, that is analytic in the real sense (a reversing diffeomorphism is the complex conjugation involution).

It is easy to see that

$$A(z)-\frac{i}{2}A(z)\overline{A(z)}^N=\lambda(z+\frac{i}{2}z\bar{z}^N),$$

whence

$$A(z)=\lambda z+\lambda i z\bar{z}^N+O(|z|^{2N+1}).$$

Thus, λ and $\bar{\lambda}$ are eigenvalues of $(A)_1$. Since $\lambda^N=1$,

$$(A(z))^N=z^N(1+iN\bar{z}^N)+O(|z|^{3N}),$$

whence

$$\operatorname{Im}(A(z))^N=\operatorname{Im}z^N+N|z|^{2N}+O(|z|^{3N}).$$

If z is small enough then

$$\operatorname{Im}(A(z))^N\geq\operatorname{Im}z^N+(N-1)|z|^{2N}\geq\operatorname{Im}z^N+(N-1)(\operatorname{Im}z^N)^2.$$

Hence, the fixed point 0 of A is unstable.

For an analogous example in the case of symplectic diffeomorphisms see, e.g., [22 (§ 31)] .

As well as in the global situation, the existence of invariant circles of a nondegenerate elliptic diffeomorphism $A:(\mathbb{R}^2,0)\to(\mathbb{R}^2,0)$ follows from the intersection property: every closed curve surrounding 0 intersects its A-image (see [22 (§§ 32-34)]).

There exist reversible smooth germs $A:(\mathbb{R}^2,0)\to(\mathbb{R}^2,0)$ for which the intersection property fails in every neighbourhood of 0, i.e. in every neighbourhood of 0, there exists such a close curve Γ surrounding 0 that $A(\Gamma)$ lies strictly inside Γ.

To construct appropriate examples introduce Cartesian coordinates

(u,v) on a plane $\mathbb{R}^2$. Denote by $[a,b,c,d]$, where $a,b,c,$ and d are arbitrary positive numbers, the rectangle with apices (a,b), $(-d,b)$, $(-d,-c)$, $(a,-c)$. Rectangles $[a,b,b,a]$ will be denoted merely by $[a,b]$.

Denote by F the following function in $C^\infty(\mathbb{R},\mathbb{R})$:

$$F(t)=\begin{cases} t+\gamma_* \exp(-\frac{1}{t^2})\sin\frac{1}{t}, & \text{for } t\neq 0 \\ 0, & \text{for } t=0 \end{cases}$$

where

$$0<\gamma_*<\left(\max_{t\neq 0}\left|\frac{d}{dt}\exp(-\frac{1}{t^2})\sin\frac{1}{t}\right|\right)^{-1}.$$

EXAMPLE 1. $A(u,v)=(F(u),F^{-1}(v))$. Note that $(A)_1=E_2$.

EXAMPLE 2. $A(u,v)=(-F(u),-F^{-1}(v))$. Note that $(A)_1=-E_2$.

In both examples $A([a,b])=[F(a),F^{-1}(b)]$. If $F(a)<a$ and $F(b)>b$ then $A([a,b])$ lies strictly inside $[a,b]$.

EXAMPLE 3. Denote by $\tilde{F}$ the following function in $C^\infty(\mathbb{R},\mathbb{R})$:

$$\tilde{F}(t)=\begin{cases} -F(t) & , \text{for } t\geq 0 \\ -F^{-1}(t) & , \text{for } t<0. \end{cases}$$

The function $\tilde{F}:\mathbb{R}\to\mathbb{R}$ is an involution.

Let $A(u,v)=(\tilde{F}(v),-u)$. Note that eigenvalues of $(A)_1$ are 1 and -1. $A([a,b,c,d])=[F^{-1}(c),d,a,F(b)]$. If $a<c<F(a)$ and $F(b)<d<b$ then $A([a,b,c,d])$ lies strictly inside $[a,b,c,d]$.

In all three examples A is reversible with respect to the involution $G:(u,v)\mapsto(v,u)$.

In all other examples known to me of reversible diffeomorphisms

$(\mathbb{R}^2, 0) \to (\mathbb{R}^2, 0)$ for which the intersection property fails in every neighbourhood of 0, eigenvalues of linearizations of these diffeomorphisms are also equal to 1 or -1, i.e. these diffeomorphisms are not elliptic.

(It is obvious that diffeomorphisms whose linearizations have a hyperbolic spectrum $\{\gamma, \gamma^{-1}\}$, $\gamma \in \mathbb{R}$, $|\gamma| > 1$, always possess the intersection property, even without the reversibility condition.)

CONJECTURE 1. Every smooth elliptic reversible diffeomorphism $A : (\mathbb{R}^2, 0) \to (\mathbb{R}^2, 0)$ possesses the intersection property (in a certain sufficiently small neighbourhood of 0).

This conjecture is a local analogue to the global one formulated in § 1.5.

CONJECTURE 2. Every analytic reversible diffeomorphism $A : (\mathbb{R}^2, 0) \to (\mathbb{R}^2, 0)$ possesses the intersection property (in a certain sufficiently small neighbourhood of 0).

In the above examples 1 - 3, the absence of the analyticity of A at 0 is essential.

§ 2.10. Invariant tori near an equilibrium of a reversible vectorfield

The local KAM-theorem for vectorfields can be established similarly to the one for diffeomorphisms.

THEOREM 2.11. Let V be the germ of an analytic vectorfield $(\mathbb{R}^{2m+k}, 0)$ $(V(0) = 0)$ that is weakly reversible with respect to the germ of analytic diffeomorphism $G : (\mathbb{R}^{2m+k}, 0) \to (\mathbb{R}^{2m+k}, 0)$. Assume the field V to be slightly elliptic, i.e. its linearization $(V)_1$ to have k eigenvalues equaling 0 and $2m$ purely imaginary nonzero eigenvalues $i\varkappa_1, \ldots, i\varkappa_m, -i\varkappa_1, \ldots, -i\varkappa_m$ $(\varkappa_j > 0)$.

Suppose all m numbers $\varkappa_1, \ldots, \varkappa_m$ are distinct.

If $\kappa > 0$ then in addition assume G to be an involution of type $(m, m+\kappa)$.

Let the field V be nondegenerate, i.e. there exists $\ell \in \mathbb{N}$ such that either $V \in \Psi_\ell$ (for $\kappa > 0$) or $V \in \Psi_\ell^*$ (for $\kappa = 0$) (for definitions of Ψ_ℓ and Ψ_ℓ^* see § 2.5 and § 2.7, respectively).

Then the following holds.

a) In any neighbourhood of $0 \in \mathbb{R}^{2m+\kappa}$, there exist $(m+\kappa)$-dimensional manifolds invariant under V and G and foliated into m-dimensional tori also invariant under V and G. The field V induces on each of these tori a quasiperiodic motion, whose frequencies are constants on every $(m+\kappa)$-dimensional manifold.

b) Moreover, one can choose neighbourhoods O_ε of $0 \in \mathbb{R}^{2m+\kappa}$ ($diam(O_\varepsilon)$ tends to zero as $\varepsilon \to 0$, $O_{\varepsilon_1} \subset O_{\varepsilon_2}$ if $\varepsilon_1 < \varepsilon_2$) in such a manner that (17) should hold.

c) The $(m+\kappa)$-dimensional manifolds in question are organized into one-parameter families. The ratios of the quasiperiodic motion frequencies are constants along every family. For $m = 1$ some neighbourhood of 0 is completely foliated into invariant $(\kappa+1)$-dimensional manifolds under consideration.

d) For $\kappa = 0$, G is an involution of type (m, m).

The proof is quite analogous to that of Theorem 2.9 (the reduction to Theorem 1.2 by means of either Proposition 2.12 (for $\kappa > 0$) or Proposition 2.16 (for $\kappa = 0$)). The results c) follow from the similar global statements (namely, Remarks 2 and 3 made after the proof of Theorem 1.2 (see § 1.10)).

REMARK 1. If $m = 1$ and $\kappa > 0$ then the nondegeneracy condition is needless. It would have been needless also for $m = 1, \kappa = 0$ provided we had required G to be an involution but not considered the involutivity property of G as one of the assertions of the theorem.

The same remark refers to the analyticity condition.

We obtain that generic (i.e. with nonzero eigenvalues of the linearization) equilibria of a smooth reversible vectorfield on a plane, that belong to the fixed point line of the involution, can be only either saddles with zero trace *) (hyperbolic fields) or centers (elliptic fields).

REMARK 2. Let a vectorfield V at $(\mathbb{R}^{2m},0)\ (V(0)=0)$ and a diffeomorphism $G:(\mathbb{R}^{2m},0)\to(\mathbb{R}^{2m},0)$ be formal (possibly not analytic). It seems very likely that if $G_*V=-V$, V is elliptic, all eigenvalues $i\varkappa_1,\dots,i\varkappa_m$ of the linearization $(V)_1$ with positive imaginary parts are distinct and $V\in\Psi^*_\ell$ for a certain $\ell\in\mathbb{N}$ then G is an involution, but I have no proof of this conjecture. If V is not resonant, it is known to be true (Corollary of Theorem 2.8).

---

*) i.e. with eigenvalues of the linearization equaling $\pm\tau$, $\tau>0$.

Chapter 3. THE BEHAVIOUR OF TRAJECTORIES OF REVERSIBLE VECTORFIELDS NEAR A SYMMETRIC CYCLE

§ 3.1. Symmetric cycles and their families

Consider a vectorfield V on a domain $D \subset \mathbb{R}^N$, that is weakly reversible with respect to a diffeomorphism $\sigma : D \to D$. Denote by F_t the phase flow of the field V, so that $\sigma F_t \sigma^{-1} = F_{-t}$ for each $t \in \mathbb{R}$.

Denote by $\mathrm{Fix}\,\sigma$ the fixed point set of the diffeomorphism σ.

Let Γ be a trajectory of the flow F_t that is not an equilibrium. We call Γ symmetric if σ maps Γ onto itself.

PROPOSITION 3.1. The restriction of σ to a symmetric trajectory is always an involution. Every symmetric trajectory contains either a unique point belonging to $\mathrm{Fix}\,\sigma$ or exactly two such points, and the second case occurs precisely when this trajectory is closed.

PROOF. Let Γ be a symmetric trajectory of the flow F_t. Consider an arbitrary point $x \in \Gamma$. Let $\sigma x = F_\tau x$. Then the restriction of σ to Γ is given by the formula

$$\sigma F_t x = F_{\tau - t}\, x.$$

Therefore, $\sigma|_\Gamma$ is an involution. Furthermore, $y = F_{\tau/2}\, x \in \mathrm{Fix}\,\sigma$. We have

$$\sigma F_t y = F_{-t}\, y\,.$$

Therefore, if Γ is inclosed then y is the only point of Γ fixed under σ, and if Γ is closed and its period equals $2T$ then $\Gamma \cap \mathrm{Fix}\,\sigma = \{y;\ F_T y\}$. X

PROPOSITION 3.2. Every trajectory intersecting $\mathrm{Fix}\,\sigma$ is symmetric.

PROOF. Let Γ be a trajectory of the flow F_t and let G keep a point $x\in\Gamma$ fixed. Then for each t $GF_t x = F_{-t} G x = F_{-t} x \in \Gamma$. X

Propositions 3.1 and 3.2 imply the following

PROPOSITION 3.3. If a trajectory Γ of the flow F_t intersects $\mathrm{Fix}\, G$ at two points then it is symmetric and closed.

It is this proposition that underlies the search for symmetric closed trajectories of weakly reversible vectorfields.

In the sequel, we shall call a closed trajectory (a periodic solution) of a phase flow a cycle.

Let us prove the Proposition at the end of § 1.10. Let V be a slightly integrable field on a domain $D\subset\mathbb{R}^{K+2}$ that is reversible with respect to an involution G (where $\dim \mathrm{Fix}\, G = K+1$). All trajectories of V are symmetric cycles. They intersect the hypersurface $\mathrm{Fix}\, G$ at two points (both intersections are transversal). If V' is a field close to V and reversible with respect to an involution G' close to G then every trajectory of V' intersects the hypersurface $\mathrm{Fix}\, G'$ (close to $\mathrm{Fix}\, G$) at (at least) two points. By Proposition 3.3 all trajectories of V' are symmetric cycles.

Let Γ be a symmetric cycle of period $2T$, $\Gamma\cap\mathrm{Fix}\, G = \{Q_1, Q_2\}$. Suppose through Q_1 and Q_2 there exist hypersurfaces Σ_1 and Σ_2 respectively, that are transversal to Γ and invariant under G. Fix a value of the index $i\in\{1;2\}$. Consider the trajectory of the flow F_t starting at a point $x\in\Sigma_i$. In a time $t(x)$ close to T this trajectory intersects the hypersurface Σ_{3-i} at a point $\pi_i(x)$, where $\pi_i : \Sigma_i \to \Sigma_{3-i}$ is the semi-Poincaré mapping. The mapping $A_i = \pi_{3-i}\circ\pi_i : \Sigma_i\to\Sigma_i$ is the complete Poincaré mapping (the return function). Note that $\pi_i(Q_i) = Q_{3-i}$, $A_i(Q_i) = Q_i$.

PROPOSITION 3.4. For each point $x\in\Sigma_i$ the following relation holds

$$\pi_{3-i}\, G \pi_i x = Gx \ .$$

Moreover, $t(x)=t(\sigma\pi_i x)$.

PROOF. $\sigma\pi_i x\in\Sigma_{3-i}$, and we have

$$F_{t(x)}(\sigma\pi_i x)=F_{t(x)}\sigma F_{t(x)}x=\sigma x\in\Sigma_i.$$

Therefore, $t(\sigma\pi_i x)\leqslant t(x)$. On the other hand,

$$F_{-t(\sigma\pi_i x)}(\pi_i x)=\sigma^{-1}F_{t(\sigma\pi_i x)}(\sigma\pi_i x)=\sigma^{-1}\pi_{3-i}\sigma\pi_i x\in\Sigma_i.$$

Therefore, $t(\sigma\pi_i x)\geqslant t(x)$.

Thus, $t(x)=t(\sigma\pi_i x)$. Now we have

$$\sigma x=F_{t(x)}\sigma F_{t(x)}x=F_{t(x)}(\sigma\pi_i x)=F_{t(\sigma\pi_i x)}(\sigma\pi_i x)=\pi_{3-i}\sigma\pi_i x. \quad X$$

As an obvious consequence, we obtain

PROPOSITION 3.5. The mapping A_i is weakly reversible with respect to the restriction of the diffeomorphism σ to the hypersurface Σ_i.

Unlike closed trajectories of generic dynamical systems (with continuous time), symmetric cycles often form smooth families.

THEOREM 3.1. Let a vectorfield V on $D\subset\mathbb{R}^{2m+k+1}$ with the phase flow F_t be weakly reversible with respect to a diffeomorphism $\sigma: D\to D$, the set $\mathrm{Fix}\,\sigma$ of fixed points of the diffeomorphism σ being a smooth manifold of dimension $m+k$. Let $k\geqslant 1$. Then generically symmetric cycles of V are not isolated, but organized into smooth k-parameter families.

PROOF. Let Γ be a symmetric cycle of the field V intersecting $\mathrm{Fix}\,\sigma$ at points Q_1 and Q_2. Denote the period of Γ by $2T$. Consider the $(m+k+1)$-dimensional surface $\Phi=\{F_\tau(x)\mid\tau$ is close to T, $x\in\mathrm{Fix}\,\sigma$, x is close to $Q_1\}$. The surface Φ passes through Q_2. Generically Φ and $\mathrm{Fix}\,\sigma$ intersect at Q_2 transversally, and, consequently, $W = \Phi \cap Fix\, G$ is a smooth k-dimensional surface. The cycle Γ intersects W at the point Q_2 at a nonzero angle. By Proposition 3.3 each trajectory of F_t passing through a point of W is a symmetric cycle. X

REMARK. For $m=0$ Theorem 3.1 is still valid and, moreover, the genericity requirement becomes needless - in this case, Φ is a neighbourhood of the point Q_2.

One can find Theorem 3.1 in [1, 2, 36]. The particular case $k=1$ is studied in [3]. The case $m=0$, $k=1$ is considered in [30, 31].

§ 3.2. Kolmogorov tori near a symmetric cycle

This section, in contrast to the preceding one, deals with not weakly reversible, but reversible vectorfields.

Let a vectorfield V on $D \subset \mathbb{R}^{2m+k+1}$ with the phase flow F_t be reversible with respect to an involution $G: D \to D$ whose fixed point manifold $Fix\, G$ is of dimension $m+k$. Here we allow m to equal 0, i.e. we suppose $m \in \mathbb{Z}_+$. Let Γ be a symmetric cycle of the field V intersecting $Fix\, G$ at points Q_1 and Q_2. Choose transversal to Γ invariant under G $(2m+k)$-dimensional hypersurfaces passing through Q_1 and Q_2 somehow and denote them by Σ_1 and Σ_2, respectively (the existence of such hypersurfaces is obvious, since G is an involution). Fix a value of the index $i \in \{1; 2\}$. Let $\pi_i : \Sigma_i \to \Sigma_{3-i}$ be the semi-Poincaré mapping and $A_i : \Sigma_i \to \Sigma_i$ be the usual Poincaré mapping. Denote $\Sigma_i \cap Fix\, G$ by Π_i. We assume Σ_1 and Σ_2 to be chosen so that $\dim \Pi_1 = \dim \Pi_2 = m+k$.

By Proposition 3.5 A_i is reversible with respect to the involution $\sigma_i = \sigma_{|\Sigma_i}$.

PROPOSITION 3.6. The reversible operator $(A_i)_1$ (the linearization of A_i at the point Q_i) has at least κ linearly independent eigenvectors with eigenvalue 1.

PROOF. The proof of this proposition is similar to that of Proposition 2.3, which guarantees only that $(A)_{i1}$ has at least κ linearly independent eigenvectors with eigenvalues 1 or -1.

Introduce the notations $a_i = (A_i)_1$, $g_i = (\sigma_i)_1$, $\zeta_i = T_{Q_i}\pi_i$ (the differential of π_i at the point Q_i). Let γ_i be the tangent plane to Π_i at Q_i.

Let $\delta_i = \gamma_i \cap \zeta_{3-i}\,\gamma_{3-i}$. Consider an arbitrary vector $x \in \delta_i$. Since $x \in \zeta_{3-i}\,\gamma_{3-i}$ if follows that $\tilde{x} = \zeta_{3-i}^{-1} x \in \gamma_{3-i}$. Taking into account $g_i x = x$, $g_{3-i}\tilde{x} = \tilde{x}$ and $\zeta_i g_i = g_{3-i}\zeta_{3-i}^{-1}$ (which follows from Proposition 3.4) we obtain

$$\zeta_i x = \zeta_i g_i x = g_{3-i}\,\zeta_{3-i}^{-1} x = g_{3-i}\tilde{x} = \tilde{x}.$$

Therefore

$$a_i x = \zeta_{3-i}\,\zeta_i x = \zeta_{3-i}\tilde{x} = x.$$

We have proved that δ_i is invariant under a_i and the restriction of a_i to δ_i is the identity mapping. But $\dim \gamma_1 = \dim \gamma_2 = m + \kappa$, and since $\dim \Sigma_i = 2m + \kappa$, we obtain $\dim \delta_i \geq \kappa$. X

REMARK. Since $\zeta_i x = \tilde{x} \in \gamma_{3-i}$ for each $x \in \delta_i$, it follows that $\zeta_i \delta_i \subset \delta_{3-i}$. But ζ_i is an isomorphism. Thus, $\zeta_i \delta_i = \delta_{3-i}$.

PROPOSITION 3.7. Let $\Xi_i = \Pi_i \cap \pi_{3-i}\Pi_{3-i}$. Then the following holds.

a) The set Ξ_i is invariant under A_i, and the restriction of A_i to Ξ_i is the identity mapping. Moreover, $\mathcal{J}_i \Xi_i = \Xi_{3-i}$.

b) Every trajectory of the field V passing through a point of Ξ_i is a symmetric cycle.

c) Generically Ξ_i is a smooth κ-dimensional surface passing through Q_i.

PROOF. The statement a) can be verified by exactly the same arguments as those ones, by means of which Proposition 3.6 was established. The statement b) is a direct consequence of Proposition 3.3, it also follows immediately from the statement a). Finally, generically the surfaces Π_i and $\mathcal{J}_{3-i}\Pi_{3-i}$ intersect at Q_i transversally (as submanifolds of Σ_i), and, hence, Ξ_i is a smooth κ-dimensional surface. X

REMARK. We proved Theorem 3.1 (for the case of reversible fields) over again.

Proceed to theorems on Kolmogorov tori. We shall suppose $m \geqslant 1$ again. Besides that, we will drop the index 1 in Q_1, Σ_1, Π_1, Ξ_1, A_1 and G_1 to simplify the notation (so that we shall denote the phase space involution G and its restriction to Σ_1 equally). We will assume the original field V and involution G to be analytic.

By Proposition 3.7 generically $\Xi = \Pi \cap \mathcal{J}_2 \Pi_2$ is an analytic κ-dimensional surface, and $A|_\Xi = id$. A is reversible with respect to the involution G, and $G|_\Xi = id$. The linearization of A at every point of Ξ has at least κ eigenvalues equaling 1. The situation, when for each $x \in \Xi$ the other $2m$ eigenvalues of the linearization of A at x lie in $\mathcal{U}(1) \setminus \{-1; 1\}$, is said to be slightly elliptic (for $\kappa = 0$ - elliptic). Generically, for almost all $x \in \Xi$ all m eigenvalues of the linearization of A at x with positive imaginary parts are distinct and nonresonant, the germ of A at x lying in the class Ψ_1.

Theorem 2.9 provides us immediately with the following statement.

PROPOSITION 3.8. In the generic slightly elliptic situation, in every neighbourhood of Ξ , there exist $(m+\kappa)$-dimensional manifolds invariant under A and G and foliated into m-dimensional tori also invariant under A and G . The action of A on these tori is quasiperiodic, and the frequencies of this action are constants on every $(m+\kappa)$-dimensional manifold.

Returning to the original field V on the phase space $D \subset \mathbb{R}^{2m+\kappa+1}$ from the Poincaré mapping $A: \Sigma \to \Sigma$ we obtain the following main result of this chapter.

THEOREM 3.2. In the generic slightly elliptic situation, in every neighbourhood of a κ-parameter family of symmetric cycles of the field V , there exist $(m+\kappa+1)$-dimensional manifolds invariant under V and G and foliated into $(m+1)$-dimensional tori also invariant under V and G . On these tori the field V induces a quasiperiodic motion, the ratios of the frequencies of this motion being constants on every fixed $(m+\kappa+1)$-dimensional manifold.

PROOF. Proposition 3.8 implies the existence of $(m+\kappa+1)$-dimensional manifolds foliated into $(m+1)$-dimensional tori invariant under V and G and possessing the following property. Let T_λ^{m+1} be one of the tori into which a given invariant $(m+\kappa+1)$-dimensional manifold is foliated (λ being a κ-dimensional coordinate on the foliation base). Then one can introduce such a coordinate system $\varphi_1, \dots, \varphi_m, \varphi_{m+1} \bmod 2\pi$ on T_λ^{m+1} that

a) on T_λ^{m+1} the vectorfield V induces a vectorfield whose $(m+1)$-th coordinate is positive everywhere;

b) the corresponding return function has the form

$$(\varphi_1, \dots, \varphi_m, 0) \longmapsto (\varphi_1 + \omega_1, \dots, \varphi_m + \omega_m, 0)$$

where numbers $\omega_1, \dots, \omega_m$ called rotation numbers do not depend on λ ;

c) $\omega = (\omega_1, \dots, \omega_m) \in \mathcal{M}_m(\varepsilon_*, 1)$ for some small $\varepsilon_* > 0$.

Recall that F_t is the phase flow of V. Denote $(\varphi_1,\dots,\varphi_m)$ by φ'.

Let

$$F_t:(\varphi_1,\dots,\varphi_m,0)\mapsto(f_t^1(\varphi'),\dots,f_t^m(\varphi'),\ f_t^{m+1}(\varphi')),$$

where

$$f^{m+1}_{\tau(\varphi')}(\varphi')=2\pi\ ,\quad f^{j}_{\tau(\varphi')}(\varphi')=\varphi_j+\omega_j\,.$$

We wish to construct on T_λ^{m+1} coordinates $\Phi_1,\dots,\Phi_m,\Phi_{m+1}$ $\mathrm{mod}\ 2\pi$ in which the equations of the motion get the form

$$\dot\Phi_1=\Omega_1,\dots,\dot\Phi_m=\Omega_m,\ \dot\Phi_{m+1}=\Omega_{m+1}.$$

One has to seek Φ expressed in terms of the initial coordinates φ by the formulas

$$\Phi_j(F_t(\varphi',0))=\varphi_j+\psi_j(\varphi')+t\Omega_j\ ,$$

$$\Phi_{m+1}(F_t(\varphi',0))=\psi_{m+1}(\varphi')+t\Omega_{m+1}\ ,$$

where $\psi_1,\dots,\psi_m,\psi_{m+1}$ are 2π-periodic in φ' functions.

These formulas define Φ well, i.e. give Φ as a single-valued continuous function in φ, if and only if

$$\begin{cases}\varphi_j+\omega_j+\psi_j(\varphi'+\omega)\equiv\varphi_j+\psi_j(\varphi')+\tau(\varphi')\Omega_j\\ \psi_{m+1}(\varphi'+\omega)+2\pi\equiv\psi_{m+1}(\varphi')+\tau(\varphi')\Omega_{m+1}\end{cases}$$

i.e. iff

$$\begin{cases} \psi_j(\varphi'+\omega)-\psi_j(\varphi') \equiv \tau(\varphi')\Omega_j-\omega_j \\ \psi_{m+1}(\varphi'+\omega)-\psi_{m+1}(\varphi') \equiv \tau(\varphi')\Omega_{m+1}-2\pi . \end{cases} \tag{1}$$

Denote by $\langle\ \rangle$ the average operator with respect to φ' and by $L: \tilde{u} \mapsto L\tilde{u}$ the operator of solving the equation

$$u(\varphi'+\omega)-u(\varphi') \equiv \tilde{u}(\varphi'), \quad \langle u\rangle = 0$$

(here $\langle\tilde{u}\rangle = 0$) with respect to u (see § 1.3, A). Then for

$$\Omega_j = \frac{\omega_j}{\langle\tau\rangle}, \quad \Omega_{m+1} = \frac{2\pi}{\langle\tau\rangle}$$

the equations (1) are solvable:

$$\psi_j = L(\Omega_j\tau-\omega_j)+const, \quad \psi_{m+1} = L(\Omega_{m+1}\tau-2\pi)+const$$

(the constants are arbitrary). The ratio

$$(\Omega_1:\ldots:\Omega_m:\Omega_{m+1}) = (\omega_1:\ldots:\omega_m:2\pi)$$

does not depend on λ. X

REMARK. The statement of Theorem 2.9 on the measure of the union of invariant manifolds implies the similar statement in the present situation.

For the case $m = 1$, Theorem 3.2 guarantees the stability of some symmetric cycles of the field V .

EXAMPLE 1. Let $m=1, k=0$. Then generically $\Xi = \{Q\}$ and in the generic elliptic situation, in every neighbourhood of Q in Σ , there exist surrounding Q circles invariant under A and G. Consequently, the original symmetric cycle Γ is stable.

EXAMPLE 2. Let $m=1$, $\kappa\geq 1$. Generically Ξ is an analytic κ-dimensional surface passing through Q. In the generic slightly elliptic situation, we obtain (in Σ) an assemblage of $(\kappa+1)$-dimensional cylinders enclosing Ξ and invariant under A and G that are foliated into circles also invariant under A and G. The rotation number of the restriction of A to these circles is a constant on a given cylinder. Consider a cylinder Cyl corresponding to rotation number θ_0. Cyl may intersect Ξ at those points where different from 1 eigenvalues of the linearization of A are $e^{\pm i\theta_0}$. By Proposition 2.6 there exists a coordinate system $(z,\xi_1,\dots,\xi_\kappa)$ on Σ (where $z\in\mathbb{C}$, $\xi_t\in\mathbb{R}$) with origin at such a point, in which

$$(A)_3:\quad \begin{matrix} z \mapsto e^{i\theta_0} z\left(1+i\sum_{t=1}^{\kappa} a_t\xi_t+i\langle B\xi,\xi\rangle-\frac{1}{2}\sum_{t=1}^{\kappa} a_t^2\xi_t^2+ic\rho\right) \\ \xi \mapsto \xi\ , \end{matrix}$$

$$G:\quad \begin{matrix} z \mapsto \bar{z} \\ \xi \mapsto \xi\ , \end{matrix} \tag{2}$$

$$\Xi=\{z=0\}\ ,$$

where $\rho=z\bar{z}$, a_t, c are real numbers, $\langle B\xi,\xi\rangle$ is a quadratic form (B is a symmetric $\kappa\times\kappa$ matrix). We suppose that

$$c\neq 0 \quad\text{and}\quad \sum_{t=1}^{\kappa} a_t^2>0$$

(generically this holds), in particular, the germ of A at 0 belongs to Ψ_1. Let, at point $(0,\xi)\in\Xi$, the eigenvalues of the linearization of A be

$$\underbrace{1,\ldots,1}_{\kappa},\ e^{\pm i\theta(\xi)}$$

where $\theta(0)=\theta_0$. Clearly, $a d\xi$ is the differential of θ at 0. As is easy to verify, the equation of the surface Cyl in a neighbourhood of the point 0 is

$$a\xi+\langle B\xi,\xi\rangle+c\rho+O_3=0$$

where O_3 indicates terms of the third order in ξ_t, z and $\bar{z}$. Hence, this surface has no singularity at 0. The intersection of Cyl and Ξ in a neighbourhood of 0 is a $(\kappa-1)$-dimensional submanifold passing through 0. If $\kappa=1$ then, in a neighbourhood of 0, Cyl looks like a paraboloid of revolution foliated into its parallels.

Generically, some isolated points of the surface Ξ are nondegenerate critical ones for the function $\theta(\xi)$. In a neighbourhood of each such point in Σ, one can choose such a coordinate system $(z,\xi_1,\ldots,\xi_\kappa)$ in which $(A)_3$, G and Ξ have the form (2). Then all $a_t=0$, but the quadratic form $\langle B\xi,\xi\rangle$ is nondegenerate.

Let one of the following two statements hold:

a) $c>0$ and the form $\langle B\xi,\xi\rangle$ is positively defined (i.e. the function $\theta(\xi)$ has a minimum at 0),

b) $c<0$ and the form $\langle B\xi,\xi\rangle$ is negatively defined (i.e. the function $\theta(\xi)$ has a maximum at 0).

Then invariant under A and G "cylinders" corresponding to rotation numbers $\theta_0 + C\Delta\theta$, where $\Delta\theta > 0$ are small, are $(k+1)$-spheres enclosing 0. Thus, in such a case the fixed point 0 of the mapping A is stable and, consequently, the symmetric cycle of the original field V passing through 0 is stable.

REMARK. For $m=k=1$ we have a reversible vectorfield in a four-dimensional phase space with an involution whose fixed point manifold is of dimension two. It is interesting to compare the behaviour of trajectories of such a field and that of a Hamiltonian system with two degrees of freedom [1] . Cycles of the Hamiltonian system, as well as symmetric cycles of the reversible one, form one-parameter families. But the Hamiltonian system has the first integral (the Hamilton function), whence the existence of Kolmogorov tori (under the usual nondegeneracy conditions) implies the stability of every cycle of a family (Kolmogorov tori divide the isoenergetic surface passing through a given cycle and enclose this cycle). At the same time, the reversible vectorfield has, generally speaking, no first integrals, and the existence of quasiperiodic motions (whose phase curves fill three-dimensional invariant manifolds foliated into invariant two-dimensional tori) does not prevent several trajectories from escaping from the original symmetric cycle along a resonant zone (cf. [40]). For reversible vectorfields, one may succeed in establishing the stability only of some individual symmetric cycles of a given family (namely, those cycles which correspond to extrema of the rotation angle of the linearization of the Poincaré mapping).

Chapter 4. NON-AUTONOMOUS REVERSIBLE DIFFERENTIAL EQUATIONS

§ 4.1. Definitions

DEFINITION 4.1. A non-autonomous differential equation

$$\dot{x} = V_t(x) \tag{1}$$

where V_t is a vectorfield depending on the time variable t is called a quasireversible equation, if there exists a family $\{G_t\}$ of the phase space diffeomorphisms, that satisfies the identity

$$T_x G_t(V_t(x)) + \frac{\partial G_t(x)}{\partial t} = -V_{-t}(G_t(x)) \ . \tag{2}$$

The field V_t is also said to be quasireversible with respect to $\{G_t\}$.

EXAMPLE. Every vectorfield V_t at $(\mathbb{R}^N, 0)$ depending on t (t varies over some neighbourhood of 0 and $V_t(0) = 0$ for all t) is quasireversible with respect to an appropriate family of diffeomorphisms $\{G_t\}$ (for all t, $G_t : (\mathbb{R}^N, 0) \to (\mathbb{R}^N, 0)$).

To prove this statement it suffices to solve the Cauchy problem for the equation (2) with respect to the unknown function $G_t(x)$, choosing an arbitrary diffeomorphism $G_0 : (\mathbb{R}^N, 0) \to (\mathbb{R}^N, 0)$ as the initial condition $G_0(x)$.

PROPOSITION 4.1. V_t is quasireversible with respect to $\{G_t\}$ if and only if the vectorfield $V^* = V_t(x)\,\partial/\partial x + \partial/\partial t$ on the extended phase space is weakly reversible (in the usual sense) with respect to the diffeomorphism $G^* : (x, t) \mapsto (G_t(x), -t)$ of the extended phase space.

One can verify this simple, but fundamental proposition directly. It implies the following statements.

PROPOSITION 4.2. If a family $\{G_t\}$ reverses V_t then the family $\{\tilde{G}_t\}$ defined by $\tilde{G}_t(G_{-t}(x)) = x$ (for all t and x) also reverses V_t.

PROPOSITION 4.3. Let $\{F_t^\tau\}$ be the family of transformations of the phase space of equation (1) (F_t^τ is the transformation for the time from t to τ). The family $\{G_t\}$ reverses V_t if and only if for each t and τ

$$G_\tau F_t^\tau = F_{-t}^{-\tau} G_t . \tag{3}$$

A submanifold of the extended phase space of the equation (1), quasireversible with respect to a family $\{G_t\}$, will be called a manifold invariant under V_t and G_t if it is invariant under the vectorfield V^* and the diffeomorphism G^* .

DEFINITION 4.2. The equation (1) quasireversible with respect to a family $\{G_t\}$ is called a weakly reversible equation if $G_t = G$ does not depend on t , and is said to be reversible if G is an involution of the phase space.

REMARK. The definitions of quasireversible, weakly reversible and reversible equations are not invariant under a shift of the time t. For instance, the vectorfield $V_t(x) = tx\partial/\partial x$ on the real line is reversible with respect to the involution $G : x \mapsto -x$ whereas the vectorfield $V_t'(x) = (t+1)\,x\partial/\partial x$ is reversed by no t-independent diffeomorphism $G' : \mathbb{R} \to \mathbb{R}$ (but then it is quasireversible with respect to, e.g., the family $\{G_t\}$, where $G_t : x \mapsto -xe^{-2t}$, the mapping G^* corresponding to this family being an involution).

Consider a non-autonomous equation (1) with the phase space $D \subset \mathbb{R}^N$, quasireversible with respect to $\{G_t\}$. We shall call (1) a T-periodic equation if V_t and G_t are periodic in t with period $T > 0$. It is natural to call $D \times S^1$ (where

$S^1 = \mathbb{R}/T\mathbb{Z}$), not $D \times \mathbb{R}$, the extended phase space of such an equation. It will be $D \times S^1$ that will be considered as the extended phase space of a T-periodic equation (1) in the sequel.

Let F_t^τ be transformations of the phase space of a T-periodic equation (1) quasireversible with respect to $\{G_t\}$.

PROPOSITION 4.4. The monodromy operator F_0^T is weakly reversible with respect to the diffeomorphism G_0.

PROOF. (3) implies $G_T F_0^T G_0^{-1} = F_0^{-T}$. In virtue of the periodicity $G_T = G_0$ and $F_0^{-T} = F_T^0 = (F_0^T)^{-1}$. X

Proposition 4.4 is key in proving non-autonomous KAM-theorems.

§ 4.2. Kolmogorov tori of non-autonomous perturbations of integrable reversible differential equations

Consider an analytic vectorfield V^0 on a domain $D \subset \mathbb{R}^{2m+\kappa}$. Suppose V^0 is weakly reversible with respect to an analytic diffeomorphism $G^0 : D \to D$, and D is analytically foliated into invariant under V^0 and G^0 m-dimensional tori T^m_w, where w is an $(m+\kappa)$-dimensional parameter labeling the tori. Furthermore, suppose the field V^0 induces the quasiperiodic motion with frequencies $\omega(w)$ on each torus T^m_w. Assume the rank of the mapping $w \mapsto \omega(w)$ to be equal to m everywhere. Then by Proposition 1.2 G^0 is an involution. Fix a number $T > 0$.

Let V_t be an arbitrary sufficiently small analytic non-autonomous T-periodic perturbation of the field V^0 , which is weakly reversible with respect to an analytic diffeomorphism $G : D \to D$ sufficiently close to the involution G^0 (we assume the differences $V_t - V^0$ and $G - G^0$ to be small even if extended into $\mathbb{C}^{2m+\kappa}$ by the fixed distance from $\mathbb{R}^{2m+\kappa}$). For $\kappa>0$ suppose in addition that G is an involution.

THEOREM 4.1. By the assumptions just described the following holds.

a) In the extended phase space $D\times S^1$ of the equation (1) there is an assemblage of $(m+\kappa+1)$-dimensional manifolds invariant under V_t and G and foliated into $(m+1)$-dimensional tori also invariant under V_t and G.

b) The measure of the union of these manifolds tends to $mes(D\times S^1)=T\,mes\,D$ as the differences V_t-V° and $G-G^\circ$ tend to zero.

c) For $\kappa=0$, G is an involution.

PROOF. This theorem follows immediately from Theorem 1.1 and its corollaries 1 and 2. Indeed, the phase flow mapping $A^\circ=F_T$ of the field V° at time T is reversible with respect to the involution G°. The monodromy operator $A=F_0^T$ of the equation (1) is weakly reversible (for $\kappa>0$ - reversible) with respect to the diffeomorphism (for $\kappa>0$ - the involution) G. Applying Theorem 1.1 to the pair (A°,G°) and its perturbation (A,G) we obtain the desired statements. In more details, by Theorem 1.1 in D there is an assemblage of tori invariant under A and G, and the restrictions of A and G to these tori have the following form for a suitable parametrization by $\varphi\in T^m$:

$$A:\varphi\mapsto\varphi+T\omega\ ,\quad G:\varphi\mapsto-\varphi .$$

Moreover, tori with the same ω are organized into analytic κ-parameter families. Each of these tori T^m in D generates an invariant under V_t and G torus T^{m+1} in $D\times S^1$. Note that it is convenient to parametrize it by $\varphi\in T^m$ and $t\in S^1=\mathbb{R}/T\mathbb{Z}$ according to the following rule: a point with coordinates (φ,t) on

T^{m+1} is the point $(F_0^t(y-\omega t),t)$ in $D\times S^1$. In coordinates (y,t), the equation (1) induces the equation $\dot{y}=\omega$ on T^{m+1}. X

REMARK. In the extended phase space $D\times S^1$ of the original unperturbed equation, we obtain the slightly integrable vectorfield $V^*=V^\circ(x)\partial/\partial x+\partial/\partial t$ reversible with respect to the involution $G^*:(x,t)\mapsto(G^\circ(x),-t)$. Nevertheless, one can not deduce the theorem under consideration from Theorem 2.1 because the field V^* is degenerate: one of its frequencies is equal to 1 everywhere.

§ 4.3. Kolmogorov tori near equilibria and periodic solutions of non-autonomous reversible differential equations

Let a T-periodic equation (1) be weakly reversible with respect to a diffeomorphism G of the phase space. We will call a solution $x=x(t)$ of this equation symmetric periodic if $x(0)=x(T)$ and $G(x(0))=x(0)$.

THEOREM 4.2. Let V_t be the germ of an analytic T-periodic vectorfield at $(\mathbb{R}^{2m+\kappa},0)$ ($V_t(0)=0$ for all t) that is weakly reversible with respect to the germ of an analytic diffeomorphism $G:(\mathbb{R}^{2m+\kappa},0)\to(\mathbb{R}^{2m+\kappa},0)$. Let $A=F_0^T:(\mathbb{R}^{2m+\kappa},0)\to(\mathbb{R}^{2m+\kappa},0)$ be the monodromy operator of the equation (1). Assume eigenvalues of the linearization $(A)_1$ of A to be

$$\underbrace{1,\ldots,1}_{\kappa},\ \lambda_1,\ldots,\lambda_m,\ \bar\lambda_1,\ldots,\bar\lambda_m$$

where $\lambda_j \in \mathcal{U}(1)$, $\operatorname{Im} \lambda_j > 0$. Suppose all m numbers $\lambda_1, \ldots, \lambda_m$ are distinct.

If $\kappa > 0$ then in addition assume σ to be an involution of type $(m, m+\kappa)$.

Let the operator A be nondegenerate, i.e. there exists $\ell \in \mathbb{N}$ such that either $A \in \Psi_\ell$ (for $\kappa > 0$) or $A \in \Psi_\ell^*$ (for $\kappa = 0$) (for definitions of Ψ_ℓ and Ψ_ℓ^* see § 2.2 and § 2.4, respectively).

Then in the extended phase space $\mathcal{O}(0) \times S^1$ ($\mathcal{O}(0)$ being a neighbourhood of 0 in $\mathbb{R}^{2m+\kappa}$) in any neighbourhood of the zero solution of the equation (1), there exist manifolds of dimension $m+\kappa+1$ invariant under V_t and σ and foliated into $(m+1)$-dimensional tori also invariant under V_t and σ . Moreover, for $\kappa = 0$, σ is an involution.

This theorem is a particular case of the following theorem.

THEOREM 4.3. Let V_t be an analytic non-autonomous T-periodic vectorfield on a domain $D \subset \mathbb{R}^{2m+\kappa}$ that is weakly reversible with respect to an analytic diffeomorphism $\sigma : D \to D$. Let $x = x^*(t)$ be a symmetric periodic solution of the equation (1) $(x^*(0) = x^*(T) = x_0$, $\sigma(x_0) = x_0)$. Let A be the germ of the monodromy operator F_0^T of the equation (1) at x_0 . Assume eigenvalues of the linearization $(A)_1$ of A to be

$$\underbrace{1, \ldots, 1}_{\kappa}, \ \lambda_1, \ldots, \lambda_m, \bar{\lambda}_1, \ldots, \bar{\lambda}_m$$

where $\lambda_j \in \mathcal{U}(1)$, $\operatorname{Im} \lambda_j > 0$. Suppose all m numbers $\lambda_1, \ldots, \lambda_m$ are distinct.

If $\kappa > 0$ then in addition assume σ to be an involution (of type $(m, m+\kappa)$ at x_0).

Let the operator A be nondegenerate, i.e. there exists $\ell \in \mathbb{N}$

such that either $A \in \Psi_\ell$ (for $\kappa > 0$) or $A \in \Psi_\ell^*$ (for $\kappa = 0$).

Then in the extended phase space $D \times S^1$ in any neighbourhood of the solution $x = x^*(t)$, there exist manifolds of dimension $m + \kappa + 1$ invariant under V_t and G and foliated into $(m+1)$-dimensional tori also invariant under V_t and G. Moreover, for $\kappa = 0$, G is an involution.

PROOF. One may deduce these two theorems from Theorem 2.9 in exactly the same way as we have deduced Theorem 4.1 from Theorem 1.1.

REMARK 1. The statement of Theorem 2.9 on the measure of the union of invariant manifolds implies similar statements in the situations described in Theorems 4.2 and 4.3.

REMARK 2. For $m = 1$, $\kappa = 0$ we obtain that under the assumptions of Theorems 4.2 and 4.3 the zero solution and solution $x = x^*(t)$, respectively, of the equation (1) are stable. This result is analogous to the theorem on the stability of a Hamiltonian equilibrium on a plane (with the Hamilton function periodic in t) in the general elliptic case.

REMARK 3. In fact, for $\kappa > 0$ Theorems 4.2 and 4.3 are particular cases of Theorem 3.2 to be applied to the vectorfield $V^* = V_t(x)\,\partial/\partial x + \partial/\partial t$ in the extended phase space (reversible with respect to the involution $G^* : (x, t) \mapsto (G(x), -t)$) and to symmetric cycles $x = 0$ and $x = x^*(t)$, respectively. Proposition 3.7 implies (under the assumptions of Theorems 4.2 and 4.3) that the zero solution and the solution $x = x^*(t)$, respectively, of the equation (1) are embedded in κ-parameter families of symmetric periodic solutions of the equation (1).

REMARK 4. We have obtained the theorems on invariant tori of periodic reversible differential equations as corollaries to the theorems on invariant tori of reversible mappings. A priori one may propose generalizing the theorems on invariant tori of autonomous reversible vectorfields to the non-autonomous case and deducing the theorems on mappings from those on periodic differential equations. To fulfil this program it is necessary to verify that each reversible diffeomorphism close to nondegenerate (slightly) integrable one is the monodromy operator of some reversible periodic in time vectorfield close to nondegenerate (slightly) integrable autonomous one (and to verify the similar local statement as well).

I don't know whether this proposition holds in the analytic realm we are interested in (cf. [28]) but in the C^∞ -case it is almost trivial.

PROPOSITION 4.5. Let $x \bmod 2\pi$ be angular coordinates on T^m, y and η vary over some domains in spaces $\mathbb{R}^m$ and $\mathbb{R}^K$, respectively. Given an arbitrary smooth mapping

$$A:(x,y,\eta)\mapsto(x+y+\overset{1}{f}(x,y,\eta),\ y+\overset{2}{f}(x,y,\eta),\ \eta+\overset{3}{f}(x,y,\eta)) \tag{4}$$

(with $\overset{\tau}{f}$ sufficiently small) reversible with respect to the involution

$$G:(x,y,\eta)\mapsto(-x,y,\eta),$$

there exists a differential equation

$$\dot{x}=\frac{y}{2\pi}+\overset{1}{h}(x,y,\eta,t),\ \dot{y}=\overset{2}{h}(x,y,\eta,t),\ \dot{\eta}=\overset{3}{h}(x,y,\eta,t) \tag{5}$$

(with $\overset{\tau}{h}$ 2π -periodic in the time variable t, smooth and small) which is also reversible with respect to G and for which the initial mapping A is the monodromy operator.

PROOF. Fix an arbitrary smooth function $\varkappa=\varkappa(t):\mathbb{R}\to[0,1]$

vanishing for $t \leqslant \pi/3$ and equaling 1 for $t \geqslant 2\pi/3$. E.g., set

$$\varkappa(t) = \begin{cases} \dfrac{\exp\left(\frac{1}{\pi-3t}\right)}{\exp\left(\frac{1}{\pi-3t}\right)+\exp\left(\frac{1}{3t-2\pi}\right)}, & \text{for } \frac{\pi}{3} < t < \frac{2\pi}{3} \\ \frac{1}{2}+\frac{1}{2}\operatorname{sgn}(2t-\pi), & \text{for } t \notin \left(\frac{\pi}{3}, \frac{2\pi}{3}\right). \end{cases}$$

Let a mapping (4) be reversible with respect to G. On $[0,\pi]$ consider the differential equation associated with the family of transformations

$$F_0^t : \begin{array}{l} x \\ y \\ \eta \end{array} \mapsto \begin{array}{l} x + \frac{ty}{2\pi} + \frac{t-\pi}{4\pi}\varkappa(t)f^2 + \frac{1}{2}\varkappa(t)f^1 \\ y + \frac{1}{2}\varkappa(t)f^2 \\ \eta + \frac{1}{2}\varkappa(t)f^3 \end{array} \qquad 0 \leqslant t \leqslant \pi$$

(where $f^\tau = f^\tau(x,y,\eta)$).

This differential equation has the form (5) with h^τ smooth and small. Moreover, $h^\tau = 0$ for $t \notin (\pi/3, 2\pi/3)$.

Extend this differential equation to $(\pi, 2\pi)$ by setting

$$\begin{array}{l} h^1(x,y,\eta,t) = h^1(-x,y,\eta,2\pi-t) \\ h^2(x,y,\eta,t) = -h^2(-x,y,\eta,2\pi-t) \\ h^3(x,y,\eta,t) = -h^3(-x,y,\eta,2\pi-t). \end{array} \qquad \pi < t < 2\pi$$

We have obtained a smooth 2π-periodic in time differential equation reversible with respect to G. Let $F_{t_1}^{t_2}$ be the corresponding family of the phase space transformations. According to (3), $F_{\pi}^{2\pi} = F_{-\pi}^{0} = GF_{\pi}^{0}G$, i.e. $F_0^{2\pi} = G(F_0^{\pi})^{-1}GF_0^{\pi}$. Besides, $F_0^{\pi} = B$, where

$$B:(x,y,z)\mapsto\left(x+\frac{1}{2}y+\frac{1}{2}f^1,\ y+\frac{1}{2}f^2,\ z+\frac{1}{2}f^3\right).$$

As is easy to verify, $AGA = G$ implies $GB^{-1}GB = A$. X

Proposition 4.5 is proved. The analogous local statement can be proved in the similar manner.

I don't know whether one can generalize Proposition 4.5 to weakly reversible mappings.

Chapter 5. STRUCTURE OF RESONANT ZONES OF REVERSIBLE DIFFEOMORPHISMS AND VECTORFIELDS

§ 5.1. Statement of the problem

On a domain $D \subset \mathbb{R}^{2m+\kappa}$, consider a nondegenerate slightly integrable diffeomorphism $A : D \to D$ or a nondegenerate slightly integrable vectorfield V that are weakly reversible with respect to a diffeomorphism $G : D \to D$ (the dimension of invariant tori equaling m). By Proposition 1.1 (respectively Proposition 1.2) G is an involution and one can choose such a coordinate system (x, y, η) ($x \in T^m$, x is defined $\mathrm{mod}\ 2\pi$, $y \in \mathbb{R}^m$, $\eta \in \mathbb{R}^\kappa$) in a neighbourhood of every invariant torus, in which

$$A : (x, y, \eta) \mapsto (x + y, y, \eta)$$

(respectively

$$V = y \frac{\partial}{\partial x})$$

and

$$G : (x, y, \eta) \mapsto (-x, y, \eta).$$

The KAM-theory of such diffeomorphisms and vectorfields, set up in Chapter 1, guarantees that under sufficiently small analytic reversible (for $\kappa = 0$ - weakly reversible) perturbations of the diffeomorphism A (the field V respectively), κ-parameter families of invariant tori $y=const$, $\eta=const$ (η being a parameter), where $y \in \mathfrak{M}_m(C,1)$ (respectively $y \in \mathfrak{N}_m(C,1)$), do not disintegrate, but only undergo a slight deformation. Here C is a fixed number in $(0,1]$. The "small denominator" condition $y \in \mathfrak{M}_m(C,1)$ (respectively $y \in \mathfrak{N}_m(C,1)$) means that numbers $y_1,\dots,y_m$, π (respectively $y_1,\dots,y_m$) are "strongly" rationally independent.

The situation, when numbers $y_1,\dots,y_m,\pi$ (respectively $y_1,\dots,y_m$) are rationally dependent, is called "the limiting degeneration".

In this chapter, we study only the strongest "limiting degeneration" (the case opposite to that considered in the KAM-theory), when frequencies $y_1,\dots,y_m$ are rational multiples of π (respectively of one of them, note that for $m=1$ this case coincides with that in the KAM-theory!)

It turns out that

a) under small reversible perturbations of the diffeomorphism A, $(m+k)$ -dimensional invariant under A cylinders $y=const$ with $y_j/\pi \in \mathbb{Q}$ disintegrate into some k-parameter families of cycles of the perturbed diffeomorphism of the same length (a cycle of a mapping F of length $q \in \mathbb{N}$ is a set of q points $(w, F(w), F^2(w),\dots,F^{q-1}(w))$ provided $F^q(w)=w$ and $F^l(w) \neq w$ for each $l \in \mathbb{N}$, $l<q$);

b) under small reversible perturbations of the field V, $(m+k)$-dimensional invariant under V cylinders $y=const$ (where all ratios $y_{j'}/y_j \in \mathbb{Q}$, if $y_j \neq 0$) disintegrate into some k-parameter families of cycles of the perturbed field of the same period (recall that a cycle of a vectorfield is its closed trajectory).

§ 5.2. Principal theorem for diffeomorphisms and its corollaries

Let I be a domain in $\mathbb{R}^m$, $B = B_{R_0}(b)$ be a closed ball in $\mathbb{R}^k$ with an arbitrary centre b and radius R_0, O be a certain neighbourhood of B. Suppose on $\tilde{D} = \mathbb{R}^m \times I \times O$ the following mapping is given:

$$\tilde{A}: \begin{matrix} x \\ y \\ \eta \end{matrix} \longmapsto \begin{matrix} x + y + f^1(x,y,\eta) \\ y + f^2(x,y,\eta) \\ \eta + f^3(x,y,\eta) \end{matrix}$$

(x, y_τ and η being coordinates on $\mathbb{R}^m$, I and O respectively), where f^τ are smooth 2π-periodic in $x_1, \ldots, x_m$ functions.

Denote by $\tilde{G}: \tilde{D} \to \tilde{D}$ the involution

$$\tilde{G}: (x, y, \eta) \longmapsto (-x, y, \eta).$$

Let $\tilde{A}\tilde{G}\tilde{A} = \tilde{G}$ throughout $\tilde{D}$ where $\tilde{A}\tilde{G}\tilde{A}$ is defined.

Let a vector

$$\frac{2\pi p}{q} = \left(\frac{2\pi p_1}{q}, \ldots, \frac{2\pi p_m}{q}\right) \in I$$

be fixed, where $p_j \in \mathbb{Z}$ and $q \in \mathbb{N}$. Assume the greatest common divisor of $m+1$ numbers $p_1, \ldots, p_m$, q to equal 1.

One can lower the mappings $\tilde{A}$ and $\tilde{G}$ onto $D = T^m \times I \times O$, where $T^m = (\mathbb{R}/2\pi\mathbb{Z})^m$, we will denote the obtained mappings on D by A and G respectively.

Let $\sigma^1, \ldots, \sigma^{2^m}$ be all ordered collections of m numbers $(x_1, \ldots, x_m)$ with x_j equal to either 0 or π. We shall always suppose that the index ν will have the range from 1 to 2^m and the index s will have the range from 1 to $2^m q$.

Denote by $\operatorname{Fix} G$ the fixed point set of the involution G, i.e. the union of 2^m planes $\{(\sigma^\nu, y, \eta) \mid y \in I, \eta \in O\}$ of dimension $m+\kappa$.

Denote by Λ_q^p the set of such fixed points $(x, y, \eta) \in D$ of the mapping A^q that $\tilde{A}^q(x, y, \eta) = (x + 2\pi p, y, \eta)$. Λ_q^p consists of cycles of A of length q. Denote by $S\Lambda_q^p$ the union of symmetric (i.e. G-invariant) cycles of A of length q lying in Λ_q^p.

THEOREM 5.1. Let the situation just described take place. Then, if the functions f^τ are small enough in the C^1-norm, the following holds.

a) The set $S\Lambda_q^p$ consists of 2^m smooth κ-parameter families of symmetric cycles of the mapping A of length q. If q is odd then each of these cycles contains exactly one point lying on $\operatorname{Fix} G$. If q is even then 2^{m-1} families consist of cycles that do not contain points in $\operatorname{Fix} G$ at all while other 2^{m-1} families consist of cycles containing exactly two points in $\operatorname{Fix} G$.

b) From the coordinate point of view, the set $S\Lambda_q^p$ consists of $2^m q$ smooth surfaces $\mathcal{O}_s = \{x = x^s(\eta),\ y = y^s(\eta)\}$ of dimension κ which do not intersect each other (η varies over a certain neighbourhood $O' \subset O$ of the ball B). The smaller f^τ, the closer (in the C^1-norm) to the constant $2\pi p/q$ are functions $y^s(\eta)$ and the closer to the (nonordered) collection of constants

$$\left(\sigma^\nu + \frac{2\pi p \tau}{q},\ \nu = 1, \ldots, 2^m,\ \tau = 0, \ldots, q-1\right) \tag{1}$$

for q odd and

$$(\sigma^\nu + \frac{\pi p}{q} i + \frac{2\pi p r}{q},\ \nu=1,\ldots,2^m,\ i=0,1,\ r=0,\ldots,q/2-1) \tag{2}$$

for q even is the (nonordered) collection of functions $(x^s(\eta), s=1,\ldots,2^m q)$ (as is easy to verify, for each q this collection of constants consists of $2^m q$ distinct numbers in T^m).

Moreover, those 2^m functions $x^s(\eta)$, that are close to constants σ^ν , in fact coincide with them. We shall always number the surfaces $\mathcal{O}_s$ in such a way that the surface consisting of points with the x-coordinate equal to σ^ν should receive the index ν: $x^\nu(\eta) \equiv \sigma^\nu$.

Thus, 2^m of the surfaces $\mathcal{O}_s$ lie on $\mathrm{Fix}\,G$ and the other $2^m(q-1)$ surfaces $\mathcal{O}_s$ do not intersect $\mathrm{Fix}\,G$.

c) In a neighbourhood of each of the surfaces $\mathcal{O}_s$, there acts an involution G_s keeping every point on $\mathcal{O}_s$ fixed and reversing A^q (besides that, $G_\nu = G$). The type of the involution G_s is $(m, m+k)$ at every point on $\mathcal{O}_s$.

REMARK. In a neighbourhood of a point in $\Lambda_q^p \setminus S\Lambda_q^p$, generally speaking, no involution keeping it fixed and reversing A^q acts.

PROOF. If f^r are sufficiently small (in the C^0-norm) then in a domain $\tilde{D}_1 = \mathbb{R}^m \times I_1 \times O_1$, where I_1 is a domain in $\mathbb{R}^m$, $2\pi p/q \in I_1 \subset I$, O_1 is a neighbourhood of B in $\mathbb{R}^k$, $O_1 \subset O$, the qth iteration $\tilde{A}^q$ of the mapping $\tilde{A}$ is defined (and, consequently, in the domain $D_1 = T^m \times I_1 \times O_1$, the q-th iteration A^q of the mapping A is defined).

LEMMA 1. If f^r are sufficiently small (in the C^1-norm) then for each $x \in \mathbb{R}^m$ and $\eta \in O'$ (where $O' \subset O_1$ is a certain neighbourhood of B) there exists a unique number $y \in Y(x,\eta) \in I_1$, such that the first m coordinates of the point $\tilde{A}^q(x, y, \eta)$

equal $x+2\pi\rho$. The function $y=Y(x,\eta)$ is smooth and 2π-periodic in x . The smaller f^{τ} , the closer to the constant $2\pi\rho/q$ (in the C^1-norm) is this function.

PROOF. We have

$$\tilde{A}^q : \begin{matrix} x \\ y \\ \eta \end{matrix} \longmapsto \begin{matrix} x+qy+f^1_{(q)}(x,y,\eta) \\ y+f^2_{(q)}(x,y,\eta) \\ \eta+f^3_{(q)}(x,y,\eta) \end{matrix}$$

where functions $f^{\tau}_{(q)}$ are small in the C^1-norm as functions f^{τ} are. The equation $qy+f^1_{(q)}(x,y,\eta)=2\pi\rho$ (with respect to y) has a unique in I_1 solution $y=Y(x,\eta)$ for all x and η provided $f^1_{(q)}$ is small enough. This solution is obviously smoothly dependent on x and η and 2π-periodic in x . The smaller f^{τ} , the closer to $2\pi\rho/q$ is $Y(x,\eta)$. X

One can lower the function $Y(x,\eta)$ onto $T^m \times O'$, we will denote the obtained function by the same letter Y . Denote the surface $y=Y(x,\eta)$ in D by Γ . It is clear that $\Lambda^{\rho}_{q}\subset\Gamma$.

In the sequel, we shall not, as a rule, pay attention to domains over which the variables y and η will vary in this or that relation. We always suppose $y\in\tilde{I}$, $\eta\in\tilde{O}$, where $2\pi\rho/q\in\tilde{I}\subset I$, $B\subset\tilde{O}\subset O$, domains $\tilde{I}$ and $\tilde{O}$ differ only slightly from I and O respectively, and the smaller f^{τ} , the less is this difference.

LEMMA 2. The surface Γ is invariant under the involution GA^q . The sets Λ^{ρ}_{q} and $S\Lambda^{\rho}_{q}$ are invariant under both mappings A and G .

PROOF. Let $w=(x,y,\eta)\in\Gamma$ $(y=Y(x,\eta))$. Then $w' =\tilde{G}\tilde{A}^q w=(-x-2\pi\rho,\hat{y},\hat{\eta})$. Now $\tilde{A}^q w'=\tilde{A}^q\tilde{G}\tilde{A}^q w=\tilde{G}w=(-x,y,\eta)$.

Therefore, $\hat{y} = Y(-x, \hat{\eta})$ and $w' \in \Gamma$.

The set Λ_q^p is invariant under A by definition, since it consists of cycles of A. Let $w=(x,y,\eta) \in \Lambda_q^p$. Then $\tilde{G}w = (-x,y,\eta)$. We have $\tilde{A}^q(-x,y,\eta) = \tilde{A}^q\tilde{G}w = \tilde{G}\tilde{A}^{-q}w = \tilde{G}(x-2\pi p, y,\eta) = (-x+2\pi p, y, \eta)$. This means that $\tilde{G}w \in \Lambda_q^p$, i.e. Λ_q^p is invariant under G.

The set $S\Lambda_q^p$ is invariant under A and G by definition since it consists of symmetric cycles of A. X

Fix $\nu \in \{1,\ldots,2^m\}$. Let

$$\mathcal{O}_\nu = \Gamma \cap \{(x,y,\eta) \in D \mid x = \sigma^\nu\} = \{(\sigma^\nu, Y(\sigma^\nu,\eta),\eta) \mid \eta \in O'\}.$$

LEMMA 3. $\mathcal{O}_\nu \subset S\Lambda_q^p$ provided f^τ are small enough.

PROOF. It suffices to prove that A^q keeps each point of $\mathcal{O}_\nu$ fixed, i.e. that $\mathcal{O}_\nu \subset \Lambda_q^p$. The G-invariance of cycles follows from $\mathcal{O}_\nu \subset \mathrm{Fix}\, G$. Indeed, if $w \in \mathcal{O}_\nu$, then $GA^\tau w = A^{-\tau}Gw = A^{-\tau}w$.

Consider a point $w = (\sigma^\nu, Y(\sigma^\nu,\eta),\eta) \in \mathcal{O}_\nu$. We have $A^q w = w' = (\sigma^\nu, Z(\eta), H(\eta))$, where $Z(\eta)$ and $H(\eta)$ are certain functions. Since $A^q w' = A^q G w' = A^q G A^q w = Gw = w$, it follows that $w' \in \mathcal{O}_\nu$ and the identities

$$Z(\eta) = Y(\sigma^\nu, H(\eta)), \quad Z(H(\eta)) = Y(\sigma^\nu,\eta), \quad H(H(\eta)) = \eta$$

hold. Thus, the function $H(\eta) = \eta + f^3_{(q)}(\sigma^\nu, Y(\sigma^\nu,\eta),\eta)$ is an involution, and since it differs little (in the C^1-norm) from the identity function $H_0(\eta) = \eta$ (for f^τ small enough), it coincides with $H_0(\eta)$.

Indeed, let the function $W(\eta) = H(\eta) - \eta$ satisfy a Lipschitz inequality with constant less than 2. Then the identity $H(H(\eta)) = \eta$

transcribed in the form $W(\eta)-W(H(\eta))=2(H(\eta)-\eta)$ implies $H(\eta)=\eta$.

Thus, $H(\eta)=\eta$. Consequently, $Z(\eta)=Y(\sigma^\nu,\eta)$ and $w'=w$. X

REMARK. If $\kappa=0$ then Lemma 3 is almost trivial, because $Z=Y(\sigma^\nu)$ immediately implies $w'=w$.

Now consider the mapping $\tilde{A}\tilde{\sigma}$. As well as $\tilde{\sigma}$, it is an involution reversing $\tilde{A}$. The involution $\tilde{A}\tilde{\sigma}$ is given by

$$\tilde{A}\tilde{\sigma}: \begin{matrix} x \\ y \\ \eta \end{matrix} \mapsto \begin{matrix} -x+y+f^1(-x,y,\eta) \\ y+f^2(-x,y,\eta) \\ \eta+f^3(-x,y,\eta) \end{matrix} .$$

For sufficiently small f^1, the equation $-x+y+f^1(-x,y,\eta)=x$ (with respect to x) has on the torus T^m 2^m solutions $x=\sigma^\nu+y/2+F^\nu(y,\eta)$ smoothly dependent on y and η (where functions F^ν are small (in the C^1-norm) as f^1 is), and there are no other solutions of this equation. The union of 2^m surfaces $\Pi_\nu=\{(\sigma^\nu+y/2+F^\nu(y,\eta),\ y,\ \eta)\}$ of dimension $m+\kappa$ is the set $Fix\, A\sigma$ of fixed points of the involution $A\sigma$.

Denote by $\psi_{y,\eta}$ an arbitrary autodiffeomorphism of the torus T^m depending smoothly on y and η that satisfies the condition $\psi_{y,\eta}(\sigma^\nu+y/2+F^\nu(y,\eta))=\sigma^\nu$ for all ν. One can lift $\psi_{y,\eta}$ to a diffeomorphism $\tilde{\psi}_{y,\eta}:\mathbb{R}^m\to\mathbb{R}^m$. Introduce the new coordinate system (x^*,y,η) on $\tilde{D}$, where $x^*=\tilde{\psi}_{y,\eta}(x)$. Repeating the arguments of Lemma 1, we obtain the following statement.

LEMMA 1*. If f^τ are sufficiently small (in the C^1-norm) then for each $x^*\in\mathbb{R}^m$ and η there exists a unique number $y=Y^*(x^*,\eta)$ such that the first m coordinates of the point $\tilde{A}^q(x^*,y,\eta)$ equal

$x^* + 2\pi\rho$. The function $y = Y^*(x^*, \eta)$ is smooth and 2π-periodic in x^*. The smaller f^τ, the closer to the constant $2\pi\rho/q$ (in the C^1-norm) is this function.

One can lower the function $Y^*(x^*, \eta)$ onto $T^m \times \tilde{O}$, we will denote the obtained function by the same symbol Y^*. Denote the surface $y = Y^*(x^*, \eta)$ in D by Γ^*. It is clear that $\Lambda_q^\rho \subset \Gamma^*$.

Fix $\nu \in \{1, \dots, 2^m\}$. Let

$$\alpha_\nu^* = \Gamma^* \cap \{(x^*, y, \eta) \in D \mid x^* = \sigma^\nu\} = \{(\sigma^\nu, Y^*(\sigma^\nu, \eta), \eta) \mid \eta \in \tilde{O}\}.$$

Repeating the arguments of Lemma 3, we obtain the following statement.

LEMMA 3*. $\alpha_\nu^* \subset S\Lambda_q^\rho$ provided f^τ are small enough.

Return to the original coordinate system.

If f^τ are sufficiently small then each set $A^\tau \alpha_\nu$ or $A^\tau \alpha_\nu^*$, where $1 \leq \nu \leq 2^m$, $0 \leq \tau \leq q-1$, is a smooth κ-dimensional surface, whose projecting onto the η-axis is smooth, too. By Lemma 2 all these surfaces lie in $S\Lambda_q^\rho$.

Surfaces $A^\tau \alpha_\nu$ and $A^\tau \alpha_\nu^*$ are C^1-close to κ-dimensional planes $x = \sigma^\nu + 2\pi\rho\tau/q$, $y = 2\pi\rho/q$ and $x = \sigma^\nu + \pi\rho/q + 2\pi\rho\tau/q$, $y = 2\pi\rho/q$, respectively.

In a neighbourhood of each of the surfaces $A^\tau \alpha_\nu$ and $A^\tau \alpha_\nu^*$, there act involutions $A^\tau G A^{-\tau}$ and $A^{\tau+1} G A^{-\tau}$, respectively, which reverse A, keep every point of the corresponding surface fixed and have type $(m, m+\kappa)$ at these points.

LEMMA 4. Among $2^{m+1}q$ surfaces $A^\tau \alpha_\nu$, $A^\tau \alpha_\nu^*$, there are exactly $2^m q$ distinct ones. Besides that, these $2^m q$ distinct surfaces do not intersect each other.

PROOF. Define the transposition $\{1, \dots, 2^m\} \to \{1, \dots, 2^m\}, \nu \mapsto \nu'$ by the condition $\sigma^{\nu'} = \sigma^\nu + \pi\rho \ (\mathrm{modd}\ 2\pi)$. Note that this transposition is an involution. It is identical if all ρ_j are even, and it has no fixed point if there are odd numbers among $\rho_1, \ldots, \rho_m$.

CASE 1. q is odd.

Consider $2^m q$ surfaces $A^{\tau}\mathfrak{a}_{\nu}$, $\nu = 1, \ldots, 2^m$, $\tau = 0, \ldots, q-1$. These surfaces are desired ones.

Indeed, all of them do not intersect each other, since all numbers in the collection (1) are distinct.

Now consider the surfaces $\mathfrak{a}^*_{\nu}$. All points on the surface $\mathfrak{a}^*_{\nu}$ have the x-coordinate close to $\sigma^{\nu} + \pi\rho/q$. We have

$$\sigma^{\nu} + \frac{\pi\rho}{q} = \sigma^{\nu'} + \frac{2\pi\rho}{q} \cdot \frac{q+1}{2} \ (\mathrm{modd}\ 2\pi).$$

On the other hand,

$$A^{(q+1)/2}\mathfrak{a}_{\nu'} \subset \mathrm{Fix}\, AG,$$

because if $w \in \mathfrak{a}_{\nu'}$ then

$$AGA^{(q+1)/2} w = AA^{-(q+1)/2} Gw = A^{(1-q)/2} w = A^{(1-q)/2} A^{q} w = A^{(q+1)/2} w.$$

Therefore,

$$\mathfrak{a}^*_{\nu} = A^{(q+1)/2}\mathfrak{a}_{\nu'}$$

and for $\tau = 0, \ldots, q-1$

$$A^{\tau}\mathfrak{a}^*_{\nu} = A^{\tau'}\mathfrak{a}_{\nu'},$$

where $0 \leq \tau' \leq q-1$, $\tau' \equiv \tau + (q+1)/2 \ (\mathrm{mod}\, q)$.

CASE 2. q is even.

Consider $2^m q$ surfaces $A^\tau \mathfrak{A}_\nu, A^\tau \mathfrak{A}^*_\nu, \nu=1,\ldots,2^m, \tau=0,\ldots,q/2-1$. These surfaces are desired ones.

Indeed, all of them do not intersect each other, since all numbers in the collection (2) are distinct.

Now consider the surfaces $A^{q/2}\mathfrak{A}_\nu$. All points on the surface $A^{q/2}\mathfrak{A}_\nu$ have the x-coordinate close to $\sigma^\nu + \pi p = \sigma^{\nu'} \pmod{2\pi}$. On the other hand,

$$A^{q/2}\mathfrak{A}_\nu \subset \mathrm{Fix}\, G,$$

because if $w \in \mathfrak{A}_\nu$ then

$$GA^{q/2} w = A^{-q/2} Gw = A^{-q/2} w = A^{q/2} w.$$

Therefore,

$$A^{q/2}\mathfrak{A}_\nu = \mathfrak{A}_{\nu'}.$$

Analogously

$$A^{q/2}\mathfrak{A}^*_\nu = \mathfrak{A}^*_{\nu'}.$$

X

LEMMA 5. There are no points in the set $S\Lambda^p_q$ outside the union of $2^m q$ surfaces described in Lemma 4.

PROOF. Let $w \in S\Lambda^p_q$. Then $Gw = A^\tau w$ for a certain τ, $0 \leq \tau \leq q-1$. If τ is even then

$$GA^{\tau/2} w = A^{-\tau/2} Gw = A^{\tau/2} w$$

i.e. $w' = A^{\tau/2} w \in \mathrm{Fix}\, G$, whence $w' \in \mathfrak{A}_\nu$ for a certain ν. If τ is odd then

$$AGA^{(\tau+1)/2} w = A^{(1-\tau)/2} Gw = A^{(1+\tau)/2} w$$

i.e. $w' = A^{(\tau+1)/2} w \in \mathrm{Fix}\, AG$, whence $w' \in \mathfrak{A}^*_\nu$ for a certain

ν . X

Thus, if q is odd then

$$S\Lambda_q^p = \bigcup_{\nu,\tau} A^\tau \mathfrak{a}_\nu$$

where $1 \leq \nu \leq 2^m$, $0 \leq \tau \leq q-1$. $S\Lambda_q^p$ consists of 2^m κ-parameter families of symmetric cycles $\{(w, Aw, \ldots, A^{q-1}w) | w \in \mathfrak{a}_\nu\}, \nu \in \{1,\ldots,2^m\}$. Each such cycle has the only point $w \in \mathfrak{a}_\nu$ lying on $Fix\, G$. If q is even then

$$S\Lambda_q^p = (\bigcup_{\nu,\tau} A^\tau \mathfrak{a}_\nu) \cup (\bigcup_{\nu,\tau} A^\tau \mathfrak{a}_\nu^*)$$

where $1 \leq \nu \leq 2^m$, $0 \leq \tau \leq q/2 - 1$. There are odd numbers among $p_1, \ldots, p_m$ without fail. Choose an arbitrary subset $R \subset \{1,\ldots,2^m\}$ such that $\nu \in R \Leftrightarrow \nu' \notin R$ (R contains 2^{m-1} elements). $S\Lambda_q^p$ consists of 2^{m-1} κ-parameter families of symmetric cycles $\{(w, Aw, \ldots, A^{q-1}w) | w \in \mathfrak{a}_\nu\}$, $\nu \in R$ (each such cycle has exactly two points $w \in \mathfrak{a}_\nu$ and $A^{q/2} w \in \mathfrak{a}_{\nu'}$ lying on $Fix\, G$) and 2^{m-1} κ-parameter families of symmetric cycles $\{(w, Aw, \ldots, A^{q-1}w) | w \in \mathfrak{a}_\nu^*\}$, $\nu \in R$ (each such cycle has no points lying on $Fix\, G$).

This completes the proof of Theorem 5.1. X

REMARK 1. Note that while symmetric cycles of reversible differential equations contain always exactly two points fixed under the reversing involution (Proposition 3.1), symmetric cycles of reversible diffeomorphisms may contain 0,1 or 2 such points, as Theorem 5.1 asserts. On the other hand, symmetric cycles of reversible diffeomorphisms can not contain more than two points fixed under the reversing involution. More precisely, the following statement holds.

PROPOSITION 5.1. Let a diffeomorphism A be weakly reversible with respect to a diffeomorphism G, and let $Fix\, G$ denote the fixed point set of G. Any trajectory of A (i.e. an assemblage of points $A^n w,\ n \in \mathbb{Z}$) containing a point on $Fix\, G$ is symmetric (G-invariant). The restriction of G to any symmetric trajectory is an involution. Symmetric cycles of A of an even length either have no points on $Fix\, G$ at all or have exactly two such points. Symmetric cycles of A of an odd length have a unique point on $Fix\, G$.

PROOF. Let a point w of a trajectory Γ of A lie on $Fix\, G$. Then $GA^{\tau}w = A^{-\tau}Gw = A^{-\tau}w$, so Γ is symmetric.

Let Γ be a symmetric trajectory of A, and let $w \in \Gamma$. Then $Gw = A^{\tau}w$ implies $GA^{\tau}w = A^{-\tau}Gw = w$. Therefore, $G_{|\Gamma}$ is an involution.

Let Γ be a symmetric cycle of A that does not contain points on $Fix\, G$. The involution $G_{|\Gamma}$ acting on Γ has no fixed point. So the length of Γ is even.

If Γ is a symmetric cycle of A containing a unique point on $Fix\, G$, then the length of Γ is odd for the same reason.

Finally, let Γ be a symmetric cycle of A of length q, and two its distinct points w and $A^{\tau}w$ lie on $Fix\, G\ (1 \leq \tau \leq q-1)$. Since $GA^{\tau}w = A^{-\tau}w$, $\tau \equiv -\tau \pmod q$, i.e. $q \mid (2\tau)$. Since $\tau < q$, $q = 2\tau$. Thus, the length of Γ is even. If a point $A^{l}w$ of the cycle Γ lies on $Fix\, G\ (0 \leq l \leq q-1)$ then $q \mid (2l)$, i.e. either $l = 0$ or $l = \tau$. Thus, the cycle Γ contains exactly two points on $Fix\, G$. X

REMARK 2. If functions f^{τ} in Theorem 5.1 are analytic then all other objects involved in the formulation and proof of Theorem 5.1 are also analytic.

REMARK 3. All statements of Theorem 5.1 remain true (up to obvious modifications of some formulas) if the mapping $\tilde{A}$ on $\tilde{D}$ has the form

$$\tilde{A}: \begin{array}{ccc} x & & x + \theta + \gamma y + f^1(x,y,\eta) \\ y & \longmapsto & y + f^2(x,y,\eta) \\ \eta & & \eta + f^3(x,y,\eta) \end{array}$$

with arbitrary $\theta \in \mathbb{R}^m$, $\gamma \in \mathbb{R}$, $\gamma \neq 0$. One has to require $2\pi p/(q\gamma) - \theta/\gamma \in I$ instead of $2\pi p/q \in I$.

REMARK 4. If the operator A^q is slightly elliptic at some points in $S\Lambda_q^p$ then generically there exist κ-parameter families of invariant tori of this operator in a neighbourhood of such points (Theorem 2.9). The motions on these tori are called phase oscillations.

REMARK 5. Theorem 5.1 has obvious applications to the situations described in Theorems 1.1 and 4.1.

REMARK 6. If the number of cycles in Λ_q^p is finite (for $\kappa=0$) then it is even, since $S\Lambda_q^p$ contains 2^m cycles and cycles belonging to $\Lambda_q^p \setminus S\Lambda_q^p$ are naturally divided into pairs.

Now assume the functions f^τ to be not merely small but to smoothly depend on a small real parameter ε, i.e. $f^\tau = f^\tau(x,y,\eta,\varepsilon)$ (where $f^\tau(x,y,\eta,0) \equiv 0$). Otherwise speaking, consider a smooth family of mappings $\tilde{A}_\varepsilon$ reversible with respect to $\tilde{G}$:

$$\tilde{A}_\varepsilon: \begin{array}{ccc} x & & x + y + \varepsilon a^1(x,y,\eta) + O(\varepsilon^2) \\ y & \longmapsto & y + \varepsilon a^2(x,y,\eta) + O(\varepsilon^2) \\ \eta & & \eta + \varepsilon a^3(x,y,\eta) + O(\varepsilon^2) \end{array} \qquad (3)$$

In the sequel, for more concise notations we shall use the index ψ, whose value may be equal to either 2 or 3.

Since $\tilde{A}_\varepsilon \tilde{G} \tilde{A}_\varepsilon = \tilde{G}$ it follows that the identities

$$\begin{aligned} &\overset{1}{a}(x,y,\eta)-\overset{1}{a}(-x-y,y,\eta)=\overset{2}{a}(x,y,\eta)\\ &\overset{\psi}{a}(x,y,\eta)+\overset{\psi}{a}(-x-y,y,\eta)=0 \end{aligned} \tag{4}$$

hold.

REMARK. For any smooth 2π-periodic in x functions $\overset{\tau}{a}$ satisfying (4), there exists a family of $\tilde{G}$-reversible mappings $\tilde{A}_\varepsilon$ of the form (3). Show this in two ways. Let a^τ be arbitrary functions satisfying (4).

a) Consider the mapping

$$H_\varepsilon: \begin{array}{ll} x & x+\frac{y}{2}+\varepsilon \overset{1}{h}(x,y,\eta) \\ y \mapsto & y+\varepsilon \overset{2}{h}(x,y,\eta) \\ \eta & \eta+\varepsilon \overset{3}{h}(x,y,\eta) \end{array}$$

where

$$\overset{1}{h}(x,y,\eta)=\frac{1}{4}(\overset{1}{a}(x,y,\eta)+\overset{1}{a}(-x-y,y,\eta))=\frac{1}{4}(2\overset{1}{a}(x,y,\eta)-\overset{2}{a}(x,y,\eta))$$

$$\overset{\psi}{h}(x,y,\eta)=\frac{1}{4}(\overset{\psi}{a}(x,y,\eta)-\overset{\psi}{a}(-x-y,y,\eta))=\frac{1}{2}\overset{\psi}{a}(x,y,\eta).$$

As is easy to verify, the mapping $\tilde{A}_\varepsilon = \tilde{G} H_\varepsilon^{-1} \tilde{G} H_\varepsilon$ has the form (3). Clearly, it is reversible with respect to $\tilde{G}$.

b) Fix an arbitrary smooth function $\chi=\chi(t): \mathbb{R} \to [0,1]$ vanishing for $t \leq \pi/3$ and equaling 1 for $t \geq 2\pi/3$. Following the proof of Proposition 4.5, consider on $\tilde{D}$ the non-autonomous differential equation

$$\dot{x}=\frac{y}{2\pi}+\varepsilon \overset{1}{w}(x,y,\eta,t),\quad \dot{y}=\varepsilon \overset{2}{w}(x,y,\eta,t),\quad \dot{\eta}=\varepsilon \overset{3}{w}(x,y,\eta,t)$$

where $\overset{\tau}{w}$ are smooth functions 2π-periodic in x and t which are defined as follows:

$$\overset{1}{w}(x,y,\eta,t)=\frac{t-\pi}{4\pi}\dot{\varkappa}(t)\overset{2}{a}\left(x-\frac{ty}{2\pi},y,\eta\right)+\frac{1}{2}\dot{\varkappa}(t)\overset{1}{a}\left(x-\frac{ty}{2\pi},y,\eta\right)$$

$$\overset{\psi}{w}(x,y,\eta,t)=\frac{1}{2}\dot{\varkappa}(t)\overset{\psi}{a}\left(x-\frac{ty}{2\pi},y,\eta\right)$$

for $0\leq t\leq \pi$ and

$$\overset{1}{w}(x,y,\eta,t)=\frac{\pi-t}{4\pi}\dot{\varkappa}(2\pi-t)\overset{2}{a}(-x-y+\frac{ty}{2\pi},y,\eta)+\frac{1}{2}\dot{\varkappa}(2\pi-t)\overset{1}{a}(-x-y+\frac{ty}{2\pi},y,\eta)$$

$$\overset{\psi}{w}(x,y,\eta,t)=-\frac{1}{2}\dot{\varkappa}(2\pi-t)\overset{\psi}{a}(-x-y+\frac{ty}{2\pi},y,\eta)$$

for $\pi<t<2\pi$.

This differential equation is reversible with respect to $\tilde{G}$. As is easy to verify, its monodromy operator $\tilde{A}_\varepsilon$ has the form (3). According to Proposition 4.4 $\tilde{A}_\varepsilon$ is reversible with respect to $\tilde{G}$. X

Write down the Fourier series expansion for $\overset{\tau}{a}$:

$$\overset{\tau}{a}(x,y,\eta)=\sum_{n\in\mathbb{Z}^m}\overset{\tau}{g}_n(y,\eta)e^{i(n,x)}$$

where $g_n^\tau(y,\eta)$ are smooth functions. The identities (4) amount to

$$\overset{1}{g}_n - \overset{1}{g}_{-n} e^{i(n,y)} = \overset{2}{g}_n, \quad \overset{\psi}{g}_n + \overset{\psi}{g}_{-n} e^{i(n,y)} = 0 . \tag{5}$$

Denote by Ξ the set of those nonzero vectors $n=(n_1,\dots,n_m)\in\mathbb{Z}^m$ whose first nonzero component is positive (for $m=1$, $\Xi=\mathbb{N}$). The equalities (5) together with the identity $g_{-n}^\tau = \overline{g_n^\tau}$ mean that

$$\overset{1}{g}_0 = \overset{1}{\beta}_0, \quad \overset{\psi}{g}_0 = 0$$

and for $n\in\Xi$

$$\overset{\psi}{g}_n = i\overset{\psi}{\beta}_n e^{i(n,\frac{y}{2})}, \quad \overset{1}{g}_n = \left(\overset{1}{\beta}_n + \frac{i\overset{2}{\beta}_n}{2}\right) e^{i(n,\frac{y}{2})}$$

where $\overset{1}{\beta}_n\ (n\in\Xi\cup\{0\})$ and $\overset{\psi}{\beta}_n\ (n\in\Xi)$ are smooth real-valued functions.

In these notations

$$\overset{1}{a}(x,y,\eta) = \overset{1}{\beta}_0(y,\eta) + \sum_{n\in\Xi} \left(2\overset{1}{\beta}_n(y,\eta)\cos\left(n,x+\frac{y}{2}\right) - \overset{2}{\beta}_n(y,\eta)\sin\left(n,x+\frac{y}{2}\right)\right)$$

$$\overset{\psi}{a}(x,y,\eta) = -2\sum_{n\in\Xi} \overset{\psi}{\beta}_n(y,\eta)\sin\left(n,x+\frac{y}{2}\right).$$

Fix again a vector $2\pi p/q \in I$, where $p_j\in\mathbb{Z}, q\in\mathbb{N}$, and the greatest common divisor of $m+1$ numbers $p_1,\dots,p_m, q$ equals 1.

We have

$$\tilde{A}_\varepsilon^q : \begin{array}{lcl} x & & x + qy + O(\varepsilon) \\ y & \mapsto & y + \varepsilon \sum_{\tau=0}^{q-1} a^2(x+y\tau, y, \eta) + O(\varepsilon^2) \\ \eta & & \eta + \varepsilon \sum_{\tau=0}^{q-1} a^3(x+y\tau, y, \eta) + O(\varepsilon^2) \,. \end{array}$$

The function $Y(x,\eta) = Y(x,\eta,\varepsilon)$ defined in Lemma 1 is $2\pi p/q + O(\varepsilon)$. That is why

$$\tilde{A}_\varepsilon^q : \begin{array}{lcl} x & & x + 2\pi p \\ Y(x,\eta,\varepsilon) & \mapsto & Y(x,\eta,\varepsilon) + \varepsilon \sum_{\tau=0}^{q-1} a^2\left(x + \frac{2\pi p}{q}\tau, \frac{2\pi p}{q}, \eta\right) + O(\varepsilon^2) \\ \eta & & \eta + \varepsilon \sum_{\tau=0}^{q-1} a^3\left(x + \frac{2\pi p}{q}\tau, \frac{2\pi p}{q}, \eta\right) + O(\varepsilon^2) \,. \end{array} \tag{6}$$

Denote the function

$$\sum_{\tau=0}^{q-1} a^\psi\left(x + \frac{2\pi p}{q}\tau, \frac{2\pi p}{q}, \eta\right)$$

$$= -2 \sum_{n\in\Xi} \beta_n^\psi\left(\frac{2\pi p}{q}, \eta\right) \sum_{\tau=0}^{q-1} \sin\left(n, x + \frac{2\pi p}{q}\tau + \frac{\pi p}{q}\right)$$

by $U^\psi(x,\eta)$.

Denote by Π the set $\{n \in \mathbb{Z}^m \mid (n,p)/q \in \mathbb{Z}\}$. Denote the set $\Xi \cap \Pi$ by Θ. Note that for $m=1$, $\Theta = \{qd \mid d \in \mathbb{N}\}$.

LEMMA 6. The group Π is isomorphic to $\mathbb{Z}^m$ and the factor $\mathbb{Z}^m/\Pi$ is isomorphic to the cyclic group $\mathbb{Z}_q$ of order q.

PROOF. Let ℓ be the greatest common divisor of numbers $p_1,\dots,p_m$. Then numbers ℓ and q are relatively prime. There exists an $m\times m$ matrix $\mathcal{M}$ with integer elements and determinant 1 whose first column is $(p_1/\ell,\dots,p_m/\ell)$. Then, considering n as a vector-row and p as a vector-column, we have

$$(n,p)=np=n\mathcal{M}\mathcal{M}^{-1}p=n\mathcal{M}\begin{pmatrix}\ell\\0\\\vdots\\0\end{pmatrix}.$$

The correspondence $n\mapsto n'=n\mathcal{M}$ is an automorphism $\mathbb{Z}^m\to\mathbb{Z}^m$. For $N\in\mathbb{Z}$ one has $N\ell q^{-1}\in\mathbb{Z}\Leftrightarrow Nq^{-1}\in\mathbb{Z}$. The group $\Pi'=\{n'\in\mathbb{Z}^m \mid n'_1q^{-1}\in\mathbb{Z}\}$ is isomorphic to $\mathbb{Z}^m$, and $\mathbb{Z}^m/\Pi'\approx\mathbb{Z}_q$. X

Since for any $\alpha\in\mathbb{R}$ the sum

$$\sum_{\tau=0}^{q-1}\sin\left(\alpha+\frac{2\pi N\tau}{q}\right)$$

equals 0, when $N\in\mathbb{Z}, Nq^{-1}\notin\mathbb{Z}$, and equals $q\sin\alpha$, when $Nq^{-1}\in\mathbb{Z}$, it follows that

$$\mathcal{U}^{\psi}(x,\eta)=-2q\sum_{n\in\Theta}\beta_n^{\psi}\left(\frac{2\pi p}{q},\eta\right)\sin\left(n,x+\frac{\pi p}{q}\right).$$

The function $\mathcal{U}^{\psi}(x,\eta)$ is equivariant (i.e. $\mathcal{U}^{\psi}(x,\eta)\equiv\mathcal{U}^{\psi}(x+2\pi p/q,\eta)$) and odd in x. As is easy to see, $\mathcal{U}^{\psi}(x,\eta)=0$, when x belongs to collection (1) (for q odd) or collection (2) (for q even) (of course, this was to be expected).

The quantity $\sqrt{|\varepsilon|}$ is called the resonance zone width. Introduce the new coordinate

$$R = \frac{1}{\sqrt{|\varepsilon|}}\left(y - \frac{2\pi p}{q}\right)$$

(i.e. make the resonance zone $1/\sqrt{|\varepsilon|}$ times broader along the radial direction). In the normalized coordinates (x, R, η) we have

$$\tilde{A}^q_\varepsilon : \begin{array}{ccl} x & & x + 2\pi p + \sqrt{|\varepsilon|}\, qR + O(\varepsilon) \\ R & \longmapsto & R + \varkappa\sqrt{|\varepsilon|}\, U^2(x,\eta) + O(\varepsilon) \\ \eta & & \eta + O(\varepsilon) \end{array}$$

where $\varkappa = \operatorname{sgn} \varepsilon$.

Thus, in normalized coordinates the mapping A^q_ε differs from the identity one by a quantity of order of $\sqrt{|\varepsilon|}$ and agrees with the phase flow mapping of the field

$$W_\varepsilon = qR\frac{\partial}{\partial x} + \varkappa U^2(x,\eta)\frac{\partial}{\partial R}$$

at time $\sqrt{|\varepsilon|}$ up to accuracy $O(\varepsilon)$.

THEOREM 5.2. a) The field W_ε is equivariant (invariant under the transformation $(x, R, \eta) \longmapsto (x + 2\pi p/q\,, R\,, \eta)$) and reversible with respect to the involution G.

b) The field W_ε is reversible with respect to the involution $G^*: (x, R, \eta) \mapsto (x, -R, \eta)$.

c) If $m=1$ then the function

$$\mathcal{H}_\varepsilon(x,R,\eta)$$

$$=\frac{qR^2}{2}+2\varkappa\sum_{d=1}^{\infty}\frac{(-1)^{pd+1}}{d}\beta^2_{qd}\left(\frac{2\pi p}{q},\eta\right)\cos q\,dx$$

is the first integral of the field W_ε, and the differential equations associated with this field(the so called equations of phase oscillations) are

$$\dot{x}=\frac{\partial\mathcal{H}_\varepsilon}{\partial R}\ ,\ \dot{R}=-\frac{\partial\mathcal{H}_\varepsilon}{\partial x}\ ,\ \dot{\eta}=0\ .$$

Thus, if $m=1$ and $\kappa=0$ then the field W_ε is Hamiltonian (with respect to the symplectic structure $dR\wedge dx$) with the Hamilton function $\mathcal{H}_\varepsilon$.

PROOF. The equivariance and σ-reversibility of the field W_ε follow from the equivariance and oddness in x of the function $\mathcal{U}^2$. The statements b) and c) of the theorem may be verified directly. X

REMARK. The involution σ^* keeps all equilibria of W_ε fixed.

PROPOSITION 5.2. Suppose that for each fixed $\eta\in B$ the equation $\mathcal{U}^2(x,\eta)=0$ has exactly $2^m q$ solutions (i.e. has no solutions not belonging to the collection (1) (for q odd) or the collection (2) (for q even)) and $\det\partial\mathcal{U}^2/\partial x\neq 0$ at them. Then for sufficiently small ε $\Lambda^p_q=S\Lambda^p_q$.

PROOF. This proposition follows from the formula (6). Indeed, by the assumptions of the proposition for sufficiently small ε the equation $\mathcal{U}^2(x,\eta)+O(\varepsilon)=0$ has exactly $2^m q$ solutions for each fixed $\eta\in B$ (we use the compactness of B). This means that $\Lambda_q^p = S\Lambda_q^p$. X

PROPOSITION 5.3. Let $\kappa = 0$ and let the equation $\mathcal{U}^2(x) = 0$ have a solution x^*. Assume

$$\det \frac{\partial \mathcal{U}^2}{\partial x}\Big|_{x^*} \neq 0 .$$

Then for sufficiently small ε the set Λ_q^p contains a point $(x(\varepsilon), Y(x(\varepsilon), \varepsilon))$, where the function $x(\varepsilon)$ is smooth and $x(0) = x^*$.

PROOF. This proposition also follows immediately from the formula (6). X

Proposition 5.2 affords the possibility of proving an interesting statement affirming that for a "generic" (in a sense to be made precise) analytic in x family $\tilde{A}_\varepsilon$ on an annulus (i.e. when $m = 1$, $\kappa = 0$, and I is a finite interval on $\mathbb{R}$) for all numbers $2\pi p/q \in I$, with the possible exception of finitely many points, for sufficiently small ε (for $|\varepsilon| < \varepsilon_0$, say) the equality $\Lambda_q^p = S\Lambda_q^p$ holds. At the same time one ought to have in view that the necessary smallness of ε depends on $2\pi p/q$: the quantity ε_0, generally speaking, tends to zero as $q \to \infty$.

Let a constant $\rho > 0$ be fixed. Denote by $\mathfrak{W}_\rho = \mathfrak{W}$ the space of smooth functions $a(x, y, \eta)$ of the form

$$-2 \sum_{n \in \Xi} \beta_n(y, \eta) \sin(n, x + \frac{y}{2}) \tag{7}$$

(where for each $n \in \Xi$ the function $\beta_n(y, \eta)$ is smooth in y and η and real-valued) which satisfy the inequality

$$\sup_{\substack{y\in I\\ \eta\in O}} \sup_{n\in\Xi} |\beta_n(y,\eta)| e^{|n|\rho} < \infty .$$

Every function $a \in \mathfrak{A}$ is analytic in x and can be extended analytically in x into the domain

$$\{x\in \mathbb{C}^m \mid |\operatorname{Im} x_j|<\rho\}\times\{y\in \mathbb{R}^m \mid y\in I\}\times\{\eta\in\mathbb{R}^k \mid \eta\in O\}.$$

On $\mathfrak{A}$ introduce the norm

$$\|a\| = \sup_{\substack{y\in I\\ \eta\in O}} \sup_{n\in\Xi} |\beta_n(y,\eta)| e^{|n|\rho} .$$

Now consider the class of such families of smooth reversible with respect to $\tilde{G}$ mappings $\tilde{A}_\varepsilon$ of the form (3) that $a^2\in\mathfrak{A}$.

THEOREM 5.3. Let $m=1$ and $k=0$. Let I be a finite interval on $\mathbb{R}$. Then the space $\mathfrak{A}$ contains an open everywhere dense subset $\mathfrak{A}'$ such that if $a^2\in\mathfrak{A}'$ then for all numbers $2\pi p/q \in I$, with the possible exception of finitely many points, for sufficiently small ε the equality $\Lambda_q^p = S\Lambda_q^p$ holds.

PROOF. Let

$$a(x,y) = -2\sum_{n=1}^{\infty} \beta_n(y)\sin\left(nx+\frac{ny}{2}\right)\in\mathfrak{A} . \tag{8}$$

Denote by $Z : \mathfrak{A}\to\mathbb{R}_+$ the functional

$$Z(a) = \inf_{\frac{2\pi p}{q}} |\beta_q(\frac{2\pi p}{q})| e^{qp},$$

where the infimum is taken over all numbers $2\pi p/q \in I$ $(q \in \mathbb{N}$, $p \in \mathbb{Z}$, p and q are relatively prime).

Set $\mathfrak{W}' = \{a \in \mathfrak{W} \mid Z(a) > 0\}$. The set $\mathfrak{W}'$ is open, since the functional Z is continuous on $\mathfrak{W}$. The set $\mathfrak{W}'$ is everywhere dense in $\mathfrak{W}$. Indeed, consider an arbitrary function (8) and number $\varepsilon > 0$. For each fixed $q \in \mathbb{N}$ and each $p \in \mathbb{Z}$ such that $2\pi p/q \in I$ and p and q are relatively prime, choose a number h_q^p satisfying the conditions

$$|h_q^p| \leq \varepsilon, \ |\beta_q(\frac{2\pi p}{q}) e^{qp} + h_q^p| \geq \varepsilon .$$

Construct such a smooth function $\tilde{\beta}_q(y)$ that

$$\sup_{y \in I} |\tilde{\beta}_q(y)| \leq \varepsilon e^{-qp}$$

and for each p

$$\tilde{\beta}_q(\frac{2\pi p}{q}) = h_q^p e^{-qp}.$$

Since the interval between any two neighbouring numbers $2\pi p/q$ on I is no less than $2\pi/q$, it suffices to take the function

$$\sum_p h_q^p \varkappa(\frac{qy}{\pi} - 2p) e^{-qp}$$

where

$$\chi(t)=\begin{cases} \exp\left(\frac{t^2}{t^2-1}\right) & , \text{ for } -1<t<1 \\ 0 & , \text{ for } |t|\geq 1 \end{cases}$$

as $\tilde{\beta}_q(y)$ (the function $\chi:\mathbb{R}\to\mathbb{R}_+$ is smooth). The function

$$\tilde{a}(x,y)=-2\sum_{q=1}^{\infty}\tilde{\beta}_q(y)\sin\left(qx+\frac{qy}{2}\right)$$

is smooth, because for each $l\in\mathbb{N}$, $q\in\mathbb{N}$, $y\in I$

$$\left|\tilde{\beta}_q^{(l)}(y)\right|<const\cdot q^l e^{-q\rho}$$

(the constant depending only on l). Therefore $\tilde{a}\in\mathfrak{A}$ and $\|\tilde{a}\|\leq\varepsilon$. On the other hand, $Z(a+\tilde{a})\geq\varepsilon$. Thus, $\mathfrak{A}'$ is everywhere dense in $\mathfrak{A}$.

Now consider an arbitrary family $\tilde{A}_\varepsilon$ of the form (3), in which $a^2\in\mathfrak{A}'$. Let us prove that if $q\in\mathbb{N}$ is large enough then for each number $2\pi p/q\in I$ for sufficiently small ε the equality $\Lambda_q^p=S\Lambda_q^p$ holds. This will imply the assertion of the theorem, since the interval I is finite and, hence, for each q there is only a finite set of numbers $2\pi p/q$ within it.

Let $\|a^2\|=K$ and $Z(a^2)=c>0$. Fix $2\pi p/q\in I$. We have

$$u^2(x)=-2q\sum_{d=1}^{\infty}\beta^2_{qd}\left(\frac{2\pi p}{q}\right)\sin(qdx+\pi pd)$$

$$=-2q\beta_q^2\left(\frac{2\pi\rho}{q}\right)\sin(qx+\pi\rho)+\Delta(x),$$

where

$$\Delta(x)=-2q\sum_{d=2}^{\infty}\beta_{qd}^2\left(\frac{2\pi\rho}{q}\right)\sin(qdx+\pi\rho d).$$

$Z(a^2)=C$ implies

$$\left|\beta_q^2\left(\frac{2\pi\rho}{q}\right)\right|\geq ce^{-q\rho}.$$

On the other hand, for all x

$$|\Delta(x)|e^{q\rho}\leq 2qK\sum_{d=1}^{\infty}e^{-qd\rho}=\frac{2qKe^{-q\rho}}{1-e^{-q\rho}}$$

and

$$\left|\frac{d}{dx}\Delta(x)\right|e^{q\rho}$$

$$\leq 2q^2K\sum_{d=1}^{\infty}(d+1)e^{-qd\rho}=\frac{2q^2K(2e^{-q\rho}+e^{-2q\rho})}{(1-e^{-q\rho})^2}.$$

Therefore, for sufficiently large q the function $u^2(x)$ has $2q$ roots and all of them are simple. Now it remains to apply Proposition 5.2. X

The assertion of Theorem 5.3 does not extend to higher dimensions.

EXAMPLE 1. Let $m=2$ and $k=0$. Using Proposition 5.3, we shall construct such an open set $\mathfrak{W}''\subset\mathfrak{W}$ for a suitable bounded domain $I\subset\mathbb{R}^2$ that if $a^2\in\mathfrak{W}''$ then there exists an infinite set of numbers $2\pi p/q\in I$ such that for arbitrary small ε $\Lambda_q^p\setminus S\Lambda_q^p \neq\emptyset$.

Let $I=\{(y_1,y_2)\in\mathbb{R}^2 \mid 0<y_j<2\pi\}$. Consider the following function $a(x,y)$:

$$a_1(x,y)=-2\sum_{l=1}^{\infty} e^{-2l\rho}\left(\sin 2l\left(x_1+\frac{y_1}{2}\right)+\sin 2(l+1)\left(x_2+\frac{y_2}{2}\right)\right),$$

$$a_2(x,y)=-2\sum_{l=1}^{\infty} e^{-2l\rho}\left(\sin 2l\left(x_1+\frac{y_1}{2}\right)-\sin 2(l+1)\left(x_2+\frac{y_2}{2}\right)\right).$$

It is clear that $a\in\mathfrak{W}$, and $\|a\|=2e^{2\rho}$.

Take the neighbourhood of a of radius c, where $c>0$ is small enough, as $\mathfrak{W}''$. Suppose that

$$a^2(x,y)=-2\sum_{n\in\Xi}\beta_n^2(y)\sin\left(n,x+\frac{y}{2}\right)\in\mathfrak{W}''.$$

Fix a number $N\in\mathbb{N}$. Consider the point $2\pi p/q=(\pi/N, \pi/(N+1))\in I$, where $p_1=N+1$, $p_2=N$, $q=2N(N+1)$. It is obvious that

$$\Pi=\left\{n\in\mathbb{Z}^2 \,\middle|\, \frac{n_1p_1+n_2p_2}{q}\in\mathbb{Z}\right\}=\left\{(Nd_1,(N+1)d_2) \,\middle|\, d_1\in\mathbb{Z}, d_2\in\mathbb{Z}, \frac{d_1+d_2}{2}\in\mathbb{Z}\right\}.$$

Therefore, $\Theta = \Xi \cap \Pi$ contains pairs $(2N,0)$, $(N,N+1)$, $(N,-N-1)$, $(0,2N+2)$, and for all other pairs $n \in \Theta$ (denote the set of these pairs by Θ') the inequality $|n| = |n_1| + |n_2| \geqslant 4N$ holds.

Denoting the function

$$-4N(N+1) \sum_{n \in \Theta'} \beta_n^2 \left(\frac{2\pi\rho}{q}\right) \sin\left(n, x + \frac{\pi\rho}{q}\right)$$

by $\Delta(x)$, we obtain

$$u_1^2(x) = 4N(N+1) e^{-2N\rho} ((1+C_1)\sin 2Nx_1 + (1+C_2)\sin 2(N+1)x_2$$

$$+ C_3 \sin(Nx_1 + (N+1)x_2) + C_4 \sin(Nx_1 - (N+1)x_2)) + \Delta_1(x),$$

(9)

$$u_2^2(x) = 4N(N+1) e^{-2N\rho} ((1+C_5)\sin 2Nx_1 - (1+C_6)\sin 2(N+1)x_2$$

$$+ C_7 \sin(Nx_1 + (N+1)x_2) + C_8 \sin(Nx_1 - (N+1)x_2)) + \Delta_2(x)$$

where numbers $C_1, \ldots, C_8$ are small as c is ($|C_1| + |C_5| \leqslant c$, $|C_2| + |C_6| \leqslant ce^{-2\rho}$, $|C_3| + |C_7| \leqslant ce^{-\rho}$, $|C_4| + |C_8| \leqslant ce^{-\rho}$).

One sees that functions $\Delta_j(x)$ and their first derivatives are bounded from above by $KN^3 e^{-4N\rho}$, where $K > 0$ is a certain N-independent constant.

The collection (2) of those values of the variable x, at which $u^2(x)$ vanishes a priori, may be transcribe in our case as follows:

$$\left\{\left(\frac{\pi d_1}{2N}, \frac{\pi d_2}{2(N+1)}\right) \middle| d_1 \in \mathbb{Z},\, d_2 \in \mathbb{Z},\, 0 \le d_1 \le 4N-1,\, 0 \le d_2 \le 4N+3,\, \frac{d_1+d_2}{2} \in \mathbb{Z}\right\}. \quad (10)$$

If numbers $C_1, \ldots, C_8$ and the function $\Delta(x)$ were equal to 0 then the function $\mathcal{U}^2(x)$ would vanish at the point $(\pi/2N, 0)$ and its Jacobian determinant at this point would equal

$$16N^2(N+1)^2 e^{-4N\rho} \begin{vmatrix} -2N & 2(N+1) \\ -2N & -2(N+1) \end{vmatrix} = 128N^3(N+1)^3 e^{-4N\rho}.$$

It is easy to prove the following lemma.

LEMMA 7. Let a constant $K>0$ be fixed. There exists $C>0$ such that for sufficiently large N for any numbers $C_1, \ldots, C_8$ and any smooth functions $\Delta_1(x)$ and $\Delta_2(x)$ (generally speaking, these numbers and functions are dependent on N) satisfying the inequalities $|C_1|, \ldots, |C_8| < C$ and

$$|\Delta_j(x)|, \quad \left|\frac{\partial \Delta_j(x)}{\partial x_1}\right|, \quad \left|\frac{\partial \Delta_j(x)}{\partial x_2}\right| < KN^3 e^{-4N\rho}$$

the function $\mathcal{U}^2(x)$ given by the formulas (9) has in the domain

$$\frac{3\pi}{8N} < x_1 < \frac{5\pi}{8N}, \quad -\frac{\pi}{8(N+1)} < x_2 < \frac{\pi}{8(N+1)}$$

a unique zero $x^{(N)}$, and the Jacobian determinant of $\mathcal{U}^2(x)$ at $x^{(N)}$ does not vanish.

If N is large enough then by Proposition 5.3 for each family

$\tilde{A}_\varepsilon$ such that $a^2 \in \mathfrak{W}''$ (i.e. $\|a^2 - a\| < c$, where the value of c is determined by Lemma 7) for sufficiently small ε the set Λ_q^ρ contains the point $(x^{(N)}(\varepsilon), Y(x^{(N)}(\varepsilon), \varepsilon))$ which is close to the point $(x^{(N)}, Y(x^{(N)}, \varepsilon))$ and therefore does not belong to $S\Lambda_q^\rho$, (since $x^{(N)}$ does not belong to the collection (10)).

The assertion of Theorem 5.3 would be also invalid if in $\mathfrak{W}$ one introduced a little more strong topology than that determined by the norm $\| \ \|$.

Let (see (7))

$$\mathcal{L}_\sigma = \{ a \in \mathfrak{W} \mid \sup_{\substack{y \in I \\ \eta \in O}} \ \sup_{n \in \Xi} |\beta_n(y,\eta)| e^{2|n|\rho} < \sigma \}$$

(where $\sigma > 0$). In $\mathfrak{W}$ define the topology $\mathcal{T}$ by taking the sequence of sets $a + \mathcal{L}_{1/\ell}$, $\ell \in \mathbb{N}$, as a fundamental system of neighbourhoods of point $a \in \mathfrak{W}$, for each a.

EXAMPLE 2. Let $m = 1$ and $\kappa = 0$. Using Proposition 5.3, we shall construct such an open with respect to the topology $\mathcal{T}$ set $\mathfrak{W}''' \subset \mathfrak{W}$ for a suitable finite interval $I \subset \mathbb{R}$ that if $a^2 \in \mathfrak{W}'''$ then there exists an infinite set of numbers $2\pi p/q \in I$ such that for arbitrary small ε $\Lambda_q^\rho \setminus S\Lambda_q^\rho \neq \emptyset$.

Let $I = (0, 3\pi)$. Consider the function

$$a(x,y) = -2 \sum_{\ell=1}^{\infty} e^{-2\ell\rho} \sin 2\ell\left(x + \frac{y}{2}\right).$$

It is clear that $a \in \mathfrak{W}$, and $\|a\| = 1$.

Take the neighbourhood $a + \mathcal{B}_c$ of a , where $c>0$ is small enough, as $\mathfrak{W}'''$. Suppose that $a^2 \in \mathfrak{W}'''$.

Fix a number $N \in \mathbb{N}$ and consider the point $2\pi/N \in I$. We have

$$\mathcal{U}^2(x) = -2Ne^{-2N\rho}(c_1 \sin Nx + (1+c_2)\sin 2Nx) + \Delta(x)$$

where the function $\Delta(x)$ and its derivative are bounded from above by $KN^2e^{-3N\rho}$, where $K>0$ is a certain N-independent constant, and numbers c_1 and c_2 are small as c is $(|c_1|<c, |c_2|<ce^{-2N\rho})$.

The collection (1) or (2) of those values of the variable x, at which $\mathcal{U}^2(x)$ vanishes a priori, is $\{\pi d/N \mid d \in \mathbb{Z}, 0 \leq d \leq 2N-1\}$.

If N is large enough then for sufficiently small c (the necessary smallness of c does not depend on N) $\mathcal{U}^2(x)$ has a simple zero close to $\pi/2N$, and we can complete the verification of our construction in the same way as in Example 1.

To conclude this section consider families (3) of reversible with respect to $\tilde{G}$ smooth mappings $\tilde{A}_\varepsilon$ on a plane (for $m=1$ and $\kappa=0$) once more. Let $2\pi p/q \in I$ be fixed. The function $\mathcal{U}^2(x)$ has the form

$$\mathcal{U}^2(x) = 2q\sum_{d=1}^{\infty}(-1)^{pd+1}\beta^2_{qd}\left(\frac{2\pi p}{q}\right)\sin q\,dx.$$

This function is equivariant (invariant under the rotation through angle $2\pi/q$) and odd. Hence generically it has $2Nq$ simple roots $(N \in \mathbb{N})$. Correspondingly the equivariant, reversible and Hamiltonian approximating field W_ε has $2Nq$ equilibria. A half of them is saddles with zero trace (i.e. with eigenvalues of the linearization equaling $\pm\zeta$) and the other half is centers. On the circle $y = 2\pi p/q$, saddles and centers of the field W_ε alternate (since W_ε has a saddle at that point, where $\varkappa(U^2)' > 0$, and a center at that point, where $\varkappa(U^2)' < 0$, here $\varkappa = \operatorname{sgn}\varepsilon$).

By Proposition 5.3, for sufficiently small ε the set Λ_q^p consists of $2Nq$ points. $2q$ points of them belong to two symmetric cycles of length q and constitute $S\Lambda_q^p$. The germ of the operator A_ε^q at these points is reversible. If the mapping A_ε^q is elliptic at points of a symmetric cycle then there exist phase oscillations round this cycle (see Remark 4 to Theorem 5.1). Elliptic fixed points of A_ε^q correspond to centers of W_ε and hyperbolic ones correspond to saddles.

Remaining $2(N-1)q$ points of the set Λ_q^p constitute $2(N-1)$ non-symmetric cycles of length q which in turn are divided into $N-1$ pairs so that the involution σ interchanges cycles of every pair.

On the circle $y = Y(x,\varepsilon)$, there lie $N-1$ point of $\Lambda_q^p \setminus S\Lambda_q^p$ between each two neighbouring points of $S\Lambda_q^p$.

If N is odd (in particular, when $N=1$), the mapping A_ε^q is elliptic at points of one of symmetric cycles and hyperbolic at points of the other symmetric cycle. If N is even, the mapping A_ε^q has the same type at all $2q$ points of $S\Lambda_q^p$.

Generally speaking, the germ of the operator A_ε^q at points of $\Lambda_q^p \setminus S\Lambda_q^p$ is not reversible. Besides that, as is easy to verify, centers of W_ε correspond to such points at which the eigenvalues of the linearization of A_ε^q have the form

$$\lambda_{1,2}(\varepsilon) = 1 - \frac{\varepsilon\sigma}{2} + \varepsilon\gamma \pm i\sqrt{\varepsilon\sigma} + O(|\varepsilon|^{3/2})$$

where $\sigma, \gamma \in \mathbb{R}$, $\varepsilon\sigma > 0$ and generically $\gamma \neq 0$. These points are called exponential foci, since

$$\ln \lambda_{1,2}(\varepsilon) = \pm i\sqrt{\varepsilon\sigma} + \varepsilon\gamma + O(|\varepsilon|^{3/2}) .$$

Saddles of W_ε correspond to such points at which the eigenvalues of the linearization of A_ε^q have the form

$$\lambda_{1,2}(\varepsilon) = 1 + \frac{\varepsilon\sigma}{2} + \varepsilon\gamma \pm \sqrt{\varepsilon\sigma} + O(|\varepsilon|^{3/2})$$

where σ and γ satisfy the same conditions. Since

$$\ln \lambda_{1,2}(\varepsilon) = \pm\sqrt{\varepsilon\sigma} + \varepsilon\gamma + O(|\varepsilon|^{3/2}) ,$$

these points are called exponential saddles.

Note that there are no (exponential) nodes among fixed points of A_ε^q .

§ 5.3. Principal theorem for vectorfields and its corollaries

Let I, B, O, $\tilde{D}$, D, x, y and η have the same meaning as in § 5.2. Suppose on $\tilde{D}$ the following vectorfield is given

$$\tilde{V} = (y + \overset{1}{f}(x,y,\eta))\frac{\partial}{\partial x} + \overset{2}{f}(x,y,\eta)\frac{\partial}{\partial y} + \overset{3}{f}(x,y,\eta)\frac{\partial}{\partial \eta}$$

where $\overset{\tau}{f}$ are smooth 2π-periodic in $x_1, \ldots, x_m$ functions.

Let $\tilde{G}_* \tilde{V} = -\tilde{V}$ on $\tilde{D}$, where $\tilde{G}: \tilde{D} \to \tilde{D}$ is the same involution as in § 5.2.

Let a vector

$$p\omega = (p_1\omega, \dots, p_m\omega) \in I$$

be fixed, where $p_j \in \mathbb{Z}$, $\omega \in \mathbb{R}$, $\omega \neq 0$. Assume the greatest common divisor of m numbers $p_1, \dots, p_m$ to equal 1. Denote the number $2\pi/\omega$ by T.

One can lower the field $\tilde{V}$ and the involution $\tilde{G}$ onto D and obtain the field V and the involution G as a result.

Let $\sigma^1, \dots, \sigma^{2^m}$ and $Fix\, G$ have the same meaning as in § 5.2 and the index ν have the range from 1 to 2^m again. Let the index μ have the range from 1 to 2^{m-1}.

We assume the numeration of $\sigma^1, \dots, \sigma^{2^m}$ to be chosen in such a way that

$$\sigma^{\mu + 2^{m-1}} = \sigma^{\mu} + \pi p \ (\mathrm{mod}\, 2\pi)$$

for each μ. This requirement is proper, since there are certainly odd numbers among $p_1, \dots, p_m$.

Denote by $\tilde{F}_t$ and F_t the phase flows of fields $\tilde{V}$ and V respectively.

Denote by Ω^p_ω the set of such fixed points $(x, y, \eta) \in D$ of the mapping F_T that $\tilde{F}_T(x, y, \eta) = (x + 2\pi p, y, \eta)$. Ω^p_ω consists of cycles of V of period T. Denote by $S\Omega^p_\omega$ the union of symmetric cycles of V of period T lying in Ω^p_ω.

THEOREM 5.4. Let the situation just described take place. Then, if the functions f^τ are small enough in the C^1-norm, the following holds.

a) The set $S\Omega^p_\omega$ consists of 2^{m-1} smooth κ-parameter families of symmetric cycles of the field V of period T.

b) From the coordinate point of view, the set $S\Omega^p_\omega$ consists of 2^{m-1} smooth surfaces $\{ F_t(\sigma^\mu, y^\mu(\eta), \eta) \mid 0 \le t < T, \eta \in O' \}$ of dimension $\kappa + 1$, where $O' \subset O$ is a certain neighbourhood of the ball B. These surfaces do not intersect each other. Furthermore,

$F_t(\sigma^\mu, y^\mu(\eta),\eta) = (x_*^\mu(\eta,t),\ y_*^\mu(\eta,t),\ \eta_*^\mu(\eta,t))$, where functions x_*^μ, y_*^μ and η_*^μ are T-periodic in t and the smaller f^τ , the closer (in the C^1-norm) to the constant $\rho\omega$, the identity function $\eta_0(\eta)=\eta$ and functions $x_0^\mu(t)=\sigma^\mu+\rho\omega t$ are functions $y_*^\mu(\eta,t)$, $\eta_*^\mu(\eta,t)$ and $x_*^\mu(\eta,t)$ respectively. Moreover,

$$x_*^\mu\left(\eta,\frac{T}{2}\right)=\sigma^{\mu+2^{m-1}} .$$

PROOF. Let us deduce Theorem 5.4 from Theorem 5.1. The mapping $\tilde F_T$ is reversible with respect to $\tilde G$ and close to the slightly integrable one $(x,y,\eta)\mapsto(x+Ty,y,\eta)$. For the mapping F_T , define the set $S\Lambda_1^\rho$ as at the beginning of § 5.2 (see Remark 3 after the proof of Theorem 5.1). It is clear that $S\Omega_\omega^\rho \cap \mathrm{Fix}\, G = S\Lambda_1^\rho$. By Theorem 5.1, for sufficiently small f^τ the set $S\Lambda_1^\rho$ is the union of 2^m smooth surfaces $\mathcal{O}\!\iota_\nu=\{(\sigma^\nu, y^\nu(\eta),\eta)\mid \eta\in O'\}$ of dimension κ . Since $F_{T/2}(S\Lambda_1^\rho)=S\Lambda_1^\rho$ it follows that $F_{T/2}\mathcal{O}\!\iota_\mu = \mathcal{O}\!\iota_{\mu+2^{m-1}}$. Therefore, $(\kappa+1)$-dimensional surfaces $\{F_t w \mid 0\le t<T,\ w\in \mathcal{O}\!\iota_\mu\}$ are desired ones. X

REMARK 1. For $m=1$ Theorem 5.4 is trivial and $S\Omega_\omega^\rho=\Omega_\omega^\rho$.

REMARK 2. If functions f^τ in Theorem 5.4 are analytic then all other objects involved in the formulation and proof of Theorem 5.4 are also analytic.

REMARK 3. All statements of Theorem 5.4 remain true (up to obvious modifications of some formulas) if the field $\tilde V$ on $\tilde D$ has the form

$$\tilde V = (\theta+\gamma y+f^1(x,y,\eta))\frac{\partial}{\partial x}+f^2(x,y,\eta)\frac{\partial}{\partial y}+f^3(x,y,\eta)\frac{\partial}{\partial \eta}$$

with arbitrary $\theta \in \mathbb{R}^m$, $\gamma \in \mathbb{R}$, $\gamma \neq 0$. One has to require $p\omega/\gamma - \theta/\gamma \in I$ instead of $p\omega \in I$.

REMARK 4. Theorem 5.4 has obvious applications to the situation described in Theorem 1.2.

REMARK 5. The set $S\Omega^p_\omega$ depends on ω smoothly.

Now assume the functions f^τ to be not merely small but to smoothly depend on a small real parameter ε, i.e. $f^\tau = f^\tau(x, y, \eta, \varepsilon)$ (where $f^\tau(x, y, \eta, 0) \equiv 0$). Otherwise speaking, consider a smooth family of fields $\tilde{V}_\varepsilon$ reversible with respect to $\tilde{G}$:

$$\tilde{V}_\varepsilon = (y + \varepsilon v^1(x, y, \eta) + O(\varepsilon^2))\frac{\partial}{\partial x}$$

$$+ (\varepsilon v^2(x, y, \eta) + O(\varepsilon^2))\frac{\partial}{\partial y} + (\varepsilon v^3(x, y, \eta) + O(\varepsilon^2))\frac{\partial}{\partial \eta}. \qquad (11)$$

We shall use the index ψ whose value may be equal to either 2 or 3, as in § 5.2.

Since $\tilde{G}_* \tilde{V}_\varepsilon = -\tilde{V}_\varepsilon$ it follows that the function v^1 is even in x and the functions v^2 and v^3 are odd in x, i.e. the identities

$$v^1(-x, y, \eta) = v^1(x, y, \eta), \quad v^\psi(-x, y, \eta) = -v^\psi(x, y, \eta) \qquad (12)$$

hold.

REMARK. For any smooth 2π-periodic in x functions v^τ satisfying (12), there exists a family of $\tilde{G}$-reversible fields $\tilde{V}_\varepsilon$ of the form (11). As an example one can consider the family

$$(y + \varepsilon v^1(x, y, \eta))\frac{\partial}{\partial x} + \varepsilon v^2(x, y, \eta)\frac{\partial}{\partial y} + \varepsilon v^3(x, y, \eta)\frac{\partial}{\partial \eta}.$$

Write down the Fourier series expansion for v^τ :

$$\overset{\tau}{v}(x,y,\eta) = \sum_{n \in \mathbb{Z}^m} \overset{\tau}{g}_n(y,\eta)\, e^{i(n,x)}$$

where $\overset{\tau}{g}_n(y,\eta)$ are smooth functions. The identities (12) amount to $\overset{1}{g}_n = \overset{1}{g}_{-n}$, $\overset{\psi}{g}_n = -\overset{\psi}{g}_{-n}$ which together with the equality $\overset{\tau}{g}_{-n} = \overline{\overset{\tau}{g}_n}$ means that

$$\overset{1}{g}_0 = \overset{1}{\beta}_0 , \quad \overset{\psi}{g}_0 = 0$$

and for $n \in \Xi$

$$\overset{1}{g}_n = \overset{1}{\beta}_n , \quad \overset{\psi}{g}_n = i\overset{\psi}{\beta}_n$$

where $\overset{1}{\beta}_n$ $(n \in \Xi \cup \{0\})$ and $\overset{\psi}{\beta}_n$ $(n \in \Xi)$ are smooth real-valued functions (the symbol Ξ has the same meaning as in § 5.2).

In these notations

$$\overset{1}{v}(x,y,\eta) = \overset{1}{\beta}_0(y,\eta) + 2\sum_{n \in \Xi} \overset{1}{\beta}_n(y,\eta)\cos(n,x)$$

$$\overset{\psi}{v}(x,y,\eta) = -2\sum_{n \in \Xi} \overset{\psi}{\beta}_n(y,\eta)\sin(n,x) .$$

Fix again a vector $\rho\omega \in I$, where $\rho_j \in \mathbb{Z}, \omega \in \mathbb{R}, \omega \neq 0$ and the greatest common divisor of m numbers $\rho_1, \dots, \rho_m$ equals 1. Let $T = 2\pi/\omega$.

We have

$$\tilde{F}_T(\varepsilon):\ \begin{aligned} x &\mapsto x + Ty + O(\varepsilon) \\ y &\longmapsto y + \varepsilon \int_0^T v^2(x+ty, y, \eta)\,dt + O(\varepsilon^2) \\ \eta &\mapsto \eta + \varepsilon \int_0^T v^3(x+ty, y, \eta)\,dt + O(\varepsilon^2) \end{aligned}$$

where $\tilde{F}_t(\varepsilon)$ is the phase flow of the field $\tilde{V}_\varepsilon$.

Define a smooth function $y = Y(x, \eta, \varepsilon)$ by the condition that the first m coordinates of the point $\tilde{F}_T(\varepsilon)(x, Y(x,\eta,\varepsilon), \eta)$ equal $x + 2\pi p$. Then $Y(x,\eta,\varepsilon) = p\omega + O(\varepsilon)$, whence

$$\tilde{F}_T(\varepsilon):\ \begin{aligned} x &\mapsto x + 2\pi p \\ Y(x,\eta,\varepsilon) &\longmapsto Y(x,\eta,\varepsilon) + \varepsilon \int_0^T v^2(x+tp\omega, p\omega, \eta)\,dt + O(\varepsilon^2) \\ \eta &\mapsto \eta + \varepsilon \int_0^T v^3(x+tp\omega, p\omega, \eta)\,dt + O(\varepsilon^2). \end{aligned}$$

Denote the function

$$\int_0^T v^\psi(x+tp\omega, p\omega, \eta)\,dt$$

$$= -2 \sum_{n \in \Xi} \beta_n^\psi(p\omega, \eta) \int_0^T \sin(n, x + tp\omega)\,dt$$

by $u^\psi(x, \eta)$.

Denote by Π the set $\{n \in \mathbb{Z}^m \mid (n,p)=0\}$. Denote the set $\Xi \cap \Pi$ by Θ. Note that for $m=1$, $\Pi=\{0\}$ and $\Theta=\emptyset$.

LEMMA 8. The group Π is isomorphic to $\mathbb{Z}^{m-1}$ and the factor $\mathbb{Z}^m/\Pi$ is isomorphic to $\mathbb{Z}$.

One may prove this lemma analogously to Lemma 6.

Since for any $\alpha \in \mathbb{R}$ the integral

$$\int_0^T \sin(\alpha + tN\omega)dt$$

equals 0, when $N \in \mathbb{Z}\setminus\{0\}$, and equals $T\sin\alpha$, when $N=0$, it follows that

$$u^\psi(x,\eta) = -2T\sum_{n\in\Theta} \beta_n^\psi(p\omega,\eta)\sin(n,x).$$

The function $u^\psi(x,\eta)$ is equivariant (i.e. $u^\psi(x,\eta) \equiv u^\psi(x+pt,\eta)$ for each $t\in\mathbb{R}$) and odd in x. For $m=1$, $u^\psi(x,\eta)\equiv 0$.

The quantity $\sqrt{|\varepsilon|}$ is called the resonance zone width (for $m=1$, this definition is nominal, since the notion of a resonance zone loses its sense: for all sufficiently small ε the field V_ε is slightly integrable, see the Proposition at the end of § 1.10). Introduce the new coordinate

$$R = \frac{1}{\sqrt{|\varepsilon|}}(y - p\omega)$$

(i.e. make the resonance zone $1/\sqrt{|\varepsilon|}$ times broader along the radial direction). In the normalized coordinates (x, R, η) we have

$$\tilde{F}_T(\varepsilon):\quad \begin{matrix} x \\ R \\ \eta \end{matrix} \longmapsto \begin{matrix} x + 2\pi p + \sqrt{|\varepsilon|}\, TR + O(\varepsilon) \\ R + \varkappa\sqrt{|\varepsilon|}\, \mathcal{U}^2(x,\eta) + O(\varepsilon) \\ \eta + O(\varepsilon) \end{matrix}$$

where $\varkappa = \operatorname{sgn}\varepsilon$.

Thus, in normalized coordinates the mapping $F_T(\varepsilon)$ differs from the identity one by a quantity of order of $\sqrt{|\varepsilon|}$ and agrees with the phase flow mapping of the field

$$W_\varepsilon = TR\frac{\partial}{\partial x} + \varkappa\,\mathcal{U}^2(x,\eta)\frac{\partial}{\partial R}$$

at time $\sqrt{|\varepsilon|}$ up to accuracy $O(\varepsilon)$.

THEOREM 5.5. The field W_ε is equivariant (invariant under transformations $(x, R, \eta) \longmapsto (x + pt, R, \eta),\ t \in \mathbb{R})$ and reversible with respect to both involutions σ and $\sigma^*: (x, R, \eta) \mapsto (x, -R, \eta)$.

PROOF. This theorem follows from the equivariance and oddness in x of the function $\mathcal{U}^2$. X

REMARK 1. For $m = 1$, $W_\varepsilon = TR\,\partial/\partial x$. Every function depending on R and η only is the first integral of the field W_ε. For $m = 1$ and $\kappa = 0$, this field is Hamiltonian (with respect to the symplectic structure $dR \wedge dx$) with the Hamilton function $TR^2/2$.

REMARK 2. The involution σ^* keeps all equilibria of W_ε fixed.

§ 5.4. Resonance zones on a plane near fixed points of diffeomorphisms

Proceed to the local theory of resonance zones. For simplicity let us confine ourselves to the case of dimension two. As the theory of reversible vectorfields on a plane is trivial, we shall study only resonance zones near fixed points of reversible diffeomorphisms.

The local theory of Kolmogorov circles of reversible diffeomorphisms on a plane considers a fixed elliptic reversible germ $A: (\mathbb{R}^2,0) \longrightarrow (\mathbb{R}^2,0)$ and an assemblage of invariant circles of this germ which contract to 0. In contrast with this, the local theory of resonance zones of reversible diffeomorphisms on a plane considers a one-parameter family of elliptic reversible germs $A_\varepsilon:(\mathbb{R}^2,0)\longrightarrow(\mathbb{R}^2,0)$ (where eigenvalues of the linearization of A_0 are roots of unity of degree q), but for each fixed value of ε no resonance zone but one (corresponding to the same for all ε rotation number $2\pi p/q$) of the mapping A_ε undergoes an investigation. As ε tends to 0, these zones contract to 0.

Thus, consider a number $2\pi p/q \in (0,\pi)$, where $p, q \in \mathbb{N}$ are relatively prime. Let us assume $q \geqslant 5$ (a so called weak resonance). Consider a smooth one-parameter family of smooth diffeomorphisms A_ε (the parameter ε varies over a neighbourhood of $0 \in \mathbb{R}$) with fixed point $0 \in \mathbb{R}^2$. The diffeomorphisms A_ε are assumed to be defined on a certain neighbourhood of $0 \in \mathbb{R}^2$ not depending on ε and to be reversible with respect to a smooth involution $G:(\mathbb{R}^2,0) \longrightarrow (\mathbb{R}^2,0)$. Let eigenvalues of the linearization of A_ε be $e^{\pm i\theta_\varepsilon}$, where $\theta_0 = 2\pi p/q$. Generically

$$\frac{d}{d\varepsilon}\theta_\varepsilon\Big|_{\varepsilon=0} \neq 0,$$

and one may take the quantity $q\theta_\varepsilon - 2\pi p$ as a new parameter. In the sequel, we shall set $\theta_\varepsilon = (2\pi p+\varepsilon)/q$.

For all sufficiently small ε, $l\theta_\varepsilon/2\pi \notin \mathbb{N}$ for $l \in \mathbb{N}$, $1 \leqslant l \leqslant q-1$. According to Proposition 2.6, there exists a coordinate system $z = z(\varepsilon) \in \mathbb{C}$ (with origin at 0) smoothly depending on ε, in which

$$(A_\varepsilon)_{q-2} : z \mapsto e^{i\theta_\varepsilon} z K_\varepsilon(\rho) \, , \quad G : z \mapsto \bar{z}$$

where $\rho = z\bar{z}$ and $K_\varepsilon(\rho)$ is a complex polynomial in ρ of degree $\leq d = [(q-3)/2]$ with constant term 1, and $(K_\varepsilon \bar{K}_\varepsilon)^{\cdot}_d = 1$ (here $(\;)^{\cdot}_\ell$ denotes the ℓ-th jet with respect to ρ). The polynomial $K_\varepsilon(\rho)$ depends on ε smoothly.

We have

$$(A_\varepsilon)_{q-1} : z \mapsto e^{i\theta_\varepsilon} z K_\varepsilon(\rho) + \sum_{n=0}^{q-1} S_n(\varepsilon) z^n \bar{z}^{q-1-n} .$$

For $\varepsilon = 0$ the monomial $z^n \bar{z}^{q-1-n}$ is resonant precisely when either $n = 0$ (if q is odd) or $n \in \{0, q/2\}$ (if q is even). Let $Q = \{1; 2; \ldots; q-1\}$ for q odd and $Q = \{1; 2; \ldots; q/2-1; q/2+1; \ldots; q-1\}$ for q even.

The condition $A_\varepsilon G A_\varepsilon = G$ implies the equality

$$\overline{S_n(\varepsilon)} + S_n(\varepsilon) e^{i(q-2-2n)\theta_\varepsilon} = 0 \tag{13}$$

for each $n \in Q \cup \{0\}$. If q is even, this condition also implies the equality

$$\left(K_\varepsilon(\rho)\overline{K_\varepsilon(\rho)} + 2\mathrm{Re}(e^{-i\theta_\varepsilon} S_{q/2}(\varepsilon))\rho^{q/2-1}\right)^{\cdot}_{q/2-1} = 1 .$$

Consider the mapping

$$H_\varepsilon : z \longmapsto z + \sum_{n \in Q} \frac{S_n(\varepsilon)}{e^{i\theta_\varepsilon} - e^{i(2n+1-q)\theta_\varepsilon}} z^n \bar{z}^{q-1-n} .$$

It depends on ε smoothly and commutes with σ by virtue of (13).

One sees that

$$(H_\varepsilon A_\varepsilon H_\varepsilon^{-1})_{q-1} : z \mapsto e^{i\theta_\varepsilon} z \left(e^{i\Omega_\varepsilon(\rho)}\right)_{q-2} + S_0(\varepsilon)\bar{z}^{q-1} \qquad (14)$$

where $\Omega_\varepsilon(\rho)$ is a real polynomial in ρ of degree $\leq d' = [(q-2)/2]$ without a constant term. This polynomial depends on ε smoothly.

In view of (13)

$$\overline{S_0(\varepsilon)} + S_0(\varepsilon) e^{i(q-2)\theta_\varepsilon} = 0$$

i.e.

$$S_0(\varepsilon) = \mu(\varepsilon) \exp\left(-i \frac{(q-2)\theta_\varepsilon + \pi}{2}\right)$$

where $\mu(\varepsilon)$ is real.

One may suppose that from the very first $(A_\varepsilon)_{q-1}$ is of the normal form (14). Then we have

$$(A_\varepsilon^q)_{q-1} : z \mapsto e^{iq\theta_\varepsilon} z \left(e^{iq\Omega_\varepsilon(\rho)}\right)_{q-2} + P(\varepsilon)\bar{z}^{q-1} .$$

The coefficient $P(\varepsilon)$ is the product of $S_0(\varepsilon)$ and a certain function in ε that does not vanish at $\varepsilon = 0$. The condition

$A_\varepsilon^q G A_\varepsilon^q = G$ implies the equality

$$\overline{p(\varepsilon)} + p(\varepsilon) e^{i(q-2)q\theta_\varepsilon} = 0 \quad ,$$

whence

$$p(\varepsilon) = \nu(\varepsilon)(-1)^{pq+1} \exp\left(-i\,\frac{(q-2)q\theta_\varepsilon + \pi}{2}\right)$$

$$= \nu(\varepsilon) \exp\left(i\,\frac{\pi-(q-2)\varepsilon}{2}\right)$$

where $\nu(\varepsilon)$ is real.

Thus,

$$(A_\varepsilon^q)_{q-1} : z \mapsto e^{i\varepsilon} z \left(e^{iq\Omega_\varepsilon(\rho)}\right)_{q-2} + \nu(\varepsilon) \exp\left(i\frac{\pi-(q-2)\varepsilon}{2}\right) \bar{z}^{\,q-1} .$$

Let $\Omega_\varepsilon(\rho) = c(\varepsilon)\rho + O(\rho^2)$.

THEOREM 5.6. Suppose in the situation just described, $C(0) \neq 0$ and $\nu(0) \neq 0$ (the generic case; the condition $\nu(0) \neq 0$ is equivalent to $S_0(0) \neq 0$). Without loss of generality we may assume that $C(0) < 0$. Then for $\varepsilon > 0$ the mapping A_ε has two symmetric cycles of length q at distance $\sim \sqrt{\varepsilon}$ from 0.

PROOF. Let $\varepsilon > 0$. The equation $\varepsilon + q\Omega_\varepsilon(\rho) = 0$ has a smooth solution of the form $\rho(\varepsilon) = \varepsilon F(\varepsilon)$, where $F(0) = -(q\,c(0))^{-1} > 0$. Introduce the variable

$$R = \left(\sqrt{\rho} - \sqrt{\varepsilon F(\varepsilon)}\right) \varepsilon^{(2-q)/4} .$$

Let R vary over a fixed, ε-independent interval. Then

$$\rho=(R\varepsilon^{(q-2)/4}+\sqrt{\varepsilon F(\varepsilon)})^2=\varepsilon F(\varepsilon)+2R\sqrt{F(0)}\varepsilon^{q/4}+o(\varepsilon^{q/4})$$

(recall that $q\geqslant 5$, whence $(q-2)/2>q/4$). Hence

$$\varepsilon+q\Omega_\varepsilon(\rho)=\varepsilon+q\Omega_\varepsilon(\varepsilon F(\varepsilon))+2qc(0)R\sqrt{F(0)}\varepsilon^{q/4}+o(\varepsilon^{q/4})$$

$$=aR\varepsilon^{q/4}+o(\varepsilon^{q/4})$$

where $a=2q\,c(0)\sqrt{F(0)}<0$.

Further, introduce the angular variable $\varphi=\arg z$. As $q\geqslant 5$ implies $(q-2)/4>1/2$,

$$\sqrt{\rho}=\sqrt{F(0)\varepsilon}+o(\sqrt{\varepsilon}).$$

Consequently

$$\nu(\varepsilon)\exp\left(i\frac{\pi-(q-2)\varepsilon}{2}\right)\bar{z}^{q-1}=i\nu(0)(F(0))^{(q-1)/2}\varepsilon^{(q-1)/2}e^{i(1-q)\varphi}+o(\varepsilon^{(q-1)/2})$$

$$=ib\varepsilon^{(q-1)/2}e^{i(1-q)\varphi}+o(\varepsilon^{(q-1)/2})$$

where $b=\nu(0)(F(0))^{(q-1)/2}\neq 0$.

It is clear that all monomials of degrees $\geqslant q$ are $o(\varepsilon^{(q-1)/2})$.

Let $\tilde{\varphi}(\varphi,R)$ and $\tilde{R}(\varphi,R)$ be components of the mapping A_ε^q in coordinates (φ,R):

$$A_\varepsilon^q:(\varphi,R)\longmapsto(\tilde{\varphi},\tilde{R})$$

(in initial coordinates,

$$A_\varepsilon^q : (\sqrt{\varepsilon F(\varepsilon)} + R\varepsilon^{(q-2)/4}) e^{i\varphi} \mapsto (\sqrt{\varepsilon F(\varepsilon)} + \tilde{R}\varepsilon^{(q-2)/4}) e^{i\tilde{\varphi}}).$$

We obtain that

$$(\sqrt{\varepsilon F(\varepsilon)} + \tilde{R}\varepsilon^{(q-2)/4}) e^{i\tilde{\varphi}}$$

$$= (\sqrt{\varepsilon F(\varepsilon)} + R\varepsilon^{(q-2)/4}) \exp(i(\varphi + aR\varepsilon^{q/4} + o(\varepsilon^{q/4})))$$

$$+ ib\varepsilon^{(q-1)/2} e^{i(1-q)\varphi} + o(\varepsilon^{(q-1)/2})$$

i.e.

$$\sqrt{\varepsilon F(\varepsilon)} + R\varepsilon^{(q-2)/4} + ib\varepsilon^{(q-1)/2} e^{-iq\varphi} + o(\varepsilon^{(q-1)/2})$$

$$= (\sqrt{\varepsilon F(\varepsilon)} + \tilde{R}\varepsilon^{(q-2)/4}) \exp(i(\tilde{\varphi} - \varphi - aR\varepsilon^{q/4} + o(\varepsilon^{q/4}))).$$

This implies that

$$\tilde{\varphi} = \varphi + aR\varepsilon^{q/4} + o(\varepsilon^{q/4}),$$

$$\tilde{R} = R + b\varepsilon^{q/4} \sin q\varphi + o(\varepsilon^{q/4}).$$

Thus, for sufficiently small positive ε the operator A_ε^q has $2q$ fixed points near the circle $R = 0$, i.e. at distance of order of $\sqrt{\varepsilon}$ from $0 \in \mathbb{R}^2$. At these points, the Jacobian determinant of A_ε^q is different from zero. It is obvious that they constitute two symmetric cycles of the mapping A_ε. X

REMARK 1. Simultaneously we have obtained that the resonance zone width equals $\varepsilon^{(q-2)/4}$.

REMARK 2. In coordinates (φ, R), the mapping A_ε^q differs from the identity one by a quantity of order of $\varepsilon^{q/4}$ and agrees with the phase flow mapping of the field

$$W = aR\frac{\partial}{\partial \varphi} + b(\sin q\varphi)\frac{\partial}{\partial R}$$

at time $\varepsilon^{q/4}$ up to accuracy $o(\varepsilon^{q/4})$.

This field is equivariant (invariant under the rotation through angle $2\pi/q$), reversible with respect to both involutions $\sigma : (\varphi, R) \longmapsto (-\varphi, R)$ and $\sigma^* : (\varphi, R) \longmapsto (\varphi, -R)$ and Hamiltonian (with respect to the symplectic structure $dR \wedge d\varphi$) with the Hamilton function $aR^2/2 + (b\cos q\varphi)/q$.

REMARK 3. Strong resonances $(q \leq 4)$ in the local theory of resonance zones deserve a separate study.

Chapter 6. FAMILIES OF SYMMETRIC CYCLES NEAR AN EQUILIBRIUM OF A REVERSIBLE VECTORFIELD

§ 6.1. Lyapunov-Devaney theorem (absence of resonances)

In this section, n is a fixed natural number.

Consider a system of differential equations in $\mathbb{R}^{2n}$, reversible with respect to some involution G whose fixed point manifold $\operatorname{Fix} G$ has dimension n. According to Theorem 3.1, symmetric cycles of this system, as well as cycles of a Hamiltonian system with n degrees of freedom, are generically organized into smooth one-parameter families. Now suppose that this system has an equilibrium lying on $\operatorname{Fix} G$. Then there arises the problem to investigate families of symmetric cycles near such an equilibrium.

A similar problem concerning Hamiltonian systems has been known for a long time. The main result here is the following classical Lyapunov theorem.

THEOREM 6.1 (Lyapunov) (see [11 (Chapter I, § 6), 22 (§§16-17)]). Let 0 be an equilibrium of a Hamiltonian vectorfield V with n degrees of freedom. Let the linearization $(V)_1$ of this field at 0 have simple purely imaginary eigenvalues $\pm i\omega$ $(\omega > 0)$; denote the other eigenvalues by $\pm\lambda_2, \ldots, \pm\lambda_n$. Suppose the nonresonance condition holds, i.e. none of the ratios $\lambda_r / i\omega$, $2 \leq r \leq n$, is an integer. Then in a neighbourhood of 0, there exists a one-parameter family of cycles γ_σ of the field V (where the parameter σ varies over a certain interval $(0, \sigma_0)$), and as σ tends to 0, cycles γ_σ shrink to the equilibrium and their period tends to $2\pi/\omega$. The dependence of γ_σ on σ is of the same smoothness (C^∞ or analytic) as V is.

An analogous theorem holds for reversible vectorfields, too. As far as I know, the first paper containing this analogue was Devaney [3] . That is why we shall call the reversible analogue to the Lyapunov theorem the Lyapunov-Devaney theorem.

Before formulating and proving this theorem let us contract for certain notations. Let $u_1,\dots,u_K$ be independent variables (real or complex) varying over a neighbourhood of 0. The symbol $O_\ell(u_1,\dots,u_K)$ (where $\ell\in\mathbb{N}$) will be understood as any smooth function depending on $u_1,\dots,u_K$ and possibly on some variables else, which belongs to the ideal generated by either all monomials

$$u_1^{d_1}\dots u_K^{d_K}\,,\quad d_1+\dots+d_K=\ell$$

(if variables $u_1,\dots,u_K$ are real) or all monomials

$$u_1^{d_1}\bar{u}_1^{\tilde{d}_1}\dots u_K^{d_K}\bar{u}_K^{\tilde{d}_K}\,,\quad d_1+\tilde{d}_1+\dots+d_K+\tilde{d}_K=\ell$$

(if these variables are complex).

In particular, a function depending on $u=(u_1,\dots,u_K)$ only is $O_\ell(u)$ precisely when its $(\ell-1)$-th jet equals 0. $O_\ell(u_1,\dots,u_K)\,O_m(\tilde{u}_1,\dots,\tilde{u}_s)$ (where $\ell,\, m\in\mathbb{N}$) will be understood as any smooth function that belongs to the ideal generated by all products fg , where $f=O_\ell(u)$ and $g=O_m(\tilde{u})$ (there may be coincidental variables among $K+s$ variables $u_1,\dots,u_K$, $\tilde{u}_1,\dots,\tilde{u}_s$). Note that if $K=1$ and the variable $u_1=u$ is real then one may write $u^\ell O_m(\tilde{u})$ instead of $O_\ell(u)O_m(\tilde{u})$.

We shall write O instead of O_1.

We shall use these notations throughout Chapter 6.

We will often use the following proposition that can be easily verified. Let $z_1,\dots,z_N$ be coordinates on $\mathbb{C}^N$. Then a vectorfield on $\mathbb{C}^N$ whose components are series in powers of $z_1,\dots,z_N$ is reversible with respect to the complex conjugation involution if and only if all coefficients of these series are purely imaginary.

Besides that, in this section, speaking on a complex coordinate system (z, Z) in $\mathbb{R}^{2n}$ we shall always suppose that $z \in \mathbb{C}$ and $Z \in \mathbb{C}^{n-1}$. We will denote $\operatorname{Re} z$ and $\operatorname{Re} Z$ by x and X respectively.

THEOREM 6.2 (Devaney) Let V be the germ of a smooth vectorfield at $(\mathbb{R}^{2n}, 0)$ $(V(0)=0)$, reversible with respect to a smooth involution $G:(\mathbb{R}^{2n},0)\to(\mathbb{R}^{2n},0)$ of type (n,n). Let the linearization $(V)_1$ of this field have simple purely imaginary eigenvalues $\pm i\omega$ $(\omega > 0)$; denote the other eigenvalues by $\pm\lambda_2, \ldots, \pm\lambda_n$. Suppose the nonresonance condition holds, i.e. none of the ratios $\lambda_r/i\omega$, $2 \le r \le n$, is an integer. Then in a neighbourhood of 0, there exists a smooth one-parameter family of symmetric cycles γ_σ of the field V (where the parameter σ varies over a certain interval $(0, \sigma_0)$), and as σ tends to 0, cycles γ_σ shrink to the equilibrium and their period tends to $2\pi/\omega$. If the field V and the involution G are analytic then one can also make γ_σ depend on σ analytically.

PROOF. There is such a complex coordinate system (z,Z) in $\mathbb{R}^{2n}$, depending on the original coordinate system smoothly (analytically if G is analytic), in which

$$(V)_1 = i\omega z\frac{\partial}{\partial z} + i(B_1 Z + B_2 \bar{Z})\frac{\partial}{\partial Z}, \quad G:(z,Z)\mapsto(\bar{z},\bar{Z}),$$

B_1 and B_2 being real $(n-1)\times(n-1)$ matrices.

The phase flow F_t of the field V has the form

$$F_t : \begin{array}{ccc} z & \longmapsto & e^{i\omega t} z + O_2(z, Z) \\ Z & & f_t(Z) + O_2(z, Z) \end{array}$$

where $f_t(Z)$ is the phase flow of the linear field $v = i(B_1 Z + B_2 \bar{Z})\partial/\partial Z$ in $\mathbb{R}^{2n-2}$.

Consider trajectories of the field V passing through points on the plane $\mathbb{R}^n = \mathrm{Fix}\, G$, i.e. points of the form (x, X). We have

$$\mathrm{Im}\, F_t(x, X) = (x \sin \omega t + \mu_t(x, X),\ \mathrm{Im} f_t(X) + \tilde{\mu}_t(x, X))$$

where $\mu_t = O_2(x, X)$, $\tilde{\mu}_t = O_2(x, X)$.

LEMMA 1. The linear operator $X \longmapsto \mathrm{Im} f_{\pi/\omega}(X)$ is nondegenerate.

PROOF. Suppose there exists a nonzero vector $a \in \mathbb{R}^{n-1} = \mathrm{Fix}\, G \cap \{x = 0\}$ such that $f_{\pi/\omega}(a)$ belongs to $\mathrm{Fix}\, G$ again. Then by Proposition 3.3 $f_{2\pi/\omega}(a) = a$. This means that 1 is an eigenvalue of the operator $f_{2\pi/\omega}$, whence the linear vectorfield v has an eigenvalue $i\omega N$, $N \in \mathbb{Z}$. This contradicts the nonresonance condition. X

Consider the mapping $\mathfrak{F} : (\mathbb{R}^{n+1}, 0) \to (\mathbb{R}^n, 0)$, $\mathfrak{F} : (\tau, x, X) \mapsto \mathrm{Im}\, F_{\pi/\omega + \tau}(x, X)$. Our goal is to find $\mathfrak{F}^{-1}(0)$. Since the linear operator $\mathrm{Im} f_{\pi/\omega}$ is nondegenerate, one can solve the equation $\mathrm{Im} f_t(X) + \tilde{\mu}_t(x, X) = 0$ for X provided t is close to π/ω: $X = g(t, x)$. The function g is smooth and $O_2(x)$. Consider the function

$$\varphi(\tau, x) = -x \sin \omega\tau + \mu_{\pi/\omega+\tau}(x, g(\tfrac{\pi}{\omega} + \tau, x)).$$

$0 \in \mathbb{R}^2$ is a critical point of this function with critical value 0, its Hessian at this point equaling $-\omega^2 < 0$. By the Morse lemma (see [37 (Chapter I, § 6, 6.2)]), $\mathcal{G}^{-1}(0)$ consists of two smooth curves that intersect at 0 at a nonzero angle. One of these curves is $x=0$. The other has the form $\tau = \frac{1}{2} T(x) - \pi/\omega$, where T is a smooth function, $T(0) = 2\pi/\omega$. Thus, $\mathcal{F}^{-1}(0)$ consists of two curves

$$x=0,\ X=0 \quad \text{and} \quad \tau=\frac{1}{2}T(x)-\frac{\pi}{\omega},\ X=g\left(\frac{\pi}{\omega}+\tau, x\right).$$

The smooth curve Γ in $\mathbb{R}^n = \operatorname{Fix} G$ given by the equation $X = g(\frac{1}{2}T(x), x)$ passes through 0 and is tangent to the coordinate line $X=0$. Consider the trajectory γ_σ of the field V starting at an arbitrary point $(\sigma, g(\frac{1}{2}T(\sigma), \sigma))$ of this curve. At time $T(\sigma)/2$ the trajectory γ_σ intersects $\operatorname{Fix} G$ again. By Proposition 3.3 γ_σ is a symmetric cycle of period $T(\sigma)$ (and both points at which γ_σ intersects $\operatorname{Fix} G$ lie on Γ). For $\sigma > 0$ we obtain the desired family of symmetric cycles. To complete the proof of Theorem 6.2 it suffices to observe that if the field V and the involution G are analytic so is the curve Γ. X

Symmetric cycles γ_σ constitute a two-dimensional surface $\mathcal{M}$ that is obviously smooth outside 0. Moreover, if the field V and the involution G are analytic so is $\mathcal{M}$ outside 0.

THEOREM 6.3. The surface $\mathcal{M}$ is smooth not only outside 0 but also at 0.

PROOF. Fix an arbitrary natural number l. By means of the standard methods of the normal forms theory which have been already used by us repeatedly in the present paper, one can pass to such a complex coordinate system (z, Z) in $\mathbb{R}^{2n}$ (via a smooth change of variables) in which

$$V=(i\omega z+O_2(z,Z))\frac{\partial}{\partial z}+(i(B_1Z+B_2\bar{Z})+O(Z)O(z,Z)$$

$$+O_{\ell+1}(z,Z))\frac{\partial}{\partial Z}\ ,\quad \sigma:(z,Z)\mapsto(\bar{z},\bar{Z}).$$

We shall use the notations introduced in the proof of Theorem 6.2. One has $\tilde{\mu}_t=O(X)O(x,X)+O_{\ell+1}(x,X)$, whence $g=O_{\ell+1}(x)$. The trajectory of the field V with initial conditions $z(0)=\sigma\geq 0$, $Z(0)=g(\frac{1}{2}T(\sigma),\sigma)$ is

$$F_t\left(\sigma,g\left(\frac{T(\sigma)}{2},\sigma\right)\right)=(e^{i\omega t}\sigma+O_2(\sigma),\ O_{\ell+1}(\sigma))\ .$$

Introduce the variable $\varphi=2\pi t/T(\sigma)$. Then this trajectory will receive the form

$$z(\varphi)=e^{i\varphi}\sigma+\sigma^2\tilde{\Phi}(\varphi,\sigma),\quad Z(\varphi)=\sigma^{\ell+1}\tilde{\Psi}(\varphi,\sigma),$$

where $\tilde{\Phi}$ and $\tilde{\Psi}$ are smooth 2π-periodic in φ functions, and $\tilde{\Phi}(0,\sigma)\equiv 0$. One can express these functions in the form $\tilde{\Phi}(\varphi,\sigma)=\Phi(e^{i\varphi},\sigma)$, $\tilde{\Psi}(\varphi,\sigma)=\Psi(e^{i\varphi},\sigma)$, where Φ and Ψ are also smooth functions(their first argument varies over $U(1)$ and the second one varies over an interval $[0,\sigma_0)$), and $\Phi(1,\sigma)\equiv 0$.

One can solve the equation $z=e^{i\varphi}\sigma+\sigma^2\Phi(e^{i\varphi},\sigma)$ for $e^{i\varphi}$ and σ and express the solutions (which are functions in the single argument z) as smooth functions in two arguments z and $\zeta=z/|z|$ (the variable ζ varies over the circle $U(1)$). Indeed, let $z=e^{i\varphi}\sigma\chi$, where χ is a new complex variable varying near 1. Then $\sigma=z/(\zeta|\chi|)$, $e^{i\varphi}=\zeta|\chi|/\chi$, and the above equation may be rewritten in the form

$$\chi = 1 + \frac{z\chi}{\zeta^2|\chi|^2}\,\Phi\left(\frac{\zeta|\chi|}{\chi}, \frac{z}{\zeta|\chi|}\right).$$

This implies

$$\chi = 1 + z h_1(z, \zeta) ,$$

and, consequently,

$$e^{i\vartheta} = \zeta + z h_2(z, \zeta) ,$$

$$\sigma = \frac{z}{\zeta} + z^2 h_3(z, \zeta)$$

where h_1 , h_2 and h_3 are smooth functions (when their first argument varies near $0 \in \mathbb{C}$ and the second one varies over $U(1)$).

Therefore, the equation of the surface $\mathcal{M}$ has the form

$$Z = z^{\ell+1}\,\Omega(z, \zeta)$$

where Ω is a smooth function.

Thus, $\mathcal{M}$ is of class C^{ℓ} at 0. But ℓ is arbitrary, and we obtain the statement of the theorem. X

Hereby, the surface $\mathcal{M}$ is diffeomorphic to a disc foliated into concentric circles.

THEOREM 6.4. If the field V and the involution σ are analytic then the surface $\mathcal{M}$ is analytic not only outside 0 but also at o.

We shall not prove this theorem here. For its proof see, e.g., [11 (Chapter I)] . The main part of the proof is verifying (by means of the majorant method) convergence of a formal change of variables taking the field V and the involution σ into the form

$$V = (i\omega z + O_2(z,Z))\frac{\partial}{\partial z} + (i(B_1 Z + B_2\bar{Z}) + O(Z)\,O(z, Z))\frac{\partial}{\partial Z} ,$$

$$\sigma : (z, Z) \mapsto (\bar{z}, \bar{Z}).$$

It is clear that after such a change of variables, the surface $\mathcal{M}$ receives the equation $Z = 0$.

REMARK 1. For $n = 1$ Theorems 6.1 - 6.4 are trivial.

REMARK 2. If in Theorems 6.3 or 6.4 the field V depends smoothly (respectively analytically) on a parameter so does the surface $\mathcal{M}$.

§ 6.2. Resonance $1:1$.

From now on and up to the end of Chapter 6 we shall assume n to be a natural number ≥ 2. Let V be a smooth vectorfield at $(\mathbb{R}^{2n}, 0)$ $(V(0) = 0)$, reversible with respect to a smooth involution $\sigma : (\mathbb{R}^{2n}, 0) \to (\mathbb{R}^{2n}, 0)$ of type (n, n). Suppose that the linearization $(V)_1$ of this field has four purely imaginary eigenvalues in resonance, namely, $\pm i\omega$, $\pm iN\omega$, where $\omega > 0$, $N \in \mathbb{N}$. Denote the other eigenvalues by $\pm\lambda_3, \ldots, \pm\lambda_n$. We assume the resonance to have codimension 1, i.e. that none of the ratios $\lambda_r / i\omega$, $3 \leq r \leq n$, is an integer.

In such a situation, we wish to describe families of symmetric cycles of the field V of periods close to $2\pi/\omega$ near 0. According to general ideas of the singularity theory due to Poincaré, one ought to study resonant systems of codimension 1 embedding them in one-parameter families of reversible systems depending on a small parameter ε (the value $\varepsilon = 0$ corresponds to the resonance). The equilibrium may be assumed to be independent of ε and situated at 0.

Thus, we will consider smooth one-parameter families V_ε of smooth vectorfields at $(\mathbb{R}^{2n}, 0)$ $(V_\varepsilon(0)=0$ for all $\varepsilon)$, reversible with respect to a smooth ε-independent involution $G:(\mathbb{R}^{2n},0)\longrightarrow(\mathbb{R}^{2n},0)$ of type (n,n) , and assume the spectrum of $(V_0)_1$ to have the structure described above. We shall call such a situation resonance $1:N$.

From this section and up to the end of Chapter 6, speaking on a complex coordinate system (z, Z) in $\mathbb{R}^{2n}$ we shall always suppose that $z=(z_1, z_2)\in\mathbb{C}^2$ and $Z\in\mathbb{C}^{n-2}$. We will denote $Re\, z$ and $Re\, Z$ by x and X respectively. Denote by $F_{\varepsilon,t}$ the phase flow of the field V_ε.

We shall consider only such complex coordinate systems (z, Z) in $\mathbb{R}^{2n}$ in which $G:(z,Z)\mapsto(\bar{z}, \bar{Z})$. In this case, the search of symmetric cycles of the field V_ε whose periods are close to $2\pi/\omega$ amounts to the search of such points $(x,X)\in\mathbb{R}^n = Fix\, G$ that $Im\, F_{\varepsilon,t}(x,X)=0$ for some t close to π/ω.

It turns out, that for each N there exist two greatly different types of the bifurcations of families of symmetric cycles of the field V_ε of periods close to $2\pi/\omega$ as ε passes through the resonant value 0 (both types are generic). We shall call these types elliptic and hyperbolic regimes.

We will not note every time that this or that function, mapping or change of variables will be smooth and depend on ε smoothly (except in the formulations of theorems), and, on the contrary, we shall specially point out those cases when it will not be so.

We will not consider the analytic case, when the fields V_ε and the involution G are analytic and V_ε depends on ε also analytically. All those objects which are smooth or depend on ε smoothly in the constructions stated below are analytic or depend on ε analytically in the analytic case.

The paper [2] contains the discussion on results obtained in this section and the next one and the pictures of bifurcations (in

[2] , only the case $n=2$ is considered but this is of no consequence because the bifurcations for $n>2$ are trivial extensions (by multiplication by $\mathbb{R}^s$ with an appropriate $s\in\mathbb{N}$) of the bifurcations for $n=2$, see Theorems 6.5 and 6.8 below).

In this section, we study resonance $1:1$. Let ωi and $-\omega i$ be eigenvalues of $(V_0)_1$ of multiplicity two.

For small ε , near 0 there is a two-dimensional surface $\mathcal{M}_\varepsilon$ invariant under the field V_ε and foliated into symmetric cycles of periods close to $2\pi/\omega$. Let $\mathcal{M}_\varepsilon \cap \mathrm{Fix}\, G = \Gamma_\varepsilon$.

Our goal is to investigate the bifurcations of the curve Γ_ε which occur as ε passes through the resonant value 0.

THEOREM 6.5. If the 3-jet of the field V_ε satisfies certain nondegeneracy conditions C_1, C_2, C_3 exposed below then the following holds.

a) In the space $\mathbb{R}^n = \mathrm{Fix}\, G$, there is a two-dimensional surface Σ_ε depending on ε smoothly, on which the curve Γ_ε lies.

b) By a suitable choice of a smoothly depending on ε coordinate system (ξ,η) on Σ_ε and, if necessary, the change of the sign of ε (i.e. multiplying ε by -1), the equation of the family of curves Γ_ε may be put into the following form:

$$(\varepsilon \pm \xi^2)\,\xi^2 = \eta^2 \qquad (1)$$

where the sign $+$ corresponds to the hyperbolic regime and the sign $-$ corresponds to the elliptic one (a regime is determined by the 3-jet of the field V_0).

REMARK 1. Actually, the conditions C_1 , C_2 and C_3 are imposed on $(V_0)_1$, $(V_\varepsilon)_1$ and $(V_0)_3$ respectively.

REMARK 2. For $n=2$ the statement a) is trivial: $\Sigma_\varepsilon = \mathrm{Fix}\, G$.

PROOF. First of all, let us verify that it suffices to reduce Γ_ε to the form (1) in that case when any smooth changes of ε

are allowed (not only multiplying ε by -1). Indeed, a family of curves

$$(\tilde{\varepsilon} \pm \tilde{\xi}^2)\tilde{\xi}^2 = \tilde{\eta}^2$$

where $\tilde{\varepsilon} = \tilde{\varepsilon}(\varepsilon) = a\varepsilon + O_2(\varepsilon)$, $a > 0$, can be put into the form (1) via the change of variables $\xi = \tilde{\xi}\sqrt{\varepsilon/\tilde{\varepsilon}}$, $\eta = \tilde{\eta}\varepsilon/\tilde{\varepsilon}$.

Hence, proving Theorem 6.5 we may use all smooth changes of ε.

Generically, what corresponds to eigenvalues $\pm\omega i$ of the field $(V_0)_1$ of multiplicity two is the generalized Jordan block $J_{i\omega}$ of order 4 (see § 2.1). It is this requirement that is the nondegeneracy condition C_1. For small ε, $(V_\varepsilon)_1$ has two eigenvalues $\lambda_1(\varepsilon)$, $\lambda_2(\varepsilon)$ close to ωi and two eigenvalues $-\lambda_1(\varepsilon)$, $-\lambda_2(\varepsilon)$ close to $-\omega i$. Of course, the dependence of λ_1 and λ_2 on ε is not smooth. The kernel of the linear operator

$$((V_\varepsilon)_1^2 - \lambda_1^2(\varepsilon)E_{2n})((V_\varepsilon)_1^2 - \lambda_2^2(\varepsilon)E_{2n})$$

is a four-dimensional space $W_\varepsilon \subset \mathbb{R}^{2n}$ smoothly depending on ε and invariant under $(G)_1$.

LEMMA 2. Let v_ε and g_ε be linear operators in $\mathbb{R}^4$ depending smoothly on ε. Suppose g_ε is an involution of type $(2,2)$ and v_ε is infinitesimally reversible with respect to g_ε. Let v_0 be conjugate to the generalized Jordan block $J_{i\omega}$ of order 4. Then in $\mathbb{R}^4$ one can choose such a linear complex coordinate system (z_1, z_2) depending on ε smoothly in which

$$v_\varepsilon : \begin{matrix} z_1 \\ z_2 \end{matrix} \mapsto \begin{matrix} i\omega z_1 + iz_2 \\ i\alpha(\varepsilon)z_1 + i(\omega+\beta(\varepsilon))z_2 \end{matrix}, \qquad g_\varepsilon : \begin{matrix} z_1 \\ z_2 \end{matrix} \mapsto \begin{matrix} \bar{z}_1 \\ \bar{z}_2 \end{matrix},$$

where α and β are smooth real-valued functions equaling $O(\varepsilon)$.

PROOF. Complexify $\mathbb{R}^4$. We will denote the complexifications of v_ε and g_ε by the same letters. Thus, on $\mathbb{C}^4$, there act $\mathbb{C}$-linear operators v_ε and g_ε and the $\mathbb{C}$-antilinear operator I of complex conjugation. We have $v_\varepsilon I = I v_\varepsilon$, $g_\varepsilon I = I g_\varepsilon$, $g_\varepsilon v_\varepsilon = -v_\varepsilon g_\varepsilon$. Operators g_ε, I and $I g_\varepsilon$ are involutions whose invariant subspaces have real dimension 4. For small ε the operator v_ε has two eigenvalues $\lambda_1(\varepsilon)$, $\lambda_2(\varepsilon)$ close to ωi and two eigenvalues $-\lambda_1(\varepsilon)$, $-\lambda_2(\varepsilon)$ close to $-\omega i$. Let

$$L_\varepsilon = \operatorname{Ker}(I g_\varepsilon - E) \cap \operatorname{Ker}(v_\varepsilon - \lambda_1(\varepsilon)E)(v_\varepsilon - \lambda_2(\varepsilon)E)$$

where E is the identity operator $\mathbb{C}^4 \to \mathbb{C}^4$.

As is easy to verify, L_ε is a subspace of $\mathbb{C}^4$ of real dimension 2 that is not invariant under I, g_ε and v_ε but is invariant under $i v_\varepsilon$. For $\varepsilon = 0$ the operator $-i v_0 : L_0 \to L_0$ is conjugate to the Jordan block J_ω of order 2.

If (e_1, e_2) is a basis of L_ε as of a linear space over $\mathbb{R}$ then the vectors b_1, c_1, b_2, c_2, where $b_\nu = e_\nu + I e_\nu$, $c_\nu = i(e_\nu - I e_\nu)$, $\nu \in \{1; 2\}$, lie in the original space $\mathbb{R}^4$ and constitute its basis. Moreover, introduce a complex coordinate system (z_1, z_2) in $\mathbb{R}^4$ as follows: a vector with coordinates (z_1, z_2) is the vector

$$\sum_{\nu=1}^{2} \left((\operatorname{Re} z_\nu) b_\nu + (\operatorname{Im} z_\nu) c_\nu \right) .$$

In coordinates (z_1, z_2) the original (non-complexified) operator $g_\varepsilon : \mathbb{R}^4 \to \mathbb{R}^4$ has the form $g_\varepsilon : (z_1, z_2) \mapsto (\bar{z}_1, \bar{z}_2)$.

If the matrix of the operator $-i v_\varepsilon : L_\varepsilon \to L_\varepsilon$ in the basis (e_1, e_2) is

$$\begin{pmatrix} a_1 & a_2 \\ a_3 & a_4 \end{pmatrix}$$

then in coordinates (z_1, z_2) the original (non-complexified) operator $V_\varepsilon : \mathbb{R}^4 \to \mathbb{R}^4$ has the form

$$V_\varepsilon : \begin{matrix} z_1 \\ z_2 \end{matrix} \longmapsto \begin{matrix} ia_1 z_1 + ia_2 z_2 \\ ia_3 z_1 + ia_4 z_2 . \end{matrix}$$

Now the statement of the lemma follows directly from the fact that the matrix

$$\begin{pmatrix} \omega & 1 \\ \varepsilon_1 & \omega + \varepsilon_2 \end{pmatrix}$$

is a real versal unfolding of the Jordan block

$$J_\omega = \begin{pmatrix} \omega & 1 \\ 0 & \omega \end{pmatrix}$$

(see [19, Chapter 6, § 30]). X

Lemma 2 implies that there is such a complex coordinate system (z', Z) in $\mathbb{R}^{2n}$ depending on ε smoothly in which

$$(V_\varepsilon)_1 = (i\omega z_1' + i z_2')\frac{\partial}{\partial z_1'} + \left(i\alpha(\varepsilon) z_1' + i(\omega + \beta(\varepsilon)) z_2'\right)\frac{\partial}{\partial z_2'} + i(B_1(\varepsilon)Z + B_2(\varepsilon)\bar{Z})\frac{\partial}{\partial Z},$$

$$\sigma : (z', Z) \mapsto (\bar{z}', Z)$$

where α and β are real-valued functions in ε equaling $O(\varepsilon)$ while B_1 and B_2 are real matrix-valued (of order $n-2$) functions in ε.

Pass to coordinates $z_1 = z_1'$, $z_2 = (2z_2' - \beta z_1')/(2\omega+\beta)$. In the coordinate system (z, Z)

$$(V_\varepsilon)_1 = \frac{2\omega+\beta}{2}\left(i(z_1+z_2)\frac{\partial}{\partial z_1} + i\left(\frac{4\alpha+\beta^2}{(2\omega+\beta)^2}z_1+z_2\right)\frac{\partial}{\partial z_2}\right) + i(B_1 Z + B_2\bar{Z})\frac{\partial}{\partial Z}.$$

Generically $\alpha(\varepsilon) \neq O_2(\varepsilon)$ (this is the nondegeneracy condition C_2), and we can take $(4\alpha+\beta^2)/(2\omega+\beta)^2$ as a new parameter. Besides that, changing the time scale we can eliminate the factor $(2\omega+\beta)/2$ (of course, this should also cause a change of B_1 and B_2).

Thus, the nondegeneracy conditions C_1 and C_2 allow us to set

$$V_\varepsilon = i(z_1+z_2+\varphi^1_\varepsilon)\frac{\partial}{\partial z_1} + i(\varepsilon z_1 + z_2 + \varphi^2_\varepsilon)\frac{\partial}{\partial z_2} + i(B_1 Z + B_2\bar{Z} + \Phi_\varepsilon)\frac{\partial}{\partial Z},$$

$$\sigma : (z, Z) \mapsto (\bar{z}, \bar{Z}) \tag{2}$$

where functions $\varphi^1_\varepsilon(z,Z)$, $\varphi^2_\varepsilon(z,Z)$ and $\Phi_\varepsilon(z,Z)$ are $O_2(z,Z)$.

Close to i eigenvalues $\lambda_{1,2}(\varepsilon)$ of the operator $(V_\varepsilon)_1$ equal

$$i \pm \sqrt{-\varepsilon} \quad \text{for} \quad \varepsilon < 0,$$
$$i(1 \pm \sqrt{\varepsilon}) \quad \text{for} \quad \varepsilon > 0.$$

Thus, for $\varepsilon<0$ $\lambda_{1,2}(\varepsilon)$ are not purely imaginary whereas for $\varepsilon>0$ $\lambda_{1,2}(\varepsilon)\in\mathbb{R}i$ and the resonance distuny $|\lambda_2(\varepsilon)-\lambda_1(\varepsilon)|$ equals $2\sqrt{\varepsilon}$.

In the Taylor series of the field V_0, all monomials of degree 2 in variables z and $\bar{z}$ in functions $\varphi_0^{1,2}$ and all monomials in these variables in functions Φ_0 are nonresonant (in the sense of the theory of Poincaré-Dulac normal forms). Therefore, for each $\ell\in\mathbb{N}$ by means of a change of variables smoothly depending on ε and commuting with G we can achieve

$$\varphi_\varepsilon^{1,2}(z,Z)=O(Z)O(z,Z)+O_3(z), \quad \Phi_\varepsilon(z,Z)=O(Z)O(z,Z)+O_{\ell+1}(z).$$

For our purposes, it will suffice to set $\ell=2$. Besides that, we shall take no interest in resonant monomials of degree 3 in variables z and $\bar{z}$ in functions $\varphi_0^{1,2}$ except the monomial $\gamma z_1^2\bar{z}_1$ in φ_0^2 (the coefficient γ is a real number). Thus, let

$$\begin{gathered}\varphi_\varepsilon^1(z,Z)=O(Z)O(z,Z)+O_3(z)\\ \varphi_\varepsilon^2(z,Z)=O(Z)O(z,Z)+(\gamma+O(\varepsilon))z_1^2\bar{z}_1+O(z_2)O_2(z)+O_4(z_1)\\ \Phi_\varepsilon(z,Z)=O(Z)O(z,Z)+O_3(z).\end{gathered}\tag{3}$$

Then, as is easy to verify,

$$\operatorname{Im}F_{\varepsilon,t}(x_1,x_2,X)=(\psi_{\varepsilon,t}^1(x,X),\ \psi_{\varepsilon,t}^2(x,X),\ \Psi_{\varepsilon,t}(x,X))$$

where

$$\overset{1}{\psi}_{\varepsilon,t}(x,X)=x_1\sin t+x_2 t\cos t+\varepsilon O(x,X)+O(X)O(x,X)+O_3(x)$$

$$\overset{2}{\psi}_{\varepsilon,t}(x,X)=\varepsilon t x_1\cos t+x_2\sin t+\gamma t x_1^3\cos t$$

$$+\varepsilon^2 O(x_1)+\varepsilon O_3(x_1)+\varepsilon O(x_2,X)+O(X)O(x,X)+x_2 O_2(x)+O_4(x_1)$$

$$\psi_{\varepsilon,t}(x,X)=\operatorname{Im} f_t(X)+\varepsilon O(X)+O(X)O(x,X)+O_3(x) \quad .$$

Here $f_t(Z)$ is the phase flow of the linear field $i(B_1(0)Z + B_2(0)\bar{Z})\,\partial/\partial Z$ in $\mathbb{R}^{2n-4}$.

Let $t=\pi+\tau$, where τ is small. Similarly to Lemma 1 it is easy to prove that the linear operator $X \mapsto \operatorname{Im} f_\pi(X)$ is non-degenerate. Now, equaling $\psi_{\varepsilon,t}(x,X)$ to zero we obtain

$$X=g(x,\tau,\varepsilon) \tag{4}$$

where $g=O_3(x)$. Substituting (4) into $\overset{1}{\psi}_{\varepsilon,t}=0$ and $\overset{2}{\psi}_{\varepsilon,t}=0$ we rewrite the equation $\operatorname{Im} F_{\varepsilon,\pi+\tau}(x,X)=0$ in the form

$$\begin{cases} x_1\tau+\pi x_2+b_1(x,\tau,\varepsilon)=0 & (5)\\ \varepsilon\pi x_1+x_2\tau+\gamma\pi x_1^3+b_2(x,\tau,\varepsilon)=0 & (6)\\ X=g(x,\tau,\varepsilon) \end{cases}$$

where

$$b_1=x_1 O_3(\tau)+x_2 O(\tau)+\varepsilon O(x)+O_3(x) \quad ,$$

$$b_2=\varepsilon x_1 O(\tau)+x_2 O_3(\tau)+x_1^3 O(\tau)+\varepsilon^2 O(x_1)+\varepsilon O_3(x_1)+\varepsilon O(x_2)$$

$$+x_2 O_2(x)+O_4(x_1) \, .$$

From equation (5) we obtain

$$x_2 = -\frac{x_1\tau}{\pi} + x_1 b_3(x_1,\tau,\varepsilon) \tag{7}$$

where

$$b_3 = O_3(\tau) + O(\varepsilon) + O_2(x_1).$$

After the substitution of (7) into (6) the equation (6) decomposes into two ones :

$$x_1 = 0$$

and

$$\varepsilon\pi - \frac{\tau^2}{\pi} + \gamma\pi x_1^2 + b_4(x_1,\tau,\varepsilon) = 0$$

where

$$b_4 = \varepsilon O(\tau) + \varepsilon O_2(x_1) + O_2(\varepsilon) + O_4(\tau) + x_1^2 O(\tau) + O_3(x_1).$$

Solve the second equation for ε :

$$\varepsilon = \frac{\tau^2}{\pi^2} - \gamma x_1^2 + R(x_1,\tau) \tag{8}$$

where $R = O_3(x_1) + x_1^2 O(\tau) + O_4(\tau)$. Substituting (8) into (7) we obtain

$$x_2 = -\frac{x_1\tau}{\pi} + x_1 S(x_1,\tau)$$

where $S = O_2(\tau) + O_2(x_1)$.

Consider the mapping $\mathcal{F} : \mathbb{R}^{n+2} \longrightarrow \mathbb{R}^n$, $\mathcal{F} : (\varepsilon, \tau, x, X) \mapsto \operatorname{Im} F_{\varepsilon,\pi+\tau}(x, X)$ defined near $0 \in \mathbb{R}^{n+2}$. We see that $\mathcal{F}^{-1}(0)$ consists of the two-dimensional plane

$$x = 0\ ,\ X = 0$$

and two-dimensional surface

$$\begin{cases} x_2 = -\dfrac{x_1 \tau}{\pi} + x_1 S(x_1, \tau) \\ \varepsilon = \dfrac{\tau^2}{\pi^2} - \gamma x_1^2 + R(x_1, \tau) \\ X = g(x, \tau, \varepsilon)\ . \end{cases} \tag{9}$$

Let $R(x_1, \tau) = R_0(\tau) + x_1 R_1(x_1, \tau)$, where $R_0 = O_4(\tau)$, $R_1 = O_2(x_1, \tau)$. Introduce the new variable

$$w = -\frac{\tau}{\pi}\sqrt{1 + \frac{\pi^2 R_0(\tau)}{\tau^2}}\ ,$$

then $\tau = wK(w)$, where $K(0) = -\pi$, and one may transcribe (9) in the form

$$x_2 = x_1(w + H_1(x_1, w)) \tag{10}$$

$$\begin{cases} \varepsilon = -\gamma x_1^2 + w^2 + x_1 H_2(x_1, w) \\ X = g(x, wK(w), \varepsilon) \end{cases} \tag{11}$$

where $H_\nu = O_2(x_1, w),\ \nu = 1, 2$.

Decompose functions H_ν into even and odd parts in w: $H_\nu(x_1, w) = \overset{1}{H}_\nu(x_1, w^2) + w\overset{2}{H}_\nu(x_1, w^2),\ \nu = 1, 2$, where functions $\overset{1}{H}_\nu$ and $\overset{2}{H}_\nu$ vanish at 0 (moreover, $\partial \overset{1}{H}_\nu / \partial x_1$ also vanishes at 0). Now from equations (10), (11) one can express $x_1 w$ and w^2 as functions in x and ε:

$$\begin{cases} x_1 w = P_1(x,\varepsilon) = x_2 + Q_1(x,\varepsilon) \\ w^2 = P_2(x,\varepsilon) = \varepsilon + \gamma x_1^2 + Q_2(x,\varepsilon) \end{cases} \tag{12}$$

where, as is easy to verify, $Q_\nu = s_\nu x_1 x_2 + \varepsilon O(x) + O_3(x)$, $\nu = 1, 2$ (s_ν are real numbers).

Thus, the system of equations (9) amounts to

$$\begin{cases} x_1 w = P_1(x,\varepsilon) \\ w^2 = P_2(x,\varepsilon) \\ X = \tilde{g}(x_1, w, \varepsilon) \end{cases}$$

where

$$\tilde{g}(x_1, w, \varepsilon) = g(x_1,\, x_1(w + H_1(x_1, w)),\, wK(w), \varepsilon).$$

We have $\tilde{g} = O_3(x_1)$.

Let

$$\tilde{g}(x_1, w, \varepsilon) = x_1^3 \mu_1(x_1, w^2, \varepsilon) + x_1^3 w \mu_2(x_1, w^2, \varepsilon).$$

It is

$$X = x_1^3 \mu_1(x_1, P_2(x,\varepsilon), \varepsilon) + x_1^2 P_1(x,\varepsilon) \mu_2(x_1, P_2(x,\varepsilon), \varepsilon) \tag{13}$$

that is the equation of the desired surface Σ_ε on which the curve Γ_ε lies.

Now return to equations (10), (11). In the space

$$\mathbb{R}^3 = \bigcup_\varepsilon (\Sigma_\varepsilon \times \{\varepsilon\}) \quad ,$$

where coordinates on Σ_ε are x_1 and x_2 , we obtain a surface Π (more precisely, the germ of a surface) which is the image of the mapping

$$\Lambda : (\mathbb{R}^2, 0) \to (\mathbb{R}^3, 0)$$

given by the formulas

$$\begin{aligned} x_1 &= y \\ x_2 &= y(w + H_1(y, w)) \\ \varepsilon &= -\gamma y^2 + w^2 + y H_2(y, w) \end{aligned} \tag{14}$$

(y and w are coordinates on the space-preimage $\mathbb{R}^2$). This surface is dissected by the level planes of the coordinate function $\varepsilon : (\mathbb{R}^3, 0) \to (\mathbb{R}, 0)$. It is these sections that are the curves Γ_ε. Thus, we must reduce the diagram

$$\Pi \hookrightarrow \mathbb{R}^3 \xrightarrow{\varepsilon} \mathbb{R}$$

to a normal form (by means of diffeomorphisms of $\mathbb{R}^3$ preserving the line $x_1 = x_2 = 0$ which corresponds to the origin for various values of ε).

By virtue of (12) the equations (14) are equivalent to

$$y = x_1$$

$$yw = x_2 + Q_1(x, \varepsilon)$$

$$w^2 = \varepsilon + \gamma x_1^2 + Q_2(x, \varepsilon) .$$

In $\mathbb{R}^3$ introduce the new coordinate system

$$u_1 = x_1 \ , \ u_2 = x_2 + Q_1(x, \varepsilon), \ \ u_3 = \varepsilon + \gamma x_1^2 + Q_2(x, \varepsilon) .$$

In coordinates (u_1, u_2, u_3) the mapping Λ takes the form

$$u_1 = y$$

$$u_2 = yw$$
$$u_3 = w^2 .$$

Thus, Λ is the Whitney mapping and the surface Π is the Whitney umbrella (without "the handle", or "the stick") [37 (Chapter I, § 1, 1.9)] . Note that the relation $x_1 = x_2 = 0$ amounts to $u_1 = u_2 = 0$, since $Q_1 = O(x)$. The function ε in the new coordinates is

$$\varepsilon = u_3 - \gamma u_1^2 - s_2 u_1 u_2 + u_3 O(u_1, u_2) + O_3(u) . \tag{15}$$

Now it remains to reduce the function ε (15) to a normal form by a diffeomorphism of $\mathbb{R}^3$ leaving the standard Whitney umbrella $u_2^2 = u_1^2 u_3$ invariant. Note that every diffeomorphism preserving the Whitney umbrella preserves the line $u_1 = u_2 = 0$ too, because the half-line $u_1 = u_2 = 0,\ u_3 \leq 0$ is the handle of the umbrella and the half-line $u_1 = u_2 = 0,\ u_3 \geq 0$ is its self-intersection line.

All smooth curves on the Whitney umbrella without the handle passing through its vertex 0 are tangent to each other at 0. Their common tangent is the axis u_1 . This means that the direction of the axis u_1 is invariantly connected with the umbrella. Denote by $\mathcal{Cl}$ the class of smooth functions $\rho : (\mathbb{R}^3, 0) \to (\mathbb{R}, 0)$ such that $\partial\rho/\partial u_1 = 0$ at 0. Then $\varepsilon \in \mathcal{Cl}$.

We will reduce to a normal form by diffeomorphisms of $\mathbb{R}^3$ preserving the umbrella not only the function ε but any generic function in the class $\mathcal{Cl}$. Let ρ be an arbitrary function in $\mathcal{Cl}$. Write down ρ in the form

$$\rho(u) = a_2 u_2 + a_3 u_3 + \tau u_1^2 + O(u_2, u_3) O(u) + O_3(u_1) .$$

THEOREM 6.6. Every function $\rho \in \mathcal{Cl}$ satisfying nondegeneracy conditions

$$a_3 \neq 0$$
$$\Delta = a_2^2 - 4a_3\tau \neq 0 \tag{16}$$

can be reduced to the normal form

$$\begin{aligned} &u_3 + u_1^2 , \text{ if } a_3 > 0 \text{ and } \Delta < 0 \\ &-u_3 - u_1^2 , \text{ if } a_3 < 0 \text{ and } \Delta < 0 \\ &u_3 - u_1^2 , \text{ if } a_3 > 0 \text{ and } \Delta > 0 \\ &-u_3 + u_1^2 , \text{ if } a_3 < 0 \text{ and } \Delta > 0 \end{aligned} \tag{17}$$

by a diffeomorphism $(\mathbb{R}^3, 0) \longrightarrow (\mathbb{R}^3, 0)$ leaving the umbrella invariant.

REMARK. It is easy to verify that the nondegeneracy conditions (16) are invariant under diffeomorphisms of $\mathbb{R}^3$ preserving the umbrella.

PROOF. Firstly reduce the function ρ to the form $\rho_0 = a_2 u_2 + a_3 u_3 + \tau u_1^2$. Let us use the standard homotopic method of the theory of singularities [37 (Chapter I, § 6)]. Vectorfields $v_1 = -u_1 \partial/\partial u_1 + 2u_3 \partial/\partial u_3$ (the field $u_1 v_1$ is one of so called "Hamiltonian" fields of the umbrella), $v_2 = u_2 \partial/\partial u_2 + 2u_3 \partial/\partial u_3$ (one of so called "Euler" fields of the umbrella) and $v_3 = u_1^2 \partial/\partial u_2 + 2u_2 \partial/\partial u_3$ (a "Hamiltonian" field) are tangent to the umbrella. For each smooth function $h(u) = O(u_2, u_3)O(u) + O_3(u_1)$ we must select such smooth functions $\delta_\nu (u, t)$ (where $t \in [0,1]$), $\nu = 1, 2, 3$, that the derivative of the function $\rho_0 + th$ along the vectorfield $v_t = \delta_1 v_1 + \delta_2 v_2 + \delta_3 v_3$ equals $-h$, i.e. that

$$\begin{aligned} &-\left(2\tau u_1 + t\frac{\partial h}{\partial u_1}\right) u_1 \delta_1 + \left(a_2 + t\frac{\partial h}{\partial u_2}\right)(u_2\delta_2 + u_1^2 \delta_3) \\ &+ 2\left(a_3 + t\frac{\partial h}{\partial u_3}\right)(u_3\delta_1 + u_3\delta_2 + u_2\delta_3) = -h . \end{aligned} \tag{18}$$

Then the family of diffeomorphisms $D_t : (\mathbb{R}^3, 0) \to (\mathbb{R}^3, 0)$, $D_0 = id$, associated with the field v_t (i.e.

$$v_{t_0}(D_{t_0}(u)) = \left(\frac{d}{dt} D_t(u)\right)_{|t=t_0}$$

for all u and $t_0 \in [0,1]$) , preserves the umbrella and satisfies the identity

$$(\rho_0 + th) \circ D_t = \rho_0 \;,$$

whence the diffeomorphism D_1 takes $\rho_0 + h$ into ρ_0.

In view of $a_3 \neq 0$, in $\mathbb{R}^3$ one can introduce the new t - dependent coordinate system

$$\tilde{u}_1 = u_1$$

$$\tilde{u}_2 = 2a_3 u_2 + a_2 u_1^2 + u_1^2 t \frac{\partial h}{\partial u_2} + 2u_2 t \frac{\partial h}{\partial u_3}$$

$$\tilde{u}_3 = 2a_3 u_3 + 2u_3 t \frac{\partial h}{\partial u_3} + a_2 u_2 + u_2 t \frac{\partial h}{\partial u_2}$$

in which, as is easy to verify, the equation (18) gets the form

$$(\tilde{u}_3 - \frac{a_2}{2a_3} \tilde{u}_2 + \frac{\Delta}{2a_3} \tilde{u}_1^2 + O(\tilde{u}_2, \tilde{u}_3) O(\tilde{u}) + O_3(\tilde{u}_1)) \delta_1 + \tilde{u}_3 \delta_2 + \tilde{u}_2 \delta_3 = -h \,.$$

One can solve the last equation easily, since $\Delta \neq 0$. Moreover, functions δ_ν may be chosen to equal $O(u)$ (then components of the field v_t are $O_2(u)$ and the linearization of the diffeomorphism D_1 is the identity mapping).

Thus, let $\rho=\rho_0=a_2u_2+a_3u_3+\tau u_1^2$. Now the diffeomorphism

$$\overset{*}{D}:\begin{matrix} u_1 \\ u_2 \\ u_3 \end{matrix} \longmapsto \begin{matrix} \varkappa_1 u_1 \\ \varkappa_1\varkappa_2(u_2+\varkappa_3u_1^2) \\ \varkappa_2^2(u_3+2\varkappa_3u_2+\varkappa_3^2u_1^2) \end{matrix}$$

where

$$\varkappa_1=2\sqrt{\left|\frac{a_3}{\Delta}\right|}\;,\quad \varkappa_2=\frac{1}{\sqrt{|a_3|}}\;,\quad \varkappa_3=-\frac{a_2}{\sqrt{|\Delta|}}\,\mathrm{sgn}\,a_3$$

leaves the umbrella invariant, and $\rho\circ\overset{*}{D}$ has the form (17). X

For function (15), $a_3=1$ and $\Delta=4\gamma$. Let $\gamma\neq 0$ (this is the nondegeneracy condition C_3). By Theorem 6.6 one can put the function ε into the form

$$\varepsilon=u_3-u_1^2\quad,\ \text{if}\quad \gamma>0$$
$$\varepsilon=u_3+u_1^2\quad,\ \text{if}\quad \gamma<0$$

via a diffeomorphism $(\mathbb{R}^3,0)\longrightarrow(\mathbb{R}^3,0)$ preserving the Whitney umbrella $u_2^2=u_1^2u_3$.

Now, taking $\xi=u_1$ and $\eta=u_2$ as coordinates on a level surface Σ_ε of the function ε we obtain the equation (1) for curves Γ_ε (the regime is elliptic or hyperbolic according as $\gamma<0$ or $\gamma>0$).

This completes the proof of Theorem 6.5. X

REMARK. At the beginning of the proof of Theorem 6.5 we verified directly that it suffices to reduce Γ_ε to the form (1) in that case when any smooth changes of ε are allowed. One sees this statement follow immediately from Theorem 6.6.

In the elliptic regime for $\varepsilon\leq 0$ (we suppose that ε has already been multiplied by -1 if one needed the change of the sign of ε) Γ_ε is just the origin. For $\varepsilon>0$ Γ_ε looks like a figure-of-eight (see fig. 1). The bifurcation of Γ_ε in the hyperbolic regime is shown in fig. 3 (see also fig. 2). To guide the eye, in fig.3 for $\varepsilon \neq 0$ there is depicted the curve Γ_0 by a dotted line. For $\varepsilon = 0$ the surface $\mathcal{M}_\varepsilon$ consists of two leaves $\mathcal{M}_0^\pm$ foliated into symmetric cycles and intersecting $\mathrm{Fix}\, G$ along two curves $\Gamma_0^\pm$ which are given in coordinates (ξ, η) on Σ_0 by equations $\eta = \pm \xi |\xi|$.

To find the smoothness of these leaves at 0 we shall apply the following general theorem.

THEOREM 6.7. Consider a vectorfield

$$V = (iz_1 + O(z_1, Z)\,O(z, Z) + O_\kappa(z_2))\frac{\partial}{\partial z_1}$$

$$+ (iNz_2 + O(z_2, Z)\,O(z, Z) + O_d(z_1))\frac{\partial}{\partial z_2}$$

$$+ i(B_1 Z + B_2 \bar{Z} + O(Z)O(z, Z) + O_{\ell+1}(z))\frac{\partial}{\partial Z}$$

at $(\mathbb{R}^{2n}, 0)$ with a complex coordinate system (z, Z), where $N, \kappa, d, \ell \in \mathbb{N}$, B_1 and B_2 are real $(n-2)\times(n-2)$ matrices.

Let the field V have an invariant two-dimensional surface $\mathcal{M}^*$ passing through 0 and foliated into cycles whose period is close to 2π (and tends to 2π as cycles shrink to 0). Assume $\mathcal{M}^*$ to intersect the coordinate n-dimensional half-space $\{ z_1 \in \mathbb{R}_+,\ z_2 \in \mathbb{R},\ Z \in \mathbb{R}^{n-2} \}$ along a smooth half-curve Γ^*

$$x_1 = \sigma$$

$$x_2 = \mathcal{U}(\sigma) = a\sigma^m + O_{m+1}(\sigma)$$

$$X = Y(\sigma) = O_j(\sigma)$$

where the parameter σ varies over an interval $[0, \sigma_0)$, $m, j \in \mathbb{N}$, $a \in \mathbb{R}$, $a \neq 0$.

There passes a single cycle of V through every point of this half-curve (except 0).

Suppose that

$$m\kappa \geq 2\ , \quad d \geq m+1\ , \ j \geq m\ , \ \ell \geq m-1 \tag{19}$$

and the difference $N-m$ is either positive or negative and odd.

Then at 0 the surface $\mathcal{M}^*$ is of class C^{m-1} but not of C^m.

PROOF. The proof of this theorem resembles that of Theorem 6.3. Let F_t denote the phase flow of V. By virtue of (19) the trajectory of the field V with initial conditions $z_1(0) = \sigma \geq 0$, $z_2(0) = u(\sigma)$, $Z(0) = Y(\sigma)$ is

$$F_t(\sigma, u(\sigma), Y(\sigma)) = (e^{it}\sigma + O_2(\sigma),\ e^{iNt} a\sigma^m + O_{m+1}(\sigma)\ ,\ O_m(\sigma)).$$

This trajectory is a cycle of period $T(\sigma)$, where $T(0) = 2\pi$. $T(\sigma)$ depends on σ at 0 smoothly, because $T(\sigma)$ is the second positive root of the equation $e^{it} + \psi(t, \sigma) = 0$, where the function $\psi = O(\sigma)$ is smooth. Introduce the variable $\varphi = 2\pi t / T(\sigma)$. Then the equation of the trajectory under consideration gets the form

$$z_1(\varphi) = e^{i\varphi}\sigma + \sigma^2 \Phi_1(e^{i\varphi}, \sigma)$$

$$z_2(\varphi) = a e^{iN\varphi} \sigma^m + \sigma^{m+1} \Phi_2(e^{i\varphi}, \sigma)$$

$$Z(\varphi) = \sigma^m \Psi(e^{i\varphi}, \sigma)$$

where Φ_1, Φ_2, and Ψ are smooth functions (their first argument varies over $\mathcal{U}(1)$ and the second one varies over the interval $[0, \sigma_0)$), and $\Phi_1(1, \sigma) \equiv 0$.

As well as in the proof of Theorem 6.3, one can solve the equation $z_1 = e^{i\varphi}\sigma + \sigma^2\Phi_1(e^{i\varphi}, \sigma)$ for $e^{i\varphi}$ and σ and express the solutions as smooth functions in z_1 and $\zeta = z_1/|z_1|$. The equation of the surface $\mathcal{M}^*$ receives the form

$$z_2 = a\zeta^{N-m} z_1^m + z_1^{m+1}\,\Xi(z_1, \zeta)$$

$$Z = z_1^m \Omega(z_1, \zeta)$$

where Ξ and Ω are smooth functions.

The function $z_1^{m+1}\,\Xi(z_1, z_1/|z_1|)$ has the smoothness C^m at 0; the function $z_1^m \Omega(z_1, z_1/|z_1|)$ has the smoothness C^{m-1} at 0. By virtue of our assumption concerning the difference $N-m$ the function $z_1^N |z_1|^{m-N}$ is of class C^{m-1} but not C^m at 0. X

In our case (see (2), (3)) $N=1$, $\kappa=1$, $d=3$, $\ell=2$. In the coordinate system (x, X) the equations of the half-curves $\Gamma_0^{\pm} \cap \{x_1 \geq 0\}$ have the form $x_1 \geq 0$, $x_2 = \pm\sqrt{\gamma}\, x_1^2 + O_3(x_1)$, $X = O_3(x_1)$ (see (12), (13)). Whence $a = \pm\sqrt{\gamma}$, $m=2$ and $j=3$. One sees all the conditions of Theorem 6.7 be fulfilled. Thus, the leaves $\mathcal{M}_0^{\pm}$ at 0 are of smoothness class C^1, but not of C^2.

REMARK. Applying Theorem 6.7 in future we shall encounter the case when the first component of the field V will be equal to $iz_1 + O(z_1, Z)\,O(z, Z)$. We will conventionally indicate this situation by setting $\kappa = +\infty$.

§ 6.3. Higher resonances

In this section, continuing with the study of resonant reversible fields of codimension 1, we will examine the resonances $1:N$, $N \geq 2$. Let $(V_0)_1$ have simple purely imaginary eigenvalues $\pm i\omega$ and

$\pm iN\omega$, where $N \geq 2$.

For small ε , near 0 the field V_ε has invariant two-dimensional surfaces $\mathcal{M}_\varepsilon^1$ and $\mathcal{M}_\varepsilon^2$ foliated into symmetric cycles whose periods are close to $2\pi/\omega$ (long period cycles) and $2\pi/N\omega$ (short period cycles), respectively. Let $\mathcal{M}_\varepsilon^\nu \cap Fix\, G = \Gamma_\varepsilon^\nu$, $\nu = 1, 2$.

According to Theorems 6.2 and 6.3 the surface $\mathcal{M}_\varepsilon^2$ and the curve Γ_ε^2 do not undergo a bifurcation as ε passes through 0. $\mathcal{M}_\varepsilon^2$ is a smooth two-dimensional disc depending on ε smoothly and intersecting $Fix\, G$ along the curve Γ_ε^2 passing through 0 which is also smooth and depends on ε smoothly.

Our goal is to investigate bifurcations of the curve Γ_ε^1 as ε passes through the resonant value 0.

THEOREM 6.8. If the N-jet of the field V_ε satisfies certain nondegeneracy conditions C_1, C_2, C_3 exposed below then the following holds.

a) In the space $\mathbb{R}^n = Fix\, G$, there is a two-dimensional surface Σ_ε depending on ε smoothly, on which the curves Γ_ε^1 and Γ_ε^2 lie.

b) Bifurcations of the curve Γ_ε^1 have the following normal forms.

i) Let $N=2$. Then on Σ_ε one can choose such a coordinate system (ξ, η) depending on ε smoothly in which the curve Γ_ε^2 is given by the equation $\xi = 0$ for all ε and the curve Γ_ε^1 is given by the equation

$$\eta(\varepsilon - \eta) \pm \xi^2 = 0 \tag{20}$$

where the sign + corresponds to the hyperbolic regime and the sign − corresponds to the elliptic one (a regime is determined by the 2-jet of the field V_0).

ii) Let $N=3$. Then on Σ_ε one can choose such a coordinate system (ξ, η) depending on ε smoothly in which the curve Γ_ε^2 is given by the equation

$$\xi = c\eta + \eta^2 \Theta(\eta, \varepsilon) \tag{21}$$

where c is a real constant, Θ is a smooth function, and the curve Γ_ε^1 is given by the equation

$$\eta(\varepsilon + \eta\xi\cos\theta + \eta^2\sin\theta) + \xi^3 = 0 \tag{22}$$

where θ is a defined $\mathrm{mod}\ 2\pi$ real constant determined by the 3-jet of the field V_0, and $\Delta(\theta) \neq 0$ where $\Delta(\theta) = 4\cos^3\theta + 27\sin^2\theta$ (otherwise speaking, $\theta \neq \pm\theta_0 \ \mathrm{mod}\ 2\pi$, θ_0 being the root of the equation $\Delta(\theta) = 0$ lying on $(0, \pi)$). The inequality $\Delta(\theta) > 0$ corresponds to the elliptic regime and the inequality $\Delta(\theta) < 0$ corresponds to the hyperbolic one.

iii) Let $N \geq 4$. Then on Σ_ε one can choose a coordinate system (ξ, η) depending on ε smoothly in which, after multiplying ε by a suitable nonzero constant, the curve Γ_ε^2 is given by the equation

$$\xi = \eta^2 \Theta(\eta, \varepsilon) \tag{23}$$

where Θ is a smooth function, and the curve Γ_ε^1 is given by the equation

$$\eta(\varepsilon \pm \eta^2 - \xi^2) + \xi^N = 0 \tag{24}$$

where the sign $+$ corresponds to the hyperbolic regime and the sign $-$ corresponds to the elliptic one (a regime is determined by the 3-jet of the field V_0).

REMARK 1. Actually, the conditions C_1 and C_2 are imposed on $(V_\varepsilon)_1$ and $(V_0)_N$ respectively and the condition C_3 is imposed on $(V_0)_2$ for $N = 2$ and on $(V_0)_3$ for $N \geq 3$.

REMARK 2. For $n=2$ the statement a) is trivial: $\sum_\varepsilon = Fix\,\mathcal{G}$.

REMARK 3. For $N=3$, $\Delta(\theta)$ is the discriminant of the cubic form $\xi^3+\xi\eta^2\cos\theta+\eta^3\sin\theta$.

REMARK 4. Let $N=3$. Multiplying, if necessary, the parameter ε by -1 one may achieve $\sin\theta \geqslant 0$.

PROOF. It follows from Theorems 6.9 - 6.11 formulated below (they play the same central role in the proof of Theorem 6.8 as Theorem 6.6 does in the proof of Theorem 6.5) that it suffices to reduce Γ^1_ε to the form (20), (22) or (24) (for corresponding values of N) in that case when all smooth changes of ε are allowed.

In $\mathbb{R}^{2n}$, there is such a complex coordinate system (z, Z) depending on ε smoothly in which

$$(V_\varepsilon)_1 = i(\omega+\alpha(\varepsilon))z_1\frac{\partial}{\partial z_1}+i(N\omega+\beta(\varepsilon))z_2\frac{\partial}{\partial z_2}+i(B_1(\varepsilon)Z+B_2(\varepsilon)\bar{Z})\frac{\partial}{\partial Z},$$

$$\mathcal{G}: (z, Z)\mapsto(\bar{z}, \bar{Z})$$

where α and β are real-valued functions in ε equaling $O(\varepsilon)$ while B_1 and B_2 are real matrix-valued (of order $n-2$) functions in ε.

We have $(N\omega+\beta)/(\omega+\alpha) = N+(\beta-N\alpha)/\omega+\sigma$, where $\sigma=\sigma(\varepsilon) = O_2(\varepsilon)$. Generically $\beta-N\alpha \neq O_2(\varepsilon)$ (this is the nondegeneracy condition C_1), and we can take $(\beta-N\alpha)/\omega+\sigma$ as a new parameter. Changing the time scale we can put $(V_\varepsilon)_1$ into the form

$$(V_\varepsilon)_1 = iz_1\frac{\partial}{\partial z_1}+i(N+\varepsilon)z_2\frac{\partial}{\partial z_2}+i(B_1Z+B_2\bar{Z})\frac{\partial}{\partial Z}$$

(with changed B_1 and B_2).

The surface $\mathcal{M}^2_\varepsilon$ is smooth, depends on ε smoothly, is invariant under σ and tangent to the two-dimensional plane $z_1=0, Z=0$ at 0. That is why by a suitable change of variables (with the identity linearization) depending on ε smoothly and commuting with σ one can make the equation of $\mathcal{M}^2_\varepsilon$ into $z_1=0$, $Z=0$. Then, as $\mathcal{M}^2_\varepsilon$ is invariant under V_ε ,

$$V_\varepsilon = i(z_1+\varphi^1_\varepsilon)\frac{\partial}{\partial z_1} + i((N+\varepsilon)z_2+\varphi^2_\varepsilon)\frac{\partial}{\partial z_2}$$

$$+i(B_1 Z + B_2\bar{Z} + \Phi_\varepsilon)\frac{\partial}{\partial Z} \tag{25}$$

where

$$\varphi^1_\varepsilon(z,Z) = O(z_1, Z)O(z,Z)$$

$$\varphi^2_\varepsilon(z,Z) = O_2(z,Z)$$

$$\Phi_\varepsilon(z,Z) = O(z_1, Z)O(z,Z).$$

Now, by means of the method of Poincaré-Dulac normal forms, for each $\ell \in \mathbb{N}$ by a change of variables smoothly depending on ε and commuting with σ we can achieve

$$\varphi^1_\varepsilon(z,Z) = z_1 P^1_\varepsilon(z_1\bar{z}_1, z_2\bar{z}_2) + (\gamma_1+O(\varepsilon))\bar{z}_1^{N-1} z_2$$

$$+O(Z)O(z,Z)+O(z_1)O_N(z)$$

$$\varphi^2_\varepsilon(z,Z) = z_2 P^2_\varepsilon(z_1\bar{z}_1, z_2\bar{z}_2) + (\gamma_2+O(\varepsilon))z_1^N \tag{26}$$

$$+O(Z)O(z,Z)+O_{N+1}(z)$$

$$\Phi_\varepsilon(z,Z) = O(Z)O(z,Z) + O(z_1)O_\ell(z)$$

where ρ^1_ε and ρ^2_ε are real depending on ε smoothly polynomials in 2 variables of degree $\leq [(N-1)/2]$ without a constant term (for $N=2$, $\rho^1_\varepsilon = \rho^2_\varepsilon = 0$), γ_1 and γ_2 are real numbers.

For our purposes, it will suffice to set $\ell = N-1$.

Let $(\mu^1_{\varepsilon,t}(z),\ \mu^2_{\varepsilon,t}(z))$ be the phase flow of the field

$$i(z_1 + z_1\rho^1_\varepsilon(z_1\bar z_1, z_2\bar z_2) + \gamma_1 \bar z_1^{N-1} z_2)\frac{\partial}{\partial z_1}$$

$$+ i((N+\varepsilon)z_2 + z_2\rho^2_\varepsilon(z_1\bar z_1,\ z_2\bar z_2) + \gamma_2 z_1^N)\frac{\partial}{\partial z_2}$$

in $\mathbb{R}^4$ and $f_t(Z)$ be the phase flow of the linear field $i(B_1(0)Z + B_2(0)\bar Z)\,\partial/\partial Z$ in $\mathbb{R}^{2n-4}$. Since $\mu^1_{\varepsilon,t}(z) = O(z_1)$, $\mu^1_{\varepsilon,t}(x) = O(x_1)$. Let $\operatorname{Im}\mu^1_{\varepsilon,t}(x) = x_1\mu^3_{\varepsilon,t}(x)$. Introduce also the notation $\operatorname{Im}\mu^2_{\varepsilon,t}(x) = \mu^4_{\varepsilon,t}(x)$.

Then, as is easy to verify,

$$\operatorname{Im} F_{\varepsilon,t}(x_1, x_2, X) = (\psi^1_{\varepsilon,t}(x,X),\ \psi^2_{\varepsilon,t}(x,X),\ \psi_{\varepsilon,t}(x,X))$$

where

$$\psi^1_{\varepsilon,t}(x,X) = x_1\mu^3_{\varepsilon,t}(x) + O(X)O(x,X) + x_1 O_N(x) + x_1^{N-1}x_2 O(\varepsilon)$$

$$\psi^2_{\varepsilon,t}(x,X) = \mu^4_{\varepsilon,t}(x) + O(X)O(x,X) + O_{N+1}(x) + x_1^N O(\varepsilon)$$

$$\psi_{\varepsilon,t}(x,X) = \operatorname{Im} f_t(X) + \varepsilon O(X) + O(X)O(x,X) + x_1 O_{N-1}(x).$$

Let $t = \pi + \tau$, where τ is small. Similarly to Lemma 1 it is easy to prove that the linear operator $X \mapsto \operatorname{Im} f_\pi(X)$ is nondegenerate. Now from $\psi_{\varepsilon,t}(x, X) = 0$ we obtain

$$X = x_1 g(x,\tau,\varepsilon) \tag{27}$$

where $g = O_{N-1}(x)$. Substituting (27) into $\Psi^1_{\varepsilon,t} = \Psi^2_{\varepsilon,t} = 0$ we rewrite the equation $\operatorname{Im} F_{\varepsilon,\pi+\tau}(x,X) = 0$ in the form

$$\begin{cases} x_1 \mu^3_{\varepsilon,\pi+\tau}(x) + x_1 b_1(x,\tau,\varepsilon) = 0 & (28) \\ \mu^4_{\varepsilon,\pi+\tau}(x) + b_2(x,\tau,\varepsilon) = 0 & (29) \\ X = x_1 g(x,\tau,\varepsilon) \end{cases}$$

where $b_1 = \varepsilon O_{N-1}(x) + O_N(x)$ and $b_2 = \varepsilon O_N(x) + O_{N+1}(x)$.

The equation (28) decomposes into two ones: $x_1 = 0$ and

$$\mu^3_{\varepsilon,\pi+\tau}(x) + b_1(x,\tau,\varepsilon) = 0 . \tag{30}$$

Let (30) hold. One sees that $\mu^3_{\varepsilon,\pi+\tau}(x) = -\sin\tau + O(x)$ and therefore can solve (30) for $\tau : \tau = K_1(x,\varepsilon)$, where $K_1 = O(x,\varepsilon)$. Let now $x_1 = 0$. Then from (27) $X = 0$. One sees that

$$\mu^4_{\varepsilon,\pi+\tau}(x) = (-1)^N x_2 \sin(N\tau + \varepsilon\pi + \varepsilon\tau) + O_2(x) .$$

Therefore, after the substitution of $x_1 = 0$ into (29) the equation (29) decomposes into $x_2 = 0$ and

$$\sin(N\tau + \varepsilon\pi + \varepsilon\tau) + b_3(x_2,\tau,\varepsilon) = 0$$

where $b_3 = O(x_2)$. Solving the last equation for τ we obtain $\tau = K_2(x_2,\varepsilon)$, where $K_2 = -\varepsilon\pi/(N+\varepsilon) + O(x_2)$.

Consider the mapping $\mathcal{F} : \mathbb{R}^{n+2} \to \mathbb{R}^n$, $\mathcal{F} : (\varepsilon,\tau,x,X) \mapsto \operatorname{Im} F_{\varepsilon,\pi+\tau}(x,X)$ defined near $0 \in \mathbb{R}^{n+2}$. Introduce the notation $R(x,t,\varepsilon) = \mu^4_{\varepsilon,\pi+\tau}(x) + b_2(x,\tau,\varepsilon)$. We have proved that $\mathcal{F}^{-1}(0)$ consists of the two-dimensional plane

$$x=0\ ,\ X=0$$

(corresponding to the origin), the smooth two-dimensional surface

$$x_1 = 0$$

$$\tau = K_2(x_2,\varepsilon)$$

$$X=0$$

(corresponding to Γ_ε^2) and the two-dimensional surface

$$\tau = K_1(x,\varepsilon)$$

$$R(x,\tau,\varepsilon)=0$$

$$X = x_1 g(x,\tau,\varepsilon)$$

(corresponding to Γ_ε^1).

It is

$$X = x_1 g(x, K_1(x,\varepsilon),\varepsilon) \tag{31}$$

that is the equation of the desired surface Σ_ε on which the curves Γ_ε^1 and Γ_ε^2 lie. Note that $x_1 g(x, K_1(x,\varepsilon),\varepsilon) = O_N(x)$.

In the space

$$\mathbb{R}^3 = \bigcup_\varepsilon (\Sigma_\varepsilon \times \{\varepsilon\}),$$

where coordinates on Σ_ε are x_1 and x_2 , we obtain a plane Π_2 given by the equation $x_1 = 0$ and a two-dimensional surface Π_1 given by the equation $S(x,\varepsilon)=0$ where $S(x,\varepsilon) = R(x,K_1(x,\varepsilon),\varepsilon)$.

Sections of surfaces Π_1 and Π_2 by level planes of the coordinate function $\varepsilon : (\mathbb{R}^3, 0) \to (\mathbb{R}, 0)$ are just the curves Γ^1_ε and Γ^2_ε respectively. Thus, we must reduce the diagram

$$\begin{array}{ccccc} \Pi_1 & \searrow & & & \\ & & \mathbb{R}^3 & \xrightarrow{\varepsilon} & \mathbb{R} \\ \Pi_2 & \nearrow & & & \end{array}$$

to a normal form (paying peculiar attention to the subdiagram

$$\Pi_1 \hookrightarrow \mathbb{R}^3 \xrightarrow{\varepsilon} \mathbb{R}) .$$

A. Let $N=2$.

It is easy to verify that

$$\mu^3_{\varepsilon,t}(x) = \sin t + \gamma_1 x_2 t \cos t + \varepsilon O(x) + O_2(x) \quad ,$$

$$\mu^4_{\varepsilon,t}(x) = x_2 \sin(2+\varepsilon)t + \gamma_2 x_1^2 t \cos 2t + \varepsilon O_2(x) + O_3(x).$$

Solving the equation (30) for τ we obtain

$$\tau = K_1(x,\varepsilon) = -\pi \gamma_1 x_2 + \varepsilon O(x) + O_2(x) .$$

Hence, the function $S(x,\varepsilon)$ whose zero level surface is Π_1 equals

$$S(x,\varepsilon) = x_2 \sin \pi\varepsilon - 2\pi\gamma_1 x_2^2 + \pi\gamma_2 x_1^2 + \varepsilon O_2(x) + O_3(x) . \tag{32}$$

Let $\gamma_2 \neq 0$ (this is the nondegeneracy condition C_2). Then the surface Π_1 is diffeomorphic to a cone, i.e. is a singularity of type A_1 (see [37 (Chapter II , § 17, 17.1)]). Indeed,

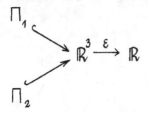

$S(x,\varepsilon)=\pi(x_2(\varepsilon-2\gamma_1 x_2)+\gamma_2 x_1^2)+O_3(\varepsilon,x)$. There is a coordinate system $u=(u_1, u_2, u_3)$ in which the cone Π_1 is given by the equation $u_1^2+u_2^2-u_3^2=0$.

In the tangent space $T_0\mathbb{R}^3$, the quadratic part of $S(x,\varepsilon)$ invariantly determines a nondegenerate quadratic form B of type either $++-$ (for $\gamma_2>0$) or $+--$ (for $\gamma_2<0$). We say that two smooth surfaces in $\mathbb{R}^3$ passing through 0 are conjugate with respect to the cone Π_1 if their tangent planes at 0 are conjugate with respect to the quadratic form B (i.e. the line which is the B - orthocomplement to one plane lies on the other plane). One sees the planes $\Pi_2=\{x_1=0\}$ and $\{\varepsilon=0\}$ be conjugate with respect to Π_1.

The cone $\{B=0\}$ intersects the tangent plane at 0 to a smooth surface in $\mathbb{R}^3$ passing through 0 along several straight lines. We call the number of these lines (0, 1, or 2) the type of a given surface with respect to the cone Π_1. Type 1 corresponds to a degenerate position of a surface in regard to Π_1.

The type of the plane Π_2 with respect to Π_1 is always equal to 2. The type of the plane $\{\varepsilon=0\}$ equals 0, 1, or 2 according as $\gamma_1\gamma_2<0$, $\gamma_1=0$, or $\gamma_1\gamma_2>0$.

Let $\gamma_1\neq 0$ (this is the nondegeneracy condition C_3).

THEOREM 6.9. In $\mathbb{R}^3$ consider a cone $u_1^2+u_2^2-u_3^2=0$, a smooth passing through 0 surface Π of type 2 with respect to this cone and a smooth function $\rho:(\mathbb{R}^3,0)\longrightarrow(\mathbb{R},0)$ whose differential at 0 is nondegenerate. Let the surface $\rho^{-1}(0)$ have type either 0 or 2 and be conjugate to the surface Π with respect to the cone.

Then the surface Π and the function ρ can be put into the normal form

$$\Pi=\{u_1=0\},\quad \rho=u_3,\quad \text{if the type of } \rho^{-1}(0) \text{ is } 0$$
$$\Pi=\{u_1=0\},\quad \rho=u_2,\quad \text{if the type of } \rho^{-1}(0) \text{ is } 2 \tag{33}$$

via a diffeomorphism $(\mathbb{R}^3, 0) \longrightarrow (\mathbb{R}^3, 0)$ leaving the cone invariant.

PROOF. At first reduce the equation of Π to the form $u_1 + O_2(u) = 0$. Let the equation of Π be $\tau_1 u_1 + \tau_2 u_2 + \tau_3 u_3 + O_2(u) = 0$, where $\tau_1^2 + \tau_2^2 + \tau_3^2 > 0$. Since Π is of type 2 with respect to the cone, $\tau_1^2 + \tau_2^2 > \tau_3^2$. The linear diffeomorphism

$$
\begin{aligned}
u_1 & \qquad (\tau_1 u_1 + \tau_2 u_2 + \tau_3 u_3)\sqrt{\tau_1^2 + \tau_2^2} \\
u_2 & \longmapsto (\tau_2 u_1 - \tau_1 u_2)\sqrt{\tau_1^2 + \tau_2^2 - \tau_3^2} \\
u_3 & \qquad \tau_1 \tau_3 u_1 + \tau_2 \tau_3 u_2 + (\tau_1^2 + \tau_2^2) u_3
\end{aligned}
$$

preserves the cone and takes the equation of Π into the form $u_1 + O_2(u) = 0$.

Now let us prove the following lemma that we shall need also in future.

LEMMA 3. Let $p, q \in \{1; 2; 3\}$ and $p \neq q$. Let a smooth function $\tilde{p} : (\mathbb{R}^3, 0) \longrightarrow (\mathbb{R}, 0)$ be $\tilde{p}(u) = u_p + O_2(u)$. Then one can put the function $\tilde{p}$ into the form $\tilde{p}(u) = u_p$ via a diffeomorphism of $\mathbb{R}^3$ preserving the cone $u_1^2 + u_2^2 - u_3^2 = 0$ and the plane $u_q = 0$.

PROOF. Without loss of generality we may assume $p = 1$ and $q = 2$. Use the homotopic method. Vectorfields $v_1 = u_1 \partial/\partial u_1 + u_2 \partial/\partial u_2 + u_3 \partial/\partial u_3$ (an "Euler" field), $v_2 = u_2 \partial/\partial u_1 - u_1 \partial/\partial u_2$ and $v_3 = u_3 \partial/\partial u_1 + u_1 \partial/\partial u_3$ ("Hamiltonian" fields) are tangent to the cone. Fields v_1, $u_2 v_2$ and v_3 are also tangent to the plane $u_2 = 0$. For each smooth function $h(u) = O_2(u)$ we must select such smooth functions $\delta_\nu(u, t)$ (where $t \in [0, 1]$), $\nu = 1, 2, 3$, that the derivative of the function $u_1 + t h(u)$ along the vectorfield $v_t = \delta_1 v_1 + u_2 \delta_2 v_2 + \delta_3 v_3$ equals $-h$, i.e. that

$$(1+t\frac{\partial h}{\partial u_1})(u_1\delta_1+u_2^2\delta_2+u_3\delta_3)$$

$$+t\frac{\partial h}{\partial u_2}(u_2\delta_1-u_1u_2\delta_2)+t\frac{\partial h}{\partial u_3}(u_3\delta_1+u_1\delta_3)=-h\ . \tag{34}$$

In the coordinate system

$$\tilde{u}_1=u_1+tu_1\frac{\partial h}{\partial u_1}+tu_2\frac{\partial h}{\partial u_2}+tu_3\frac{\partial h}{\partial u_3}$$

$$\tilde{u}_2=u_2$$

$$\tilde{u}_3=u_3+tu_3\frac{\partial h}{\partial u_1}+tu_1\frac{\partial h}{\partial u_3}$$

the equation (34) gets the form

$$\tilde{u}_1\delta_1+(\tilde{u}_2^2+O_3(\tilde{u}))\delta_2+\tilde{u}_3\delta_3=-h\ .$$

The last equation is to be solved easily. X

Applying Lemma 3 for $p=1$ (and any $q\in\{2;3\}$) we reduce Π to the normal form $\{u_1=0\}$.

See to the function ρ . Since the surface $\rho^{-1}(0)$ is conjugate to Π with respect to the cone, the function ρ has the form $\rho(u)=s_2u_2+s_3u_3+O_2(u)$, where $s_2^2+s_3^2>0$. As the type of $\rho^{-1}(0)$ does not equal 1, $|s_2|\neq|s_3|$. $\rho^{-1}(0)$ has type 0 or 2 according as $|s_2|<|s_3|$ or $|s_2|>|s_3|$. If $|s_2|<|s_3|$ then the linear diffeomorphism

$$\begin{matrix} u_1 & & u_1\sqrt{s_3^2-s_2^2} \\ u_2 & \longmapsto & s_3u_2+s_2u_3 \\ u_3 & & s_2u_2+s_3u_3 \end{matrix}$$

preserves both the cone and Π and puts ρ into the form $\rho(u) = u_3 + O_2(u)$. It remains to apply Lemma 3 for $p=3, q=1$. If $|s_2|>|s_3|$ then the linear diffeomorphism

$$\begin{matrix} u_1 & & u_1\sqrt{s_2^2-s_3^2} \\ u_2 & \longmapsto & s_2u_2+s_3u_3 \\ u_3 & & s_3u_2+s_2u_3 \end{matrix}$$

preserves both the cone and Π and puts ρ into the form $\rho(u) = u_2 + O_2(u)$. It remains to apply Lemma 3 for $p=2, q=1$. X

Theorem 6.9 is proved. Now, setting $\Pi=\Pi_2$ and $\rho=\mathcal{E}$ in Theorem 6.9, we can reduce Π_2 and $\mathcal{E}$ to the normal form (33) preserving the cone $\Pi_1=\{u_1^2+u_2^2-u_3^2=0\}$. Introducing the coordinates $\xi=u_1/2$ and $\eta=(u_2+u_3)/2$ in a level surface Σ_ε of the function $\mathcal{E}$ we obtain the equation (20) of curves Γ_ε^1 (the elliptic regime for $\gamma_1\gamma_2<0$ and the hyperbolic one for $\gamma_1\gamma_2>0$) and the equation $\xi=0$ of curves Γ_ε^2.

The case $N=2$ is examined completely. The bifurcations of Γ_ε^1 in the elliptic and hyperbolic regimes are shown in figures 4 and 5, respectively. The curve Γ_ε^2 coincides with the ordinate $\xi=0$.

Note that for $\varepsilon=0$ in the elliptic regime Γ_ε^1 is just the origin whereas in the hyperbolic regime the surface $\mathcal{M}_\varepsilon^1$ consists of two leaves foliated into symmetric cycles and intersecting $\mathrm{Fix}\,G$ along two curves which are given in coordinates (ξ,η) on Σ_0 by equations $\eta=\pm|\xi|$. In the coordinate system (x,X) half-curves $\eta=\pm\xi$, $\xi\geqslant 0$ have the form $x_1\geqslant 0$, $x_2=\pm x_1\sqrt{\gamma_2/2\gamma_1}$

$+ O_2(x_1)$, $X = O_2(x_1)$ (see (31), (32)). Applying Theorem 6.7 (in this case in the notations of Theorem 6.7 one has $N=2$, $\kappa=+\infty$, $d=2$, $\ell=1$ (see (25), (26)), $m=1$, $j=2$ and sees all the conditions of Theorem 6.7 be fulfilled) we obtain that at 0 the leaves in question do not possess even the smoothness C^1.

Proceed to the case $N \geqslant 3$. Let in (26) $\overset{\nu}{\rho}_0(y_1, y_2) = \overset{\nu}{Q}_1 y_1 + \overset{\nu}{Q}_2 y_2 + O_2(y)$, $\nu = 1, 2$, where $\overset{\nu}{Q}_1$ and $\overset{\nu}{Q}_2$ are real numbers.

B. Let $N=3$.

It is easy to verify that

$$\overset{3}{\mu}_{\varepsilon,t}(x) = \sin t + (\overset{1}{Q}_1 \overset{2}{x}_1 + \overset{1}{Q}_2 \overset{2}{x}_2 + \gamma_1 x_1 x_2) t \cos t + \varepsilon O_2(x) + O_3(x),$$

$$\overset{4}{\mu}_{\varepsilon,t}(x) = x_2 \sin(3+\varepsilon)t + (\overset{2}{Q}_1 \overset{2}{x}_1 x_2 + \overset{2}{Q}_2 \overset{3}{x}_2 + \gamma_2 \overset{3}{x}_1) t \cos 3t$$

$$+ \varepsilon O_3(x) + O_4(x).$$

Solving the equation (30) for τ we obtain

$$\tau = K_1(x, \varepsilon) = -\pi(\overset{1}{Q}_1 \overset{2}{x}_1 + \overset{1}{Q}_2 \overset{2}{x}_2 + \gamma_1 x_1 x_2) + \varepsilon O_2(x) + O_3(x).$$

Hence, the function $S(x, \varepsilon)$ whose zero level surface is Π_1 equals

$$\begin{aligned} -S(x,\varepsilon) &= x_2 \sin \pi\varepsilon + \pi(\overset{2}{Q}_1 - 3\overset{1}{Q}_1) \overset{2}{x}_1 x_2 - 3\pi\gamma_1 x_1 \overset{2}{x}_2 \\ &+ \pi(\overset{2}{Q}_2 - 3\overset{1}{Q}_2) \overset{3}{x}_2 + \pi\gamma_2 \overset{3}{x}_1 + \varepsilon O_3(x) + O_4(x). \end{aligned} \tag{35}$$

Let $\gamma_2 \neq 0$ (this is the nondegeneracy condition C_2). Then we have

$$-\frac{S(x,\varepsilon)}{\pi\gamma_2} = \frac{x_2}{\gamma_2}\Big(\frac{\sin \pi\varepsilon}{\pi} + (\overset{2}{Q}_1 - 3\overset{1}{Q}_1) \overset{2}{x}_1 - 3\gamma_1 x_1 x_2 + (\overset{2}{Q}_2 - 3\overset{1}{Q}_2) \overset{2}{x}_2$$

$$+\varepsilon O_2(x)+O_3(x))+x_1^3(1+O(\varepsilon,x)) .$$

Consequently, one can introduce such a coordinate system $u=(u_1,u_2,u_3)$, where

$$x_1=u_1(1+O(u))$$

$$x_2=\gamma_2 u_2$$

$$\varepsilon=u_3+(3Q_1^1-Q_1^2)u_1^2+3\gamma_1\gamma_2 u_1 u_2+(3Q_2^1-Q_2^2)\gamma_2^2 u_2^2$$

$$+u_3 O(u)+O_3(u) ,$$

in which the surfaces Π_1 and Π_2 are given by equations $u_2 u_3+u_1^3=0$ and $u_1=0$ respectively. The surface Π_1 is a singularity of type A_2. In the tangent space $T_0\mathbb{R}^3$, the quadratic part of the equation of Π_1 invariantly determines a degenerate quadratic form of type $+-0$. This form has two isotropic planes on which it vanishes. The tangent plane to the surface $\varepsilon^{-1}(0)$ at 0 is one of these planes.

The line $u_1=u_2=0$ corresponds to the equilibrium of the original field V_ε for various values of ε.

THEOREM 6.10. In the space $\mathbb{R}^3$ with coordinates $u=(u_1,u_2,u_3)$ consider the surface $\Pi_1=\{u_2u_3+u_1^3=0\}$, the plane $\Pi_2=\{u_1=0\}$ and a smooth function

$$\rho(u)=su_3+\tau_1 u_1^2+\tau_2 u_1 u_2+\tau_3 u_2^2+u_3 O(u)+O_3(u)$$

where $s\neq 0$. Let the cubic form

$$su_1^3-\tau_1 u_1^2 u_2-\tau_2 u_1 u_2^2-\tau_3 u_2^3$$

be nondegenerate (as is easy to verify, this condition is invariant under diffeomorphisms of $\mathbb{R}^3$ preserving the surface Π_1).

Then via a diffeomorphism of $\mathbb{R}^3$ leaving both the surface Π_1 and the line $u_1 = u_2 = 0$ invariant one can put the function ρ into the form

$$\rho = u_3 - p u_1 u_2 - q u_2^2 , \tag{36}$$

where $p^2 + q^2 = 1$ and $4p^3 + 27q^2 \neq 0$, and simultaneously the equation of the surface Π_2 into the form

$$u_1 = c u_2 + u_2^2 \Theta(u_2, u_3) , \tag{37}$$

where Θ is smooth.

Moreover, multiplying, if necessary, the function ρ by -1, one can achieve $q \geq 0$ in (36).

PROOF. Firstly reduce the function ρ to the form

$$\rho_0 = s u_3 + \tau_1 u_1^2 + \tau_2 u_1 u_2 + \tau_3 u_2^2 .$$

Use the homotopic method. Vectorfields $v_1 = u_2 \partial/\partial u_1 - 3u_1^2 \partial/\partial u_3$ (a "Hamiltonian" field), $v_2 = u_1 \partial/\partial u_1 + 3u_2 \partial/\partial u_2$, $v_3 = u_1 \partial/\partial u_1 + 3u_3 \partial/\partial u_3$ ("Euler" fields) are tangent to both the surface Π_1 and the line $u_1 = u_2 = 0$. Let $h(u)$ be an arbitrary function equaling $u_3 O(u) + O_3(u)$. We must find such smooth functions $\delta_\nu(u,t)$ (where $t \in [0,1]$), $\nu = 1,2,3,$ that the derivative of the function $\rho_0 + th$ along the vectorfield $v_t = \delta_1 v_1 + \delta_2 v_2 + \delta_3 v_3$ equals $-h$, i.e. that

$$\left(\frac{\partial \rho_0}{\partial u_1} + t\frac{\partial h}{\partial u_1}\right)(u_2\delta_1 + u_1\delta_2 + u_1\delta_3) + 3\left(\frac{\partial \rho_0}{\partial u_2} + t\frac{\partial h}{\partial u_2}\right)u_2\delta_2$$
$$+ 3\left(s + t\frac{\partial h}{\partial u_3}\right)(-u_1^2\delta_1 + u_3\delta_3) = -h . \tag{38}$$

Introduce the new coordinate system $\tilde{u}=(u_1, u_2, \tilde{u}_3)$, where

$$\tilde{u}_3 = 3su_3 + \frac{\partial \rho_0}{\partial u_1} u_1 + t u_1 \frac{\partial h}{\partial u_1} + 3t u_3 \frac{\partial h}{\partial u_3} = 3su_3 + O_2(u).$$

The equation (38) may be rewritten in the form

$$\tilde{u}_3 \delta_3 + \left(\frac{\partial \rho_0}{\partial u_1} u_2 - 3su_1^2 + \tilde{u}_3 O(\tilde{u}) + O_3(\tilde{u}) \right) \delta_1$$

$$+ \left(\frac{\partial \rho_0}{\partial u_1} u_1 + 3 \frac{\partial \rho_0}{\partial u_2} u_2 + \tilde{u}_3 O(\tilde{u}) + O_3(\tilde{u}) \right) \delta_2 = \tilde{u}_3 O(\tilde{u}) + O_3(\tilde{u}) .$$

It suffices to solve the following equation assuming functions δ_1 and δ_2 to be independent of $\tilde{u}_3$:

$$(\Lambda_1(u_1, u_2) + \mu_1(u_1, u_2, t))\delta_1$$

$$+ (\Lambda_2(u_1, u_2) + \mu_2(u_1, u_2, t))\delta_2 = \mu_0(u_1, u_2, t) \tag{39}$$

where

$$\Lambda_1 = \frac{\partial \rho_0}{\partial u_1} u_2 - 3su_1^2 , \quad \Lambda_2 = \frac{\partial \rho_0}{\partial u_1} u_1 + 3 \frac{\partial \rho_0}{\partial u_2} u_2$$

are quadratic forms, whereas $\mu_0, \mu_1, \mu_2 = O_3(u_1, u_2)$.

The last equation is solvable always, which is a consequence of the following general lemma.

LEMMA 4. Let Λ_1 and Λ_2 be two quadratic forms in u_1 and u_2 which have no common linear factor (over $\mathbb{C}$). Then for any functions μ_0, μ_1, μ_2 in u_1, u_2, t equaling $O_3(u_1, u_2)$ the equation (39) is solvable for δ_1 and δ_2 .

PROOF. If $\Lambda_1 = u_1 u_2$, $\mu_1 = 0$ and $\Lambda_2 = s_1 u_1^2 + s_2 u_2^2$, where $s_1 s_2 \neq 0$, then one can solve the equation (39) easily. The general case can be reduced to this special one as follows. First of all, since Λ_1 and Λ_2 are linearly independent, there exists their linear combination $d_1 \Lambda_1 + d_2 \Lambda_2$ of type $+-$. By the Morse lemma, one may put the function $d_1(\Lambda_1 + \mu_1) + d_2(\Lambda_2 + \mu_2)$ into the form $u_1 u_2$ by means of a t-dependent diffeomorphism $(\mathbb{R}^2, 0) \to (\mathbb{R}^2, 0)$. Thus, we may suppose $\Lambda_1 = u_1 u_2$ and $\mu_1 = 0$. Then $\Lambda_2 = s_1 u_1^2 + s_3 u_1 u_2 + s_2 u_2^2$, where $s_1 s_2 \neq 0$ (otherwise Λ_1 and Λ_2 would have a common linear factor). Replacing Λ_2 by the linear combination $\Lambda_2 - s_3 \Lambda_1$ we shall obtain the desired special case. X

In our situation

$$\Lambda_1 = \frac{\partial \rho_0}{\partial u_1} u_2 - 3 s u_1^2 = -\frac{\partial}{\partial u_1}(s u_1^3 - u_2 \lambda),$$

$$\Lambda_2 = \frac{\partial \rho_0}{\partial u_1} u_1 + 3 \frac{\partial \rho_0}{\partial u_2} u_2 = 2\left(\lambda + u_2 \frac{\partial \lambda}{\partial u_2}\right) = -2 \frac{\partial}{\partial u_2}(s u_1^3 - u_2 \lambda)$$

where $\lambda(u_1, u_2) = \rho_0(u_1, u_2, u_3) - s u_3$ (we have used the Euler formula $u_1 \partial\lambda/\partial u_1 + u_2 \partial\lambda/\partial u_2 = 2\lambda$). Since the cubic form $s u_1^3 - u_2 \lambda$ is nondegenerate according to assumptions, Λ_1 and Λ_2 have no common linear factor and, therefore, the equation (39) is solvable.

Note that the solution of the equation (38) constructed by us satisfies the conditions

$$\delta_1 = \delta_1(u_1, u_2, t) = O(u_1, u_2)$$

$$\delta_2 = \delta_2(u_1, u_2, t) = O(u_1, u_2)$$

$$\delta_3 = \delta_3(u_1, u_2, u_3, t) = O(u) .$$

Hence, the field v_t is of the form

$$(u_1 O(u)+O_2(u_2))\frac{\partial}{\partial u_1}+u_2 O(u_1,u_2)\frac{\partial}{\partial u_2}+O_2(u)\frac{\partial}{\partial u_3}.$$

Therefore the family of diffeomorphisms $D_t:(\mathbb{R}^3,0)\to(\mathbb{R}^3,0)$, $D_0=id$, associated with the field v_t, has the form

$$D_t:\begin{matrix} u_1 \\ u_2 \\ u_3 \end{matrix}\mapsto\begin{matrix} u_1+tu_1 O(u)+tO_2(u_2) \\ u_2+tu_2 O(u_1,u_2) \\ u_3+tO_2(u). \end{matrix}$$

Consequently, the diffeomorphism D_1 maps the plane $\Pi_2=\{u_1=0\}$ onto a surface $u_1=u_2^2\Theta(u_2,u_3)$ where Θ is a smooth function.

Thus, let

$$\rho=\rho_0=su_3+\tau_1 u_1^2+\tau_2 u_1 u_2+\tau_3 u_2^2,$$

$$\Pi_2=\{u_1=u_2^2\Theta(u_2,u_3)\}.$$

Consider a diffeomorphism

$$D^*:\begin{matrix} u_1 \\ u_2 \\ u_3 \end{matrix}\mapsto\begin{matrix} \varkappa_1\varkappa_3 u_1+\varkappa_2 u_2 \\ \varkappa_1^3 u_2 \\ \varkappa_3^3 u_3-\dfrac{3\varkappa_2\varkappa_3^2}{\varkappa_1}u_1^2-\dfrac{3\varkappa_2^2\varkappa_3}{\varkappa_1^2}u_1u_2-\dfrac{\varkappa_2^3}{\varkappa_1^3}u_2^2 \end{matrix}$$

where $\varkappa_1$, $\varkappa_2$, $\varkappa_3$ are arbitrary real numbers, $\varkappa_1\neq 0$, $\varkappa_3\neq 0$. This diffeomorphism leaves both the surface Π_1 and the line $u_1=u_2=0$ invariant and puts the equation of the surface Π_2 into the form (37) with $C = -\varkappa_2/(\varkappa_1 \varkappa_3)$.

The function $\rho \circ D^*$ equals

$$\tilde{s} u_3 + \tilde{\tau}_1 u_1^2 + \tilde{\tau}_2 u_1 u_2 + \tilde{\tau}_3 u_2^2 ,$$

where

$$\tilde{s} = \varkappa_3^3 s$$

$$\tilde{\tau}_1 = -\frac{3\varkappa_2 \varkappa_3^2}{\varkappa_1} s + \tau_1 \varkappa_1^2 \varkappa_3^2$$

$$\tilde{\tau}_2 = -\frac{3\varkappa_2^2 \varkappa_3}{\varkappa_1^2} s + 2\tau_1 \varkappa_1 \varkappa_2 \varkappa_3 + \tau_2 \varkappa_1^4 \varkappa_3$$

$$\tilde{\tau}_3 = -\frac{\varkappa_2^3}{\varkappa_1^3} s + \tau_1 \varkappa_2^2 + \tau_2 \varkappa_1^3 \varkappa_2 + \tau_3 \varkappa_1^6 .$$

Set $\varkappa_3 = s^{1/3}$ and $\varkappa_2 = \tau_1 \varkappa_1^3 / 3s$. Then $\tilde{s} = 1$, $\tilde{\tau}_1 = 0$, $\tilde{\tau}_2 = -\tilde{p} \varkappa_1^4$, $\tilde{\tau}_3 = -\tilde{q} \varkappa_1^6$, where $\tilde{p}$ and $\tilde{q}$ are some functions in $s, \tau_1, \tau_2, \tau_3$. The nondegeneracy condition imposed on the cubic form $u_1^3 - \tilde{\tau}_2 u_1 u_2^2 - \tilde{\tau}_3 u_2^3$ gives $-4\tilde{\tau}_2^3 + 27\tilde{\tau}_3^2 \neq 0$. Selecting $\varkappa_1$ we can achieve $\tilde{\tau}_2^2 + \tilde{\tau}_3^2 = 1$. Now setting $p = -\tilde{\tau}_2$, $q = -\tilde{\tau}_3$ we obtain (36).

If $q < 0$ then changing the sign of the function ρ , of the coordinate u_3 and of one of the coordinates u_1 or u_2 , we will change the sign of q. X

Theorem 6.10 is proved. Setting $\rho = \varepsilon$ in it and supposing that the cubic form

$$u_1^3 + (Q_1^2 - 3Q_1^1) u_1^2 u_2 - 3\gamma_1 \gamma_2 u_1 u_2^2 + (Q_2^2 - 3Q_2^1) \gamma_2^2 u_2^3$$

is nondegenerate (this is the nondegeneracy condition C_3) we may reduce ε and Π_2 to normal forms (36) and (37) preserving Π_1.

Taking $\xi = u_1$ and $\eta = u_2$ as coordinates on the surface Σ_ε we obtain equations (22) and (21) of curves Γ_ε^1 and Γ_ε^2 respectively.

REMARK 1. Let $q > 0$ in the normal form (36). Then the diffeomorphism

$$(u_1, u_2, u_3) \mapsto (q^{-1/6} u_1, q^{-1/2} u_2, u_3)$$

leaving Π_1 invariant puts the function ρ into the form $u_3 - C_1 u_1 u_2 - u_2^2$, where $C_1 = p q^{-2/3}$.

REMARK 2. One sees the normal form of curves Γ_ε^1 and Γ_ε^2 for $N=3$ contain (not to mention the function Θ) two moduli: θ and C. Their origin is the following one. On the tangent plane $T_0 \Sigma_0$, we have 5 straight lines passing through 0, namely, the line $\xi = C\eta$ tangent to Γ_0^2 at 0, the line $\eta = 0$ along which $T_0 \Sigma_0$ intersects the isotropic plane $u_2 = 0$, and 3 lines given by the equation

$$\eta(\eta \xi \cos\theta + \eta^2 \sin\theta) + \xi^3 = 0 \tag{40}$$

(two of them are complex in the elliptic regime but this is of no consequence). Cross ratios of any two of the quadruplets of these 5 straight lines are just two muduli in our problem.

The case $N=3$ is examined completely. The bifurcations of Γ_ε^1 in the elliptic and hyperbolic regimes are shown in figures 6 and 7 for $\theta = \pi/2$ and $\cos\theta = -\sqrt{24}/5$ respectively. To guide the eye, in both figures for $\varepsilon \neq 0$ there is depicted the curve Γ_0^1 by a dotted line. The curve Γ_ε^2 (for $C = 1/2$) is drawn by a dashed line.

Note that if in addition to the nondegeneracy conditions C_1, C_2, C_3, the condition $Q_2^2 \neq 3Q_2^1$ holds then the line $\xi = C\eta$ coincides with none of the lines given by the equation (40) (as in figures 6 and 7). Find the smoothness of leaves of $\mathcal{M}_0^1$ at 0 in the case $Q_2^2 \neq 3Q_2^1$. In the elliptic regime the curve Γ_0^1 is a straight line (in coordinates (ξ, η)) passing through 0, while in the hyperbolic regime it is the union of 3 such lines. In the coordinate system (x, X) these lines have the form $x_2 = C_* x_1 + O_2(x_1)$, $X = O_3(x_1)$, where $C_* \neq 0$ (see (31), (35)). Applying Theorem 6.7 (in this case in the notations of Theorem 6.7 one has $N=3$, $\kappa=+\infty$, $d=3$, $\ell=2$ (see (25), (26)), $m=1$, $j=3$ and sees all the conditions of Theorem 6.7 be fulfilled) we obtain that in the elliptic regime the surface $\mathcal{M}_0^1$ consists of a single leaf whereas in the hyperbolic regime it consists of 3 leaves and in both regimes these foliated into symmetric cycles leaves do not possess even the smoothness C^1 at 0.

C. Let $N \geq 4$.

It is easy to verify that

$$\mu_{\varepsilon,t}^3(x) = \sin t + (Q_1^1 x_1^2 + Q_2^1 x_2^2) t \cos t + \varepsilon O_2(x) + O_3(x),$$

$$\mu_{\varepsilon,t}^4(x) = x_2 \sin(N+\varepsilon)t + (Q_1^2 x_1^2 x_2 + Q_2^2 x_2^3) t \cos Nt + x_2 O_3(x)$$

$$+ \gamma_2 x_1^N t \cos Nt + \varepsilon x_2 O_2(x) + \varepsilon O_N(x) + O_{N+1}(x).$$

Solving the equation (30) for τ we obtain

$$\tau = K_1(x,\varepsilon) = -\pi(Q_1^1 x_1^2 + Q_2^1 x_2^2) + \varepsilon O_2(x) + O_3(x).$$

Hence, the function $S(x, \varepsilon)$ whose zero level surface is Π_1 equals

$$(-1)^N S(x,\varepsilon) = x_2 \sin \pi\varepsilon + \pi(Q_1^2 - NQ_1^1) x_1^2 x_2 + \pi(Q_2^2 - NQ_2^1) x_2^3$$

$$+ x_2 O_3(x) + \pi \gamma_2 x_1^N + \varepsilon x_2 O_2(x) + \varepsilon O_N(x) + O_{N+1}(x). \tag{41}$$

Let $\gamma_2 \neq 0$ (this is the nondegeneracy condition C_2). Then we have

$$(-1)^N \frac{S(x,\varepsilon)}{\pi\gamma_2} = \frac{x_2}{\gamma_2}\Big(\frac{\sin\pi\varepsilon}{\pi} + (Q_1^2 - NQ_1^1)x_1^2 + (Q_2^2 - NQ_2^1)x_2^2$$

$$+ \varepsilon O_2(x) + O_3(x)\Big) + x_1^N(1 + O(\varepsilon, x)) .$$

Consequently, one can introduce such a coordinate system $u = (u_1, u_2, u_3)$, where

$$x_1 = u_1(1 + O(u))$$

$$x_2 = \gamma_2 u_2$$

$$\varepsilon = u_3 + (NQ_1^1 - Q_1^2)u_1^2 + (NQ_2^1 - Q_2^2)\gamma_2^2 u_2^2 + u_3 O(u) + O_3(u) ,$$

in which the surfaces Π_1 and Π_2 are given by equations $u_2 u_3 + u_1^N = 0$ and $u_1 = 0$ respectively. The surface Π_1 is a singularity of type A_{N-1}. The tangent plane to the surface $\varepsilon^{-1}(0)$ at 0, i.e. the plane $u_3 = 0$, is one of two isotropic planes of the quadratic form $u_2 u_3$.

The line $u_1 = u_2 = 0$ corresponds to the equilibrium of the original field V_ε for various values of ε.

THEOREM 6.11. In the space $\mathbb{R}^3$ with coordinates $u = (u_1, u_2, u_3)$ consider the surface $\Pi_1 = \{u_2 u_3 + u_1^N = 0\}$, where $N \geq 4$, the plane $\Pi_2 = \{u_1 = 0\}$ and a smooth function

$$\rho(u) = s u_3 + \tau_1 u_1^2 + \tau_2 u_2^2 + u_3 O(u) + O_3(u) ,$$

where $s \neq 0$, $\tau_1 \neq 0$, $\tau_2 \neq 0$.

Then via a diffeomorphism of $\mathbb{R}^3$ leaving both the surface Π_1 and the line $u_1 = u_2 = 0$ invariant one can put the function ρ into the form

$$\rho = c(u_3 + u_1^2 + \varkappa u_2^2), \tag{42}$$

where $c \in \mathbb{R}$, $c \neq 0$, $\varkappa \in \{-1; 1\}$, and simultaneously the equation of the surface Π_2 into the form

$$u_1 = u_2^2 \Theta(u_2, u_3), \tag{43}$$

where Θ is smooth.

PROOF. Firstly reduce the function ρ to the form

$$\rho_0 = s u_3 + \tau_1 u_1^2 + \tau_2 u_2^2 .$$

Again use the homotopic method. Vectorfields $v_1 = u_2 \partial/\partial u_1 - N u_1^{N-1} \partial/\partial u_3$ (a "Hamiltonian" field), $v_2 = u_1 \partial/\partial u_1 + N u_2 \partial/\partial u_2$, $v_3 = u_1 \partial/\partial u_1 + N u_3 \partial/\partial u_3$ ("Euler" fields) are tangent to both the surface Π_1 and the line $u_1 = u_2 = 0$. Let $h(u)$ be an arbitrary function equaling $u_3 O(u) + O_3(u)$. We must find such smooth functions $\delta_\nu(u,t)$ (where $t \in [0,1]$), $\nu = 1,2,3$, that the derivative of the function $\rho_0 + th$ along the vectorfield $v_t = \delta_1 v_1 + \delta_2 v_2 + \delta_3 v_3$ equals $-h$, i.e. that

$$(2\tau_1 u_1 + t\frac{\partial h}{\partial u_1})(u_2\delta_1 + u_1\delta_2 + u_1\delta_3) + N(2\tau_2 u_2 + t\frac{\partial h}{\partial u_2})u_2\delta_2$$

$$+N\left(s + t\frac{\partial h}{\partial u_3}\right)\left(-u_1^{N-1}\delta_1 + u_3\delta_3\right) = -h. \tag{44}$$

Introduce the new coordinate system $\tilde{u} = (u_1, u_2, \tilde{u}_3)$, where

$$\tilde{u}_3 = N s u_3 + 2\tau_1 u_1^2 + t u_1 \frac{\partial h}{\partial u_1} + N t u_3 \frac{\partial h}{\partial u_3} = N s u_3 + O_2(u).$$

The equation (44) may be rewritten in the form

$$\tilde{u}_3\delta_3 + (2\tau_1 u_1 u_2 + \tilde{u}_3 O(\tilde{u}) + O_3(\tilde{u}))\delta_1$$

$$+2(\tau_1 u_1^2 + N\tau_2 u_2^2 + \tilde{u}_3 O(\tilde{u}) + O_3(\tilde{u}))\delta_2 = \tilde{u}_3 O(\tilde{u}) + O_3(\tilde{u}).$$

As well as in the case $N=3$, we have come to the equation (39) with $\Lambda_1 = 2\tau_1 u_1 u_2$ and $\Lambda_2 = 2\tau_1 u_1^2 + 2N\tau_2 u_2^2$. By Lemma 4 this equation is solvable.

We have constructed a diffeomorphism $(\mathbb{R}^3,0)\longrightarrow(\mathbb{R}^3,0)$ reducing ρ to ρ_0. This diffeomorphism puts the equation Π_2 into the form (43), which can be established in the same way as for the case $N=3$.

Thus, let

$$\rho = \rho_0 = s u_3 + \tau_1 u_1^2 + \tau_2 u_2^2 ,$$

$$\Pi_2 = \{ u_1 = u_2^2 \Theta(u_2, u_3) \} .$$

Consider the diffeomorphism

$$D^* : \begin{array}{ccc} u_1 & & \varkappa_1 u_1 \\ u_2 & \longmapsto & \varkappa_2 u_2 \\ u_3 & & \dfrac{\varkappa_1^N}{\varkappa_2} u_3 \end{array}$$

where

$$\varkappa_1 = \left|\frac{\tau_1^3}{\tau_2 s^2}\right|^{\frac{1}{2N-6}} , \qquad \varkappa_2 = \frac{s}{\tau_1}\left|\frac{\tau_1^3}{\tau_2 s^2}\right|^{\frac{N-2}{2N-6}} .$$

This diffeomorphism leaves both the surface Π_1 and the line $u_1=u_2=0$ invariant, the surface $D^*\Pi_2$ still has the form (43) and the function $\rho\circ D^*$ is $C(u_3+u_1^2+\varkappa u_2^2)$, where

$$C=\tau_1\left|\frac{\tau_1^3}{\tau_2 s^2}\right|^{\frac{1}{N-3}}, \quad \varkappa=\operatorname{sgn}\tau_1\tau_2 .$$

X

Theorem 6.11 is proved. Setting $\rho=\varepsilon$ in it and supposing that $\Delta=(NQ_1^1-Q_1^2)(NQ_2^1-Q_2^2)\neq 0$ (this is the nondegeneracy condition C_3) we may reduce ε and Π_2 to normal forms (42) and (43) preserving Π_1. Taking $\xi=u_1$ and $\eta=u_2$ as coordinates on the surface Σ_ε we obtain equations (24) and (23) of curves Γ_ε^1 and Γ_ε^2 respectively. The regime is elliptic or hyperbolic according as $\Delta>0$ or $\Delta<0$.

The case $N\geq 4$ is examined completely. The bifurcations of Γ_ε^1 are shown in figures 8 - 11.

$N\geq 4$	The regime	Figure
even	elliptic	8
odd	elliptic	9
even	hyperbolic	10
odd	hyperbolic	11

The dotted line for $\varepsilon>0$ is the circle $\xi^2+\eta^2=\varepsilon$ in figures 8 and 9 and the hyperbola $\xi^2-\eta^2=\varepsilon$ in figures 10 and 11. The curve Γ_ε^2 is drawn by a dashed line. The distances d_1 and d_2 for $\varepsilon>0$ are of order of $\varepsilon^{(N-1)/4}$.

Find the smoothness of leaves of $\mathcal{M}_0^1$ at 0.

In the elliptic regime in coordinates (ξ,η) the equation of the curve Γ_0^1 is $\eta=\xi^{N-2}(1+\overset{+}{H}_N(\xi))$.

In the hyperbolic regime the surface $\mathcal{M}_0^1$ consists of 3 leaves foliated into symmetric cycles and intersecting $Fix\,G$ along 3 curves, the union of which is just Γ_0^1. For N even these curves are given by equations

$$\eta=\xi^{N-2}(1+H_N^-(\xi)),\quad \eta=W_N(|\xi|),\quad \eta=W_N(-|\xi|),$$

for N odd they are given by equations

$$\eta=\xi^{N-2}(1+H_N^-(\xi)),\quad \eta=W_N^+(\xi),\quad \eta=-W_N^-(\xi).$$

(Here everywhere $H_N^+(\xi)$ and $H_N^-(\xi)$ are certain even functions equaling $O_2(\xi)$, $W_N(\xi)$ is some function equaling $\xi+O_2(\xi)$, $W_N^+(\xi)$ and $W_N^-(\xi)$ are certain odd functions equaling $\xi+O_3(\xi)$.)

In coordinates (x,X) $\Gamma_0^1\cap\{x_1\geq 0\}$ is a half-curve

$$x_1\geq 0,\quad x_2=\frac{\gamma_2}{NQ_1^1-Q_1^2}\,x_1^{N-2}+O_{N-1}(x_1),\quad X=O_N(x_1) \tag{45}$$

in the elliptic regime and the union of three half-curves, one of them is given by relations (45) and two other are given by the relations

$$x_1\geq 0,\quad x_2=\pm\sqrt{\frac{Q_1^2-NQ_1^1}{NQ_2^1-Q_2^2}}\,x_1+O_2(x_1),\quad X=O_N(x_1),$$

in the hyperbolic regime (see (31), (41)). Applying Theorem 6.7 (in this case in the notations of Theorem 6.7 one has $\kappa=+\infty$, $d=N$, $\ell=N-1$ (see (25), (26)), $m\in\{1;\,N-2\}$, $j=N$ and sees all the conditions of Theorem 6.7 be fulfilled) we obtain that in the elliptic regime the surface $\mathcal{M}_0^1$ is of class C^{N-3} rather than C^{N-2} at 0 whereas in the hyperbolic regime it consists of 3 leaves, one of them is of class C^{N-3} at 0 rather than C^{N-2} while two others do not possess even the smoothness C^1 at 0.

This completes the proof of Theorem 6.8. X

REMARK. For $N \geq 3$ the singularities of the pair (the surface $\Pi_1 \subset \mathbb{R}^3$ of type A_{N-1}, the function $\mathcal{E}:(\mathbb{R}^3,0)\longrightarrow(\mathbb{R},0)$) are real versions of critical points of a function on a manifold with singular boundary of type $\tilde{A}_3$ for $N=3$ and type $I_3(N)$ for $N \geq 4$ in Lyashko's classification [32].

O.V.Lyashko has informed me kindly, that the list of unimodal singularities in [32 (Theorem 1)] is not complete: one must add the singularity

$$xy = z^3 + Q\ ,\ f_\lambda = x + yz + \lambda_2 y + \lambda_1 z + \lambda_0\ ,\ \mu = 3,\ \ m = 1$$

(we use the notations of [32]) to the case of critical points of type $\tilde{A}_3$ (on a manifold with the boundary of type A_2) there.

§ 6.4. Subharmonic resonances

Let V_ε be a smooth one-parameter family of smooth vectorfields at $(\mathbb{R}^{2n},0)$ $(V_\varepsilon(0)=0$ for all ε) reversible with respect to a smooth involution $\sigma:(\mathbb{R}^{2n},0)\longrightarrow(\mathbb{R}^{2n},0)$ of type (n,n). Suppose that the linearization $(V_0)_1$ of the field V_0 has simple purely imaginary eigenvalues $\pm ip\omega,\ \pm iq\omega$, where $\omega>0,\ p,q\in\mathbb{N},\ 1<p<q$, p and q are relatively prime. Denote the other eigenvalues of $(V_0)_1$ by $\pm\lambda_3,\dots,\pm\lambda_n$. Assume that none of the ratios $\lambda_r/i\omega,\ 3\leq r\leq n,$ is an integer.

In this situation the family of fields V_ε is said to pass through the subharmonic resonance $p:q$ (of codimension 1) at $\varepsilon=0$.

For a subharmonic resonance the Lyapunov-Devaney theorem describes both short period and long period cycles, but such a resonance allows so called very long period cycles to exist.

For small ε, near 0 the field V_ε has invariant two-dimensional surfaces $\mathcal{M}_\varepsilon^1$, $\mathcal{M}_\varepsilon^2$ and $\mathcal{M}_\varepsilon^3$ foliated into symmetric cycles whose periods are close to $2\pi/\omega$ (very long period cycles), $2\pi/(p\omega)$ (long period cycles) and $2\pi/(q\omega)$ (short period cycles), respectively. Let $\mathcal{M}_\varepsilon^\nu \cap \operatorname{Fix} G = \Gamma_\varepsilon^\nu$, $\nu=1,2,3$.

According to Theorems 6.2 and 6.3 the surfaces $\mathcal{M}_\varepsilon^2$, $\mathcal{M}_\varepsilon^3$ and the curves Γ_ε^2, Γ_ε^3 do not undergo a bifurcation as ε passes through 0. $\mathcal{M}_\varepsilon^2$ and $\mathcal{M}_\varepsilon^3$ are smooth two-dimensional discs depending smoothly on ε and intersecting $\operatorname{Fix} G$ along the curves Γ_ε^2 and Γ_ε^3, respectively, which are also smooth and depend smoothly on ε. These curves pass through 0 and at 0 intersect at a nonzero angle.

Our goal is to investigate the bifurcations of the curve Γ_ε^1 as ε passes through the resonant value 0.

As well as in the case of strict resonances $1:N$, for each p and q there exist two greatly different types of bifurcations of $\mathcal{M}_\varepsilon^1$ (both types are generic). We shall call these types elliptic and hyperbolic regimes again.

THEOREM 6.12. If the 3-jet of the field V_ε satisfies certain nondegeneracy conditions C_1 and C_2 exposed below then the following holds.

a) In the space $\mathbb{R}^n = \operatorname{Fix} G$, there is a two-dimensional surface Σ_ε depending on ε smoothly, on which the curves Γ_ε^ν, $\nu=1,2,3$, lie.

b) By a suitable choice of a smoothly depending on ε coordinate system (ξ,η) on Σ_ε and, if necessary, the change of the sign of ε (i.e. multiplying ε by -1), the equations of the families of curves Γ_ε^1, Γ_ε^2, Γ_ε^3 may be simultaneously put into the form

$$\xi^2 \pm \eta^2 = \varepsilon \quad , \quad \eta = 0 \quad , \quad \xi = 0 \tag{46}$$

respectively, where the sign $+$ corresponds to the elliptic regime and the sign $-$ corresponds to the hyperbolic one (a regime is determined by the 3-jet of the field V_0).

REMARK 1. Actually, the conditions C_1 and C_2 are imposed on $(V_\varepsilon)_1$ and $(V_0)_3$ respectively.

REMARK 2. For $n=2$ the statement a) is trivial: $\Sigma_\varepsilon = Fix\, G$.

PROOF. First of all, let us verify that it suffices to reduce Γ_ε^ν to the form (46) in that case when any smooth changes of ε are allowed (not only multiplying ε by -1). Indeed, a family of curves $\tilde{\xi}^2 \pm \tilde{\eta}^2 = \tilde{\varepsilon}$, where $\tilde{\varepsilon} = \tilde{\varepsilon}(\varepsilon) = a\varepsilon + O_2(\varepsilon)$, $a > 0$, can be put into the form (46) via the change of variables $\xi = \tilde{\xi}\sqrt{\varepsilon/\tilde{\varepsilon}}$, $\eta = \tilde{\eta}\sqrt{\varepsilon/\tilde{\varepsilon}}$.

Hence, proving Theorem 6.12 we may use all smooth changes of ε.

In $\mathbb{R}^{2n}$, there is such a complex coordinate system (z, Z) depending on ε smoothly in which

$$(V_\varepsilon)_1 = i(p\omega + \alpha(\varepsilon))z_1\frac{\partial}{\partial z_1} + i(q\omega + \beta(\varepsilon))z_2\frac{\partial}{\partial z_2} + i(B_1(\varepsilon)Z + B_2(\varepsilon)\bar{Z})\frac{\partial}{\partial Z},$$

$$G : (z, Z) \mapsto (\bar{z}, \bar{Z})$$

where α and β are real-valued functions in ε equaling $O(\varepsilon)$ while B_1 and B_2 are real matrix-valued (of order $n-2$) functions in ε.

We have

$$\frac{q\omega+\beta}{p\omega+\alpha}=\frac{1}{p}\left(q+\frac{p\beta-q\alpha}{p\omega}+\sigma\right)$$

where $\sigma=\sigma(\varepsilon)=O_2(\varepsilon)$. Generically $p\beta-q\alpha\neq O_2(\varepsilon)$ (this is the nondegeneracy condition C_1), and we can take $(p\beta-q\alpha)/(p\omega)+\sigma$ as a new parameter. Changing the time scale we can put $(V_\varepsilon)_1$ into the form

$$(V_\varepsilon)_1=ipz_1\frac{\partial}{\partial z_1}+i(q+\varepsilon)z_2\frac{\partial}{\partial z_2}+i(B_1Z+B_2\bar{Z})\frac{\partial}{\partial Z}$$

(with changed B_1 and B_2).

The surfaces $\mathcal{M}_\varepsilon^2$ and $\mathcal{M}_\varepsilon^3$ are smooth, depend on ε smoothly, are invariant under $\mathcal{G}$ and tangent to the two-dimensional planes $z_2=0$, $Z=0$ and $z_1=0$, $Z=0$, respectively, at 0. That is why by a suitable change of variables (with the identity linearization) depending on ε smoothly and commuting with $\mathcal{G}$ one can make the equations of these surfaces into $z_2=0, Z=0$ and $z_1=0, Z=0$ respectively. Then, as $\mathcal{M}_\varepsilon^2$ and $\mathcal{M}_\varepsilon^3$ are invariant under V_ε,

$$V_\varepsilon=i(pz_1+\varphi_\varepsilon^1)\frac{\partial}{\partial z_1}+i((q+\varepsilon)z_2+\varphi_\varepsilon^2)\frac{\partial}{\partial z_2}$$

$$+i(B_1Z+B_2\bar{Z}+\Phi_\varepsilon)\frac{\partial}{\partial Z}$$

where

$$\varphi_\varepsilon^1(z,Z)=O(z_1,Z)O(z,Z)$$

$$\varphi^2_\varepsilon(z,Z)=O(z_2,Z)O(z,Z)$$

$$\Phi_\varepsilon(z,Z)=O(Z)O(z,Z)+O(z_1)O(z_2).$$

Now, by means of the method of Poincaré-Dulac normal forms, for each $\ell\in\mathbb{N}$ by a change of variables smoothly depending on ε and commuting with σ we can achieve

$$\varphi^1_\varepsilon(z,Z)=(Q^1_1+O(\varepsilon))z_1^2\bar z_1+(Q^1_2+O(\varepsilon))z_1z_2\bar z_2+O(Z)O(z,Z)+O(z_1)O_3(z)$$

$$\varphi^2_\varepsilon(z,Z)=(Q^2_1+O(\varepsilon))z_1\bar z_1z_2+(Q^2_2+O(\varepsilon))z_2^2\bar z_2+O(Z)O(z,Z)+O(z_2)O_3(z)$$

$$\Phi_\varepsilon(z,Z)=O(Z)O(z,Z)+O(z_1)O(z_2)O_{\ell-1}(z)$$

where Q^ν_1 and Q^ν_2, $\nu=1,2$, are real numbers.

For our purposes, it will suffice to set $\ell=2$.

Then, as is easy to verify,

$$\operatorname{Im}F_{\varepsilon,t}(x_1,x_2,X)=(\psi^1_{\varepsilon,t}(x,X),\ \psi^2_{\varepsilon,t}(x,X)\ ,\ \Psi_{\varepsilon,t}(x,X)),$$

where

$$\psi^1_{\varepsilon,t}(x,X)=x_1(\sin pt+(Q^1_1x_1^2+Q^1_2x_2^2)t\cos pt+\varepsilon O_2(x)+O_3(x))$$
$$+O(X)O(x,X)$$

$$\psi^2_{\varepsilon,t}(x,X)=x_2(\sin(q+\varepsilon)t+(Q^2_1x_1^2+Q^2_2x_2^2)t\cos qt+\varepsilon O_2(x)+O_3(x))$$
$$+O(X)O(x,X)$$

$$\Psi_{\varepsilon,t}(x,X)=\operatorname{Im} f_t(X)+\varepsilon O(X)+O(X)O(x,X)+x_1x_2O(x).$$

Here $f_t(Z)$ is the phase flow of the linear field $i(B_1(0)Z + B_2(0)\bar{Z})\partial/\partial Z$ in $\mathbb{R}^{2n-4}$.

Let $t=\pi+\tau$, where τ is small. Similarly to Lemma 1 it is easy to prove that the linear operator $X\mapsto \operatorname{Im} f_\pi(X)$ is non-degenerate. Now from $\Psi_{\varepsilon,t}(x,X)=0$ we obtain

$$X=x_1x_2g(x,\tau,\varepsilon) \tag{47}$$

where $g=O(x)$. Substituting (47) into $\overset{\nu}{\Psi}_{\varepsilon,t}=0$, $\nu=1,2$, we rewrite the equation $\operatorname{Im} F_{\varepsilon,\pi+\tau}(x,X)=0$ in the form

$$\begin{cases} x_1\mu_1(x,\tau,\varepsilon)=0\\ x_2\mu_2(x,\tau,\varepsilon)=0\\ X=x_1x_2g(x,\tau,\varepsilon)\end{cases}$$

where

$$\mu_1(x,\tau,\varepsilon)=\sin p\tau+(\overset{1}{Q}_1x_1^2+\overset{1}{Q}_2x_2^2)(\pi+\tau)\cos p\tau+\varepsilon O_2(x)+O_3(x),$$

$$\mu_2(x,\tau,\varepsilon)=\sin(q\tau+\varepsilon\pi+\varepsilon\tau)+(\overset{2}{Q}_1x_1^2+\overset{2}{Q}_2x_2^2)(\pi+\tau)\cos q\tau$$
$$+\varepsilon O_2(x)+O_3(x).$$

One may solve the equations $\mu_\nu(x,\tau,\varepsilon)=0$ $(\nu=1,2)$ for τ:

$$\tau=K_\nu(x,\varepsilon),$$

where

$$K_1(x,\varepsilon) = -\frac{\pi}{p}(Q_1^1 x_1^2 + Q_2^1 x_2^2) + \varepsilon O_2(x) + O_3(x),$$

$$K_2(x,\varepsilon) = -\frac{\varepsilon\pi}{q+\varepsilon} - \frac{\pi}{q}(Q_1^2 x_1^2 + Q_2^2 x_2^2) + \varepsilon O_2(x) + O_3(x).$$

Consider the mapping $\mathcal{F} : \mathbb{R}^{n+2} \longrightarrow \mathbb{R}^n$, $\mathcal{F} : (\varepsilon, \tau, x, X) \longmapsto \operatorname{Im} F_{\varepsilon,\pi+\tau}(x,X)$ defined near $0 \in \mathbb{R}^{n+2}$. One sees that $\mathcal{F}^{-1}(0)$ consists of the following 4 smooth surfaces of dimension two: the plane

$$x = 0 \ , \ X = 0$$

(corresponding to the origin), the surface

$$x_2 = 0 \ , \ \tau = K_1(x_1, 0, \varepsilon), \ X = 0$$

(corresponding to Γ_ε^2), the surface

$$x_1 = 0 \ , \ \tau = K_2(0, x_2, \varepsilon) \ , \ X = 0$$

(corresponding to Γ_ε^3) and the surface

$$\mu_1(x,\tau,\varepsilon) = 0, \ \mu_2(x,\tau,\varepsilon) = 0, \ X = x_1 x_2 g(x,\tau,\varepsilon)$$

(corresponding to Γ_ε^1).

Each of two surfaces

$$X = x_1 x_2 g(x, K_\nu(x,\varepsilon), \varepsilon) \ , \ \nu = 1,2 \tag{48}$$

can be taken as Σ_ε.

In the space

$$\mathbb{R}^3 = \bigcup_\varepsilon (\Sigma_\varepsilon \times \{\varepsilon\}),$$

where coordinates on Σ_ε are x_1 and x_2, we obtain surfaces Π_1, Π_2, and Π_3 given by the equations

$$K_1(x,\varepsilon)=K_2(x,\varepsilon)\ ,\quad x_2=0\ ,\quad \text{and}\ x_1=0$$

respectively. Sections of surfaces Π_ν, $\nu=1,2,3$, by level planes of the coordinate function $\varepsilon:(\mathbb{R}^3,0)\longrightarrow(\mathbb{R},0)$ are just the curves Γ_ε^ν. Thus, we must reduce the diagram

$$\begin{array}{ccccc} & & \Pi_1 & & \\ & & \downarrow & & \\ \Pi_2 & \hookrightarrow & \mathbb{R}^3 & \xrightarrow{\ \varepsilon\ } & \mathbb{R} \\ & & \uparrow & & \\ & & \Pi_3 & & \end{array}$$

to a normal form.

One can transcribe the equation $K_1(x,\varepsilon)=K_2(x,\varepsilon)$ of the surface Π_1 in the form

$$\varepsilon=\frac{q}{p}\left(Q_1^1x_1^2+Q_2^1x_2^2\right)-\left(Q_1^2x_1^2+Q_2^2x_2^2\right)+O_3(x). \tag{49}$$

There exists such a coordinate system $u=(u_1,u_2,u_3)$, where $u_1=x_1$, $u_2=x_2$, $u_3=\varepsilon+O_2(x)$, in which the equations of surfaces Π_1, Π_2 and Π_3 are $u_3=0$, $u_2=0$ and $u_1=0$ respectively and the function ε has the form $\varepsilon(u)=u_3+\tau_1u_1^2+\tau_2u_2^2+P(u_1,u_2)$, where $\tau_\nu=(q/p)Q_\nu^1-Q_\nu^2$, $\nu=1,2$, and $P=O_3(u_1,u_2)$.

THEOREM 6.13. Let $u=(u_1,u_2,u_3)$ be coordinates in $\mathbb{R}^3$. Every function

$$\rho(u)=su_3+\tau_1u_1^2+\tau_2u_2^2+u_3\,O(u)+O_3(u)\ ,$$

where $s\neq0$, $\tau_1\neq0$, $\tau_2\neq0$, can be put into the form

$$\rho = \varkappa_1 (u_3 + u_1^2 + \varkappa_2 u_2^2) , \tag{50}$$

where $\varkappa_1 , \varkappa_2 \in \{-1 \; ; \; 1\}$, via a diffeomorphism of $\mathbb{R}^3$ preserving planes $u_\nu = 0$, $\nu = 1, 2, 3$.

PROOF. Consider the linear diffeomorphism

$$\overset{*}{D} : (u_1, u_2, u_3) \longmapsto \left(\frac{u_1}{\sqrt{|\tau_1|}}, \frac{u_2}{\sqrt{|\tau_2|}}, \frac{u_3 \, sgn\, \tau_1}{s} \right).$$

We have $\rho \circ \overset{*}{D}(u) = \rho_0(u) + u_3 O(u) + O_3(u)$, where ρ_0 has the form (50) with $\varkappa_1 = sgn\, \tau_1$, $\varkappa_2 = sgn(\tau_1 \tau_2)$.

Suppose $\varkappa_1 = \varkappa_2 = 1$ (i.e. $\tau_1 > 0$, $\tau_2 > 0$), the other 3 cases are entirely similar. Vectorfields $v_\nu = u_\nu \partial/\partial u_\nu$, $\nu = 1, 2, 3$, are tangent to all three planes $u_\nu = 0$. Let $h(u)$ be an arbitrary function equaling $u_3 O(u) + O_3(u)$. We must find such smooth functions $\delta_\nu(u, t)$ (where $t \in [0,1]$), $\nu = 1, 2, 3$, that the derivative of the function $\rho_0 + th$ along the vectorfield $v_t = \delta_1 v_1 + \delta_2 v_2 + \delta_3 v_3$ equals $-h$, i.e. that

$$(2u_1 + t\frac{\partial h}{\partial u_1}) u_1 \delta_1 + (2u_2 + t\frac{\partial h}{\partial u_2}) u_2 \delta_2$$

$$+ \left(1 + t\frac{\partial h}{\partial u_3}\right) u_3 \delta_3 = -h . \tag{51}$$

Introduce the new coordinate system $\tilde{u} = (u_1, u_2, \tilde{u}_3)$, where $\tilde{u}_3 = u_3 + t u_3 \, \partial h/\partial u_3$. The equation (51) may be rewritten in the form

$$\tilde{u}_3 \delta_3 + 2(u_1^2 + \tilde{u}_3 O(\tilde{u}) + O_3(\tilde{u})) \delta_1 + 2(u_2^2 + \tilde{u}_3 O(\tilde{u}) + O_3(\tilde{u})) \delta_2 = \tilde{u}_3 O(\tilde{u}) + O_3(\tilde{u}).$$

By Lemma 4 this equation is always solvable. X

Theorem 6.13 is proved. Setting $\rho = \varepsilon$ in it and supposing that $\Delta = (q Q_1^1 - p Q_1^2)(q Q_2^1 - p Q_2^2) \neq 0$ (this is the nondegeneracy condition C_2) we can reduce $\mathcal{E}$ to the normal form (50) preserving planes $u_\nu = 0$, $\nu = 1,2,3$. Taking $\xi = u_1$ and $\eta = u_2$ as coordinates on the surface Σ_ε we obtain the equations (46) of curves Γ_ε^ν, $\nu = 1,2,3$. The elliptic regime corresponds to $\Delta > 0$, the hyperbolic one corresponds to $\Delta < 0$. X

REMARK. At the beginning of the proof of Theorem 6.12 we verified directly that it suffices to reduce Γ_ε^ν, $\nu = 1,2,3$, to the form (46) in that case when any smooth changes of $\mathcal{E}$ are allowed. One sees this statement follow immediately from Theorem 6.13.

In the elliptic regime Γ_0^1 is just the origin. In the hyperbolic regime the surface $\mathcal{M}_0^1$ consists of two leaves foliated into symmetric cycles and intersecting $\operatorname{Fix} G$ along two curves which in the coordinates (ξ, η) on Σ_0 are given by equations

$$\begin{aligned} \eta &= \pm \xi && \text{for } p \text{ odd, } q \text{ odd} \\ \eta &= \pm |\xi| && \text{for } p \text{ odd, } q \text{ even} \\ \xi &= \pm |\eta| && \text{for } p \text{ even, } q \text{ odd}. \end{aligned}$$

Let us show that these leaves do not possess even the smoothness C^1 at 0. Indeed, suppose that one of the leaves (for definitiveness the one that contains the half-curve $\eta = \xi$, $\xi \geq 0$) is of class C^1 at 0. Denote this leaf by $\mathcal{M}^*$. The half-curve $\{\eta = \xi, \xi \geq 0\}$ belonging to $\mathcal{M}^*$ is given in coordinates (x, X) by

$$x_2 \geq 0, \quad x_1 = a x_2 + O_2(x_2), \quad X = O_3(x_2) \tag{52}$$

where

$$a = \sqrt{\frac{q Q_2^1 - p Q_2^2}{p Q_1^2 - q Q_1^1}}$$

(see (48), (49)). Therefore $\mathcal{M}^*$ and the plane $\{Re\, z_2=0\}$ of dimension $2n-1$ intersect at 0 transversally. Hence, $\mathcal{M}^*\cap\{Re\, z_2=0\}$ is a C^1-curve passing through 0. On the other hand, consider the trajectory $(z_1(t),\ z_2(t),\ Z(t))$ of the field V_0 passing through an arbitrary point of the half-curve (52). If $z_2(0)=x_2\in\mathbb{R}_+$ then

$$z_1(t)=e^{ipt}x_2+x_2^2R(t,x_2),\quad z_2(t)=e^{iqt}x_2+x_2^2S(t,x_2).$$

On $[0,2\pi)$ the equation $\cos qt+x_2 Re S(t,x_2)=0$ has $2q$ solutions $t_\nu(x_2)=\pi(2\nu-1)/(2q)+O(x_2)$ $(\nu=1,2,\dots,2q)$ depending smoothly on x_2. Now we have

$$z_1(t_\nu(x_2))=x_2\exp\Big(\frac{p\pi i}{2q}(2\nu-1)\Big)(1+O(x_2)),$$

$$z_2(t_\nu(x_2))=i(-1)^{\nu+1}x_2(1+O(x_2)).$$

Since p and q are relatively prime it follows that all q numbers

$$\exp\Big(\frac{p\pi i}{2q}(2\nu-1)\Big),\quad \nu=1,2,\dots,q,$$

are distinct. Thus, $\mathcal{M}^*\cap\{Re\, z_2=0\}$ contains at least $q\geqslant 3$ distinct smooth half-curves emanating from 0. The obtained contradiction shows that at 0 $\mathcal{M}^*$ does not possess even the smoothness C^1.

The behaviour of solutions of reversible systems at the instant of resonance is very much like that of resonant Hamiltonian systems. For instance, for resonance $1:3$ between two purely imaginary eigenvalues of the linearization of a Hamiltonian system with many degrees of freedom Roels [33] has found either a single two-dimensional passing through an equilibrium surface foliated into long period cycles or three such surfaces, according to the 4-jet of the Hamilton function. For resonance $1:N$, $N \geq 4$, (also in the multidimensional situation) he has found in [34] a two-dimensional surface passing through an equilibrium, foliated into long period cycles and tangent to the corresponding invariant plane of the linearization. The case of a resonant Hamiltonian system with two degrees of freedom is considered in detail in Henrard [35] (where one can find the more complete list of references as well). Henrard has shown that for resonance $1:2$ either there are no families of long period cycles near an equilibrium of a nondegenerate system or there exist two such families, whereas for resonance $1:N, N \geq 3$, the number of families of long period cycles equals either 1 or 3. Subharmonic resonances $p:q$ are also examined in [35]. It has been proved that a resonant $p:q$ nondegenerate system has either no families of very long period cycles near an equilibrium or two such families.

APPENDIX

Some further problems

In the main text of the paper, we have already mentioned some petty unsolved questions of the reversible dynamical systems theory: conjectures on the intersection property of reversible plane diffeomorphisms (for annulus mappings in § 1.5 and for the local situation at the end of § 2.9), hypothetical analogues to Theorems 2.1 and 2.2 for linear operators over an arbitrary field (§ 2.1), conjectures concerning resonant elliptic formal diffeomorphisms and vectorfields (see commentaries after formulations of Theorem 2.4 (§ 2.3) and Theorem 2.7 (§ 2.6), Remark after the proof of Theorem 2.9 (§ 2.8), and Remark 2 after the proof of Theorem 2.11 (§ 2.10)).Here we enumerate some other problems which are of more fundamental character.

1°. In all 4 reversible analytic KAM-theorems (global Theorem 1.1 for mappings, global Theorem 1.2 for vectorfields, local Theorem 2.9 for mappings, and local Theorem 2.11 for vectorfields), in the middle dimension case (i.e. when the number of frequencies equals half of the dimension of the phase space), one does not require the involutivity of the reversing diffeomorphism G but does prove it (by the positivity of the measure of the union of invariant tori, the involutivity of G on these tori, and the analyticity of G). What can one say on the C^{∞} case or on the finite (sufficiently high) smoothness case?

Throughout this paper, for simplicity we considered analytic reversible KAM-theorems only, but their smooth versions are also valid. In the smooth middle dimension case, as well as in the analytic one, the existence of Kolmogorov sets of positive measure, on which G is an involution, can be established without any assumptions about involutive properties of G to be imposed a priori . But in the smooth case the existence of such a set does not imply the involutivity of G on the whole phase space.

2°. Does a regular drift in resonant zones along directions transversal to invariant tori take place in generic reversible systems (for simplicity, with continuous time), close to integrable or slightly integrable ones (cf. the remark at the end of § 3.2)? Is the reversible version of the Nekhoroshev theorem on the exponential smallness of such a drift in the perturbations of generic integrable Hamiltonian systems ([41, 42, 43] , see [19, Chapter 4, § 19] as well) valid?

In Nekhoroshev's theory, one estimates the highest possible speed of a drift in terms of the geometrical properties of the unperturbed Hamilton function. There is no analogue to a Hamilton function for reversible vectorfields. Whereas integrable Hamiltonian systems differ by their Hamilton functions, all nondegenerate integrable reversible systems are the same near an invariant torus (see Proposition 1.2 in § 1.7). There is no analogue to the concept of the isoenergetic nondegeneracy for reversible vectorfields. All these circumstances indicate that, seemingly, Nekhoroshev's results do not carry over directly to reversible systems.

3°. (Cf. [28]). Is it true that each analytic (weakly) reversible diffeomorphism close to nondegenerate reversible slightly integrable one is the monodromy operator of some analytic (weakly) reversible periodic in time vectorfield close to nondegenerate reversible slightly integrable autonomous one? The analogous statement on reversible C^{∞}-mappings is true (see § 4.3, Proposition 4.5).

4°. [1] . Transfer Arnol'd's conjectures on intersections of Lagrangian manifolds and the number of periodic solutions of Hamiltonian systems (see [18, Appendix 9]), proved recently by C.Conley, E.Zehnder, and M.Chaperon, to the reversible case (cf. Chapter 5 of the present paper).

5°. In the case of "the limiting degeneration" (see § 5.1) study the disintegration of invariant tori with any rank of collections of frequencies over rationals under small perturbations of integrable or slightly integrable reversible systems.

CONJECTURE 1. Consider an invariant torus T^m_ω of a nondegenerate integrable reversible diffeomorphism A with frequencies $\omega = (\omega_1, \dots, \omega_m)$. Suppose that among numbers $\pi, \omega_1, \dots, \omega_m$, there exist n rationally independent ones, where $1 \leq n \leq m+1$ (without loss of generality these numbers are $\pi, \omega_1, \dots, \omega_{n-1}$), and the remaining $m+1-n$ numbers $\omega_n, \dots, \omega_m$ are linear combinations of $\pi, \omega_1, \dots, \omega_{n-1}$ with rational coefficients. For $n \geq 2$ assume in addition that $\pi, \omega_1, \dots, \omega_{n-1}$ are "strongly" rationally independent (i.e. $(\omega_1, \dots, \omega_{n-1}) \in \mathfrak{M}_{n-1}$).

Then under a small reversible perturbation of A the torus T^m_ω disintegrates into several invariant under both the perturbed mapping A' and the reversing involution collections of tori of dimension $n-1$. The numbers of these tori T^{n-1} in all collections are the same. If every collection consists of q tori then each of these tori T^{n-1} is invariant under the q-th iteration of A', and on T^{n-1} $(A')^q$ defines a quasi-periodic motion with frequencies $(q\omega_1, \dots, q\omega_{n-1})$.

REMARK. For $n=1$ (we understand a torus of dimension zero as a point) this conjecture has been proved in § 5.2 (Theorem 5.1). The number of collections (i.e. of symmetric cycles of A') is equal to 2^m. For $n = m+1$ this conjecture also holds (the KAM-theorem, §§ 1.2 - 1.4), the number of collections and the number of tori in the collection being 1.

CONJECTURE 2. Consider an invariant torus T^m_ω of a nondegenerate integrable reversible vectorfield V with frequencies $\omega = (\omega_1, \dots, \omega_m)$. Suppose that among numbers $\omega_1, \dots, \omega_m$, there exist n rationally independent ones, where $1 \leq n \leq m$ (without loss of generality these numbers are $\omega_1, \ldots, \omega_n$), and the remaining $m-n$ numbers $\omega_{n+1}, \ldots, \omega_m$ are linear combinations of $\omega_1, \ldots, \omega_n$ with rational coefficients. For $n \geq 2$ assume in addition that $\omega_1, \ldots, \omega_n$ are "strongly" rationally independent (i.e. $(\omega_1, \ldots, \omega_n) \in \mathcal{N}_n$).

Then under a small reversible perturbation of V the torus T^m_ω disintegrates into several invariant under both the perturbed vectorfield V' and the reversing involution tori of dimension n, on which V' induces a quasiperiodic motion with frequencies $(\omega_1, \ldots, \omega_n)$.

REMARK. For $n=1$ this conjecture has been proved in § 5.3 (Theorem 5.4). The number of 1-tori (i.e. of symmetric cycles of V') is equal to 2^{m-1}. For $n=m$ this conjecture also holds (the KAM-theorem, §§ 1.8 - 1.10), the number of tori being 1.

It is easy to formulate similar conjectures for perturbations of nondegenerate slightly integrable reversible diffeomorphisms and vectorfields.

6°. Study the structure of the set of invariant tori T^s of a reversible vectorfield near an elliptic equilibrium and that of a reversible diffeomorphism near an elliptic fixed point for all dimensions $s = 1, \ldots, m$, where $2m$ is the phase space dimension (see the Introduction, subsection 6°). In the present paper, we have considered the cases $s = m$ and $s = 1$ for fields (Theorem 2.11 in § 2.10 and Theorems 6.2 - 6.4 in § 6.1 respectively) and the case $s = m$ for diffeomorphisms (Theorem 2.9 in § 2.8).

The problem makes sense also for a reversible vectorfield near a symmetric cycle (we have considered the cases $s = m$ and $s = 1$, see Theorem 3.2 and Theorem 3.1 in § 3.2 and § 3.1 respectively).

7°. Construct the multidimensional local theory of resonant zones of reversible diffeomorphisms and vectorfields (cf. § 5.4).

8°. Find normal forms for the bifurcations of surfaces $\mathcal{M}_\varepsilon$ for resonance $1:1$ (see § 6.2) and of surfaces $\mathcal{M}^1_\varepsilon$ for resonances $1:N$, $N \geq 2$ (see § 6.3) and $p:q$ (see § 6.4). In Chapter 6 we obtained only normal forms for the bifurcations of intersections of these surfaces with the fixed point manifold of the reversing involution.

9°. Construct the unified theory of Hamiltonian and reversible diffeomorphisms and vectorfields, in which the close similarity between these two remarkable classes of dynamical systems would find a satisfactory explanation. V.I.Arnol'd has suggested that what would be able to shed light on the parallelism of properties of Hamiltonian and reversible objects is the superization, i.e. considering dynamical systems on sets with the superstructure. In order to realize the desired synthesis of Hamiltonian and reversible characteristic features, these systems must hypothetically be reversible with respect to even variables and be Hamiltonian with respect to odd ones.

10°. Generalize the concepts of reversibility and weak reversibility to dynamical systems with an arbitrary time group. Let us give a sketch of two possible generalizations.

The group of diffeomorphisms of a manifold generated by an involution is $\mathbb{Z}_2$. Now consider an arbitrary group H acting on some manifold $\mathcal{M}$ by diffeomorphisms.

DEFINITION 1. Fix an action of H on $\mathbb{Z}$ by automorphisms, i.e. a function $\varphi : H \to \{-1; 1\}$ such that $\varphi(g_1)\varphi(g_2) = \varphi(g_1 g_2)$ for each $g_1, g_2 \in H$. A diffeomorphism $A : \mathcal{M} \to \mathcal{M}$ is said to be (H, φ)-pseudoreversible with respect to the given action of H on $\mathcal{M}$ by diffeomorphisms, if

$$gA = A^{\varphi(g)} g$$

for each $g \in H$.

DEFINITION 2. Fix an action of H on $\mathbb{R}$ by continuous automorphisms, i.e. a function $\psi : H \to \mathbb{R} \setminus \{0\}$ such that $\psi(g_1)\psi(g_2) = \psi(g_1 g_2)$ for each $g_1, g_2 \in H$. A vectorfield V on $\mathcal{M}$ is said to be (H, ψ)-pseudoreversible with respect to the given action of H on $\mathcal{M}$ by diffeomorphisms, if

$$Tg \circ V = \psi(g) V \circ g$$

for each $g \in H$.

An (H, φ)-pseudoreversible diffeomorphism is a dynamical system whose time is the expansion of $\mathbb{Z}$ by means of H (more precisely, by means of the homomorphism $\varphi : H \to \mathrm{Aut}\, \mathbb{Z} = \mathbb{Z}_2$). An (H, ψ)-pseudoreversible vectorfield is a dynamical system whose time is the expansion of $\mathbb{R}$ by means of H (more precisely, by means of the homomorphism $\psi : H \to \mathrm{Aut}_c\, \mathbb{R} = \mathbb{R} \setminus \{0\}$).

Now consider some set S of diffeomorphisms of $\mathcal{M}$ and a bijection $f : H \setminus \{id\} \to S$.

DEFINITION 3. A diffeomorphism $A : \mathcal{M} \to \mathcal{M}$ is said to be weakly (H, φ)-pseudoreversible with respect to (S, f) if

$$f(g)\, A = A^{\varphi(g)} f(g)$$

for each $g \in H \setminus \{id\}$.

DEFINITION 4. A vectorfield V on $\mathcal{M}$ is said to be weakly (H, ψ)-pseudoreversible with respect to (S, f) if

$$Tf(g) \circ V = \psi(g) V \circ f(g)$$

for each $g \in H \setminus \{id\}$.

EXAMPLE. Suppose on $\mathcal{M}$ there acts the group of diffeomorphisms

$H_0 = \{G; id\}$, where G is an involution. Denote by $\varkappa$ the function on H_0 defined by $\varkappa(id)=1$, $\varkappa(G)=-1$. Then $(H_0,\varkappa)$-pseudoreversible diffeomorphisms and vectorfields are just ones reversible with respect to G in the usual sense. For an arbitrary diffeomorphism $G': \mathcal{M} \to \mathcal{M}$ the weak $(H_0, \varkappa)$-pseudoreversibility with respect to $(\{G'\}, G \mapsto G')$ is the usual weak reversibility with respect to G'.

More generally, a diffeomorphism $\mathcal{M} \to \mathcal{M}$ or a vectorfield on $\mathcal{M}$, weakly (H, θ)-pseudoreversible with respect to (S, f), are weakly reversible (in the usual sense) with respect to every diffeomorphism $f(g)$ such that $\theta(g) = -1$.

The following statements are trivial.

PROPOSITION 1. Let a diffeomorphism A be weakly (H, φ)-pseudoreversible with respect to (S, f). Let $S_1 = \{ R^{-1} \mid R \in S \}$. Denote by λ the bijection $\lambda : S \to S_1$ defined by $\lambda(R) = R^{-1}$ for all $R \in S$. Then the diffeomorphism A is weakly (H, φ)-pseudoreversible with respect to $(S_1, \lambda \circ f)$.

PROPOSITION 2. Let a vectorfield V be weakly (H, ψ)-pseudoreversible with respect to (S, f). Let S_1 and λ have the same meaning as in Proposition 1. Denote by $\psi_1 : H \to \mathbb{R} \setminus \{0\}$ the function given by $\psi_1(g) = 1/\psi(g)$ for all $g \in H$. Then the field V is weakly (H, ψ_1)-pseudoreversible with respect to $(S_1, \lambda \circ f)$.

PROPOSITION 3. Let F_t be the phase flow of a vectorfield V on $\mathcal{M}$. The field V is weakly (H, ψ)-pseudoreversible with respect to (S, f) if and only if for each $t \in \mathbb{R}$ and each $g \in H \setminus \{id\}$

$$f(g) F_t = F_{t\psi(g)} f(g).$$

In particular, if $\psi(g) \in \{-1; 1\}$ for all $g \in H$ then V is weakly (H, ψ) -pseudoreversible with respect to (S, f) precisely when for each t the mapping F_t is weakly (H, ψ)-pseudoreversible with respect to (S, f).

This generalization of the concepts of reversibility and weak reversibility from the group $\mathbb{Z}_2$ to an arbitrary group H seems to be somewhat empty, but it will very likely help to obtain new variants of homological equations in §§ 1.3 and 1.9 and, hence, new types of the cohomology of appropriate algebraical systems.

Another possible generalization of the concept of reversibility consists in the following. A reversible diffeomorphism is a dynamical system whose time is the symmetry group of $\mathbb{Z}$. A reversible vectorfield is a dynamical system whose time is the symmetry group of $\mathbb{R}$ (i.e. the group of mappings $\mathbb{R} \longrightarrow \mathbb{R}$ generated by translations and the multiplication by -1). A reversible dynamical system in the generalized sense is by definition a dynamical system whose time is the symmetry group (in a sense to be made precise) of an arbitrary Lie group.

FIGURES

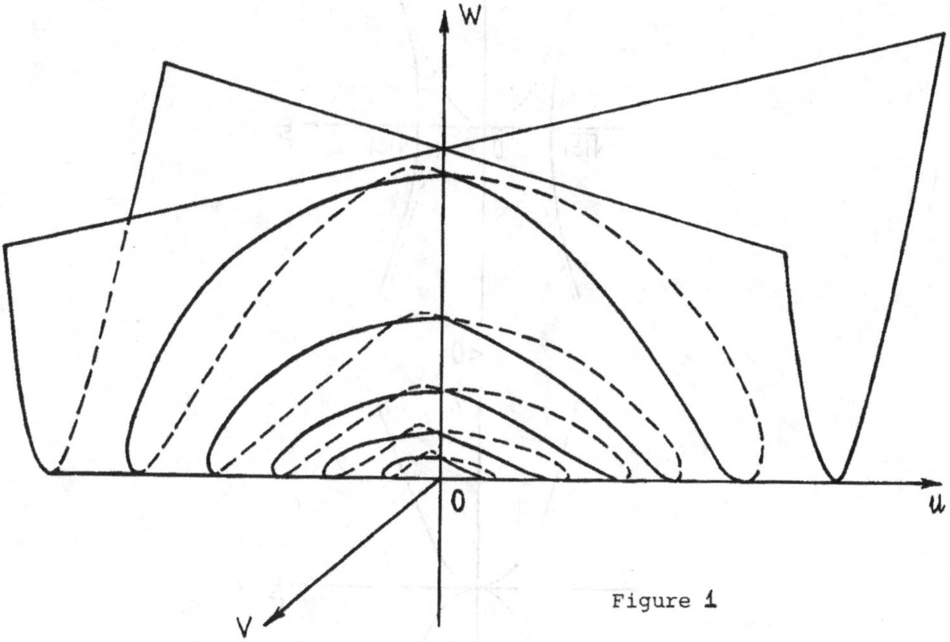

Figure 1

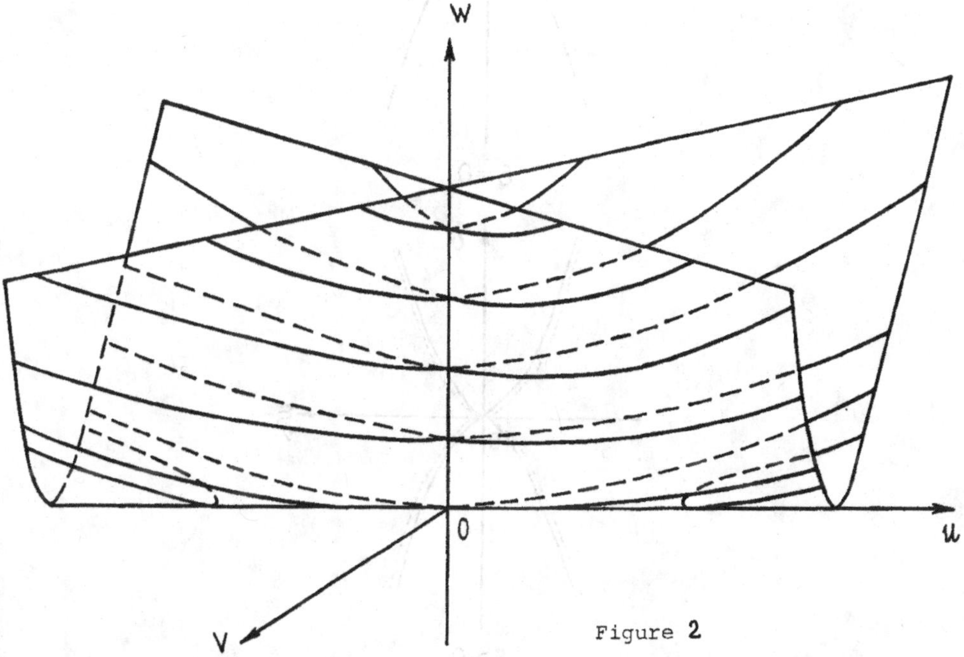

Figure 2

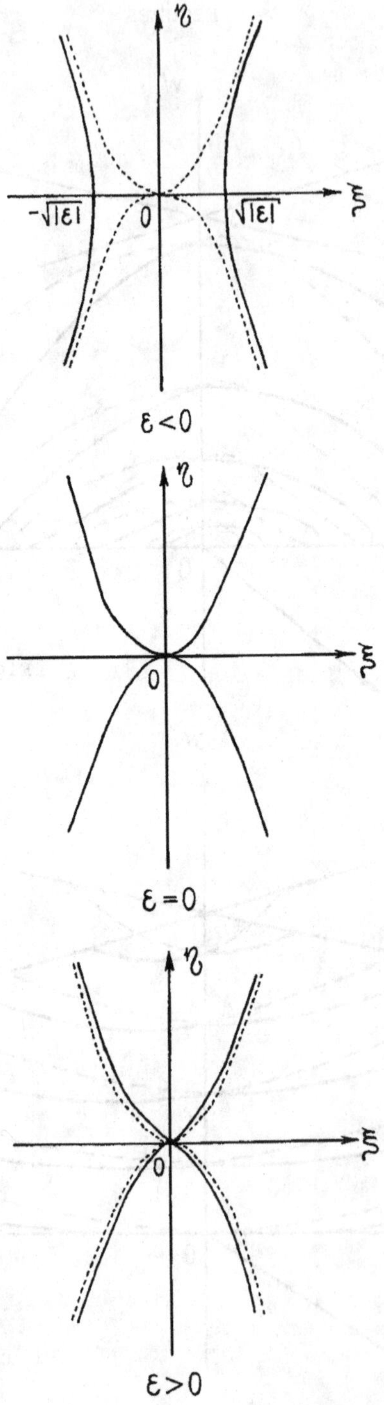

Figure 3

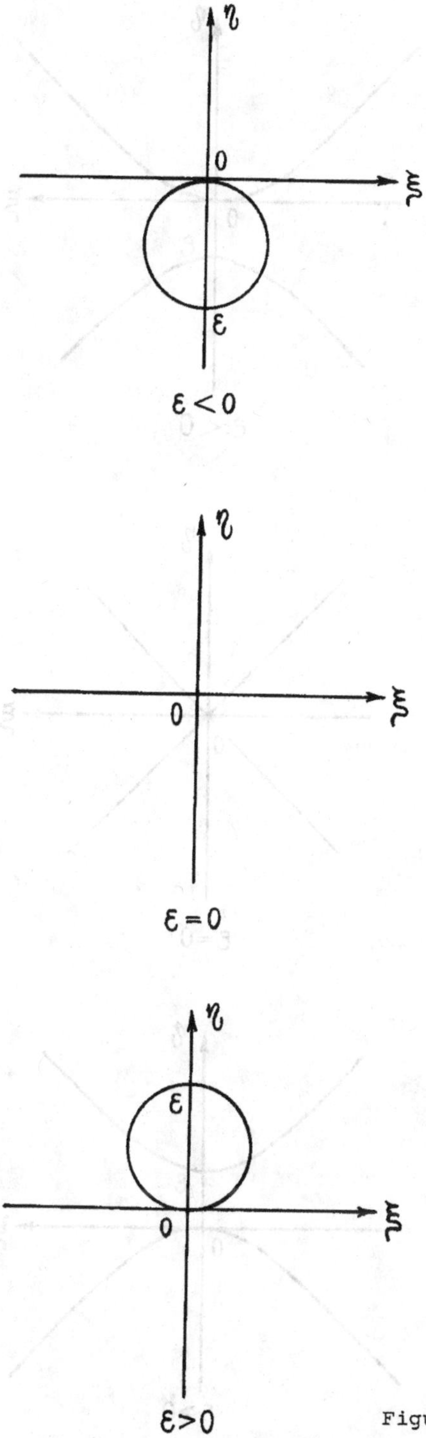

Figure 4

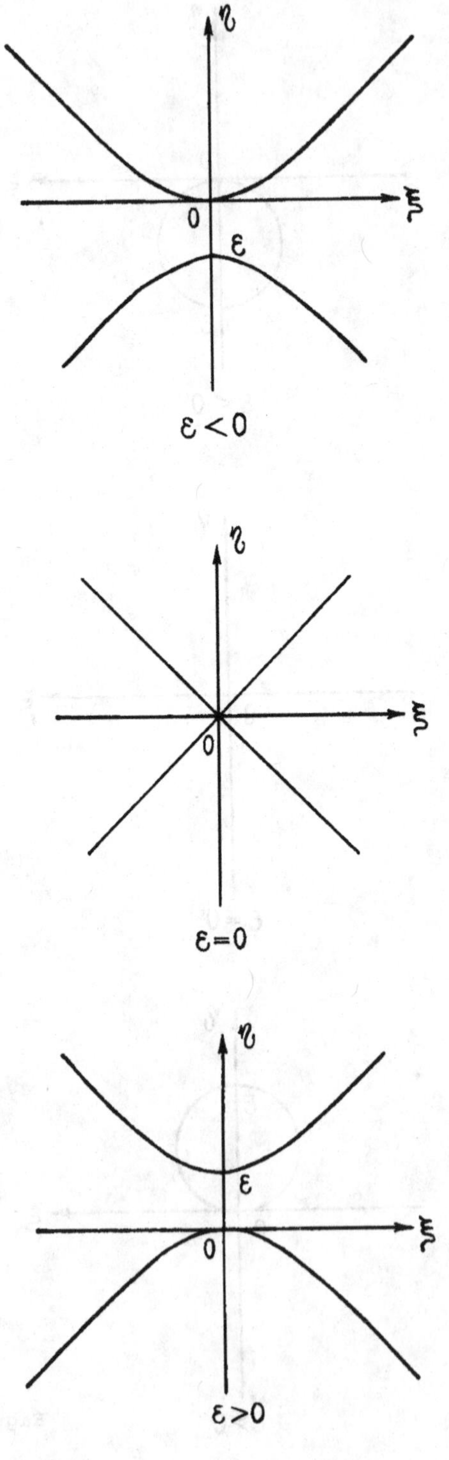

Figure 5

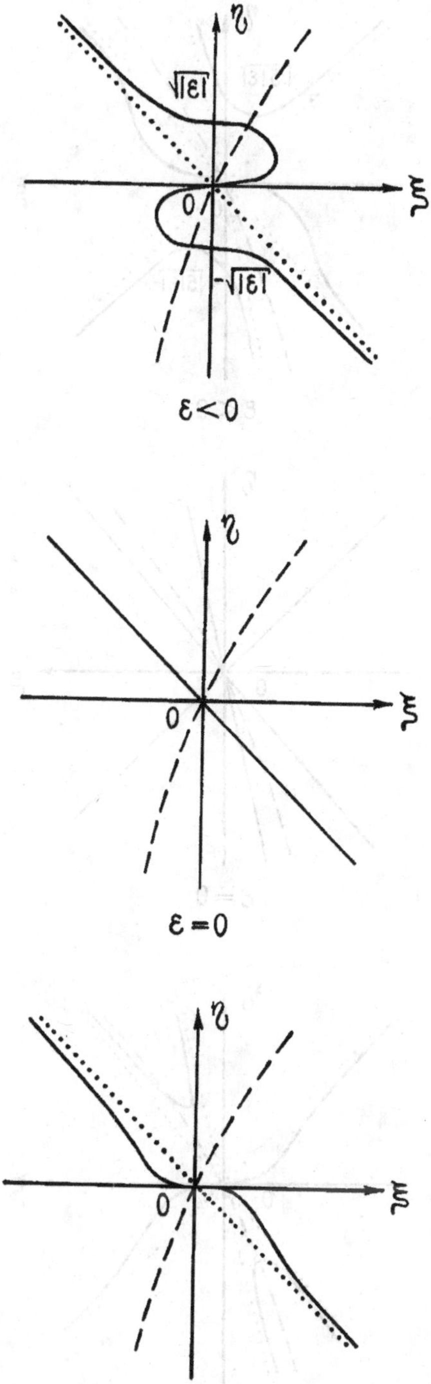

Figure 6

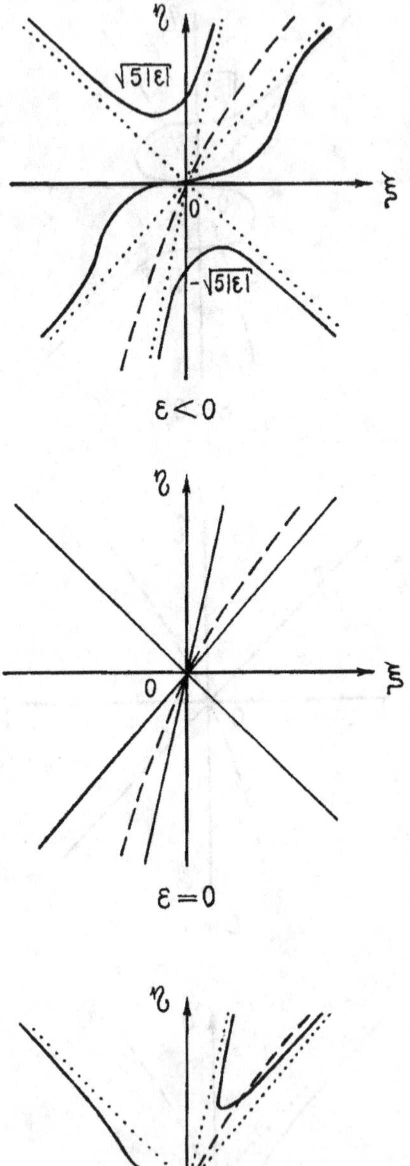

η
ξ
0
$\sqrt{5|\varepsilon|}$
$-\sqrt{5|\varepsilon|}$
$\varepsilon<0$
η
ξ
0
$\varepsilon=0$
η
ξ
0
$\varepsilon>0$

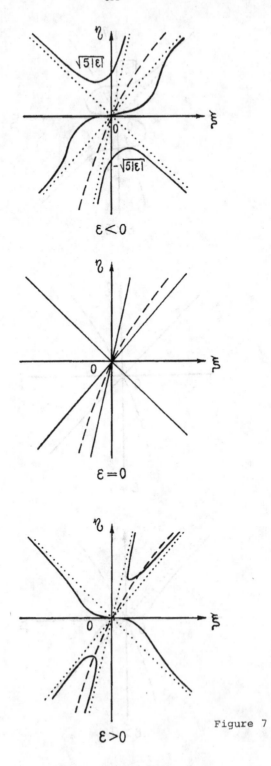

Figure 7

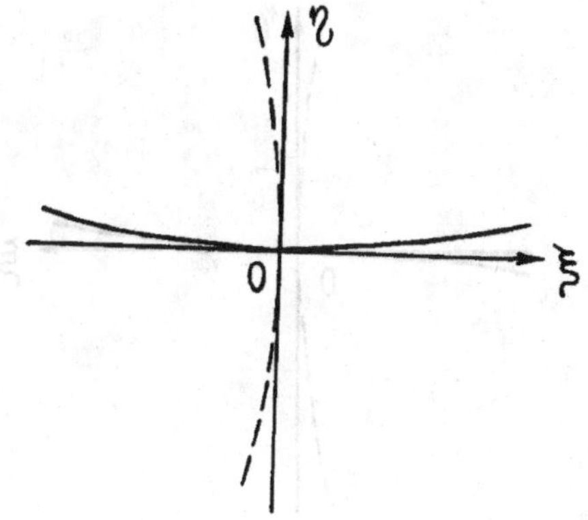

$\varepsilon < 0$

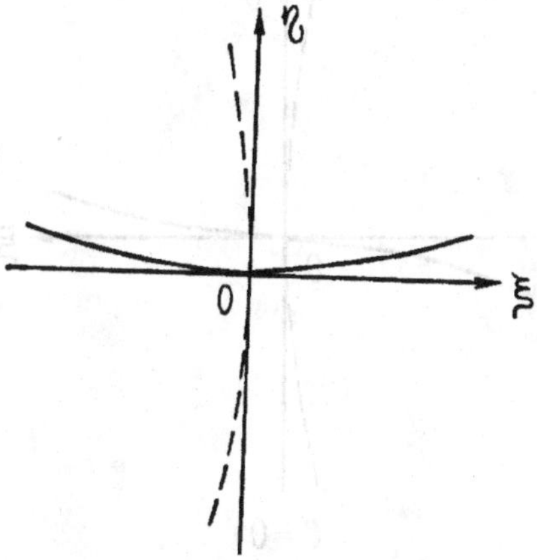

$\varepsilon = 0$

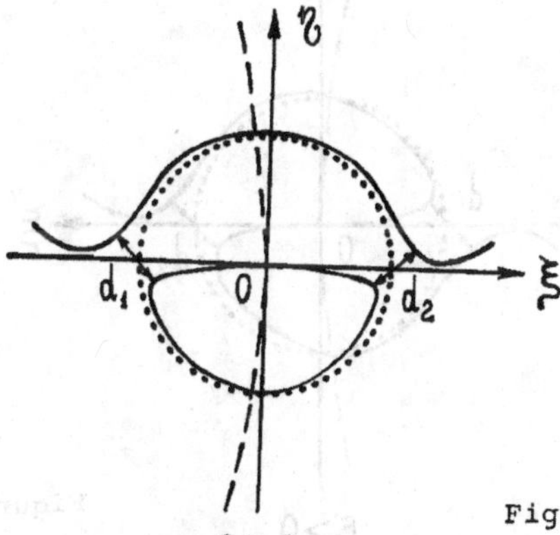

$\varepsilon > 0$

Figure 8

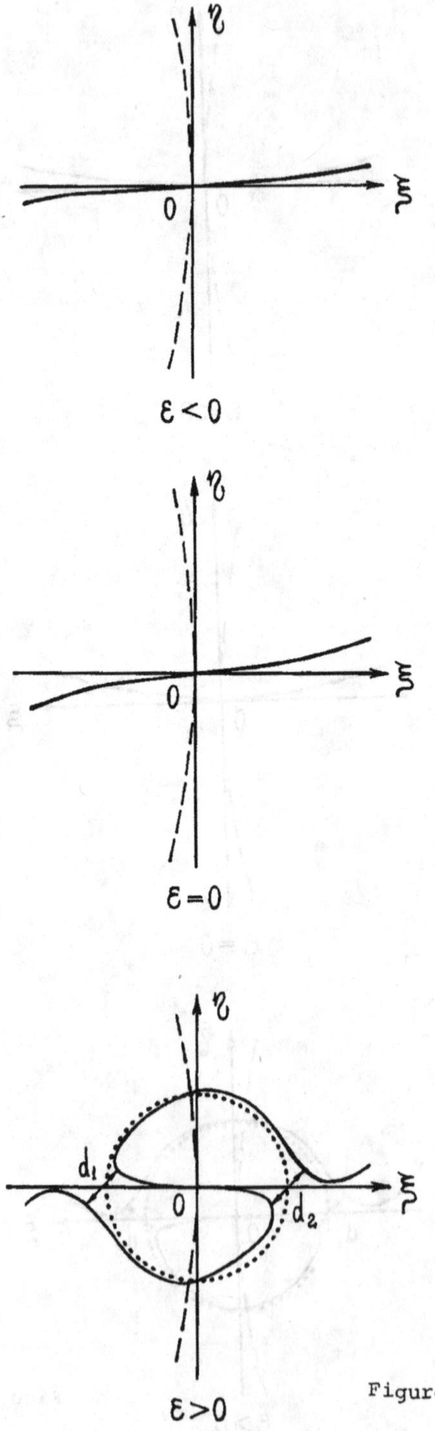

Figure 9

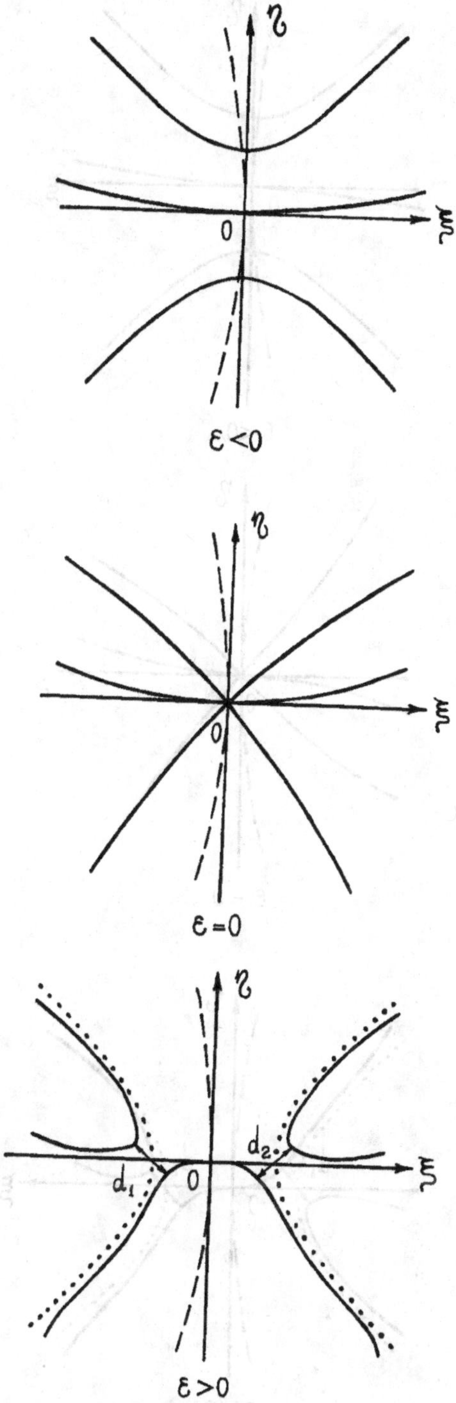

Figure 10

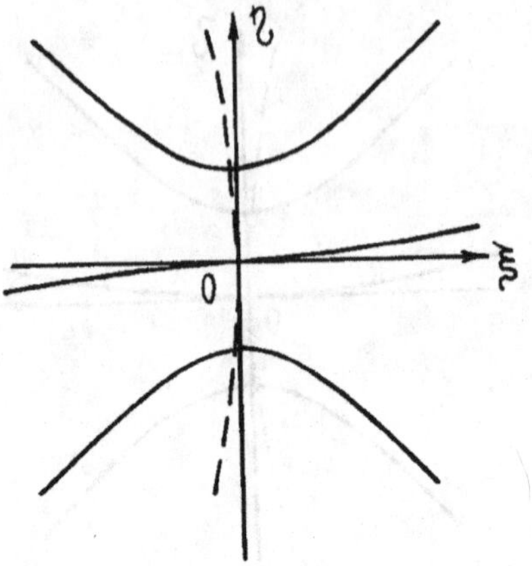

ε<0

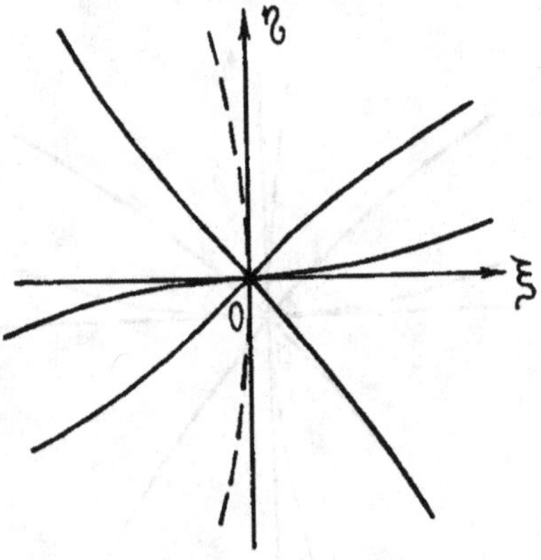

ε=0

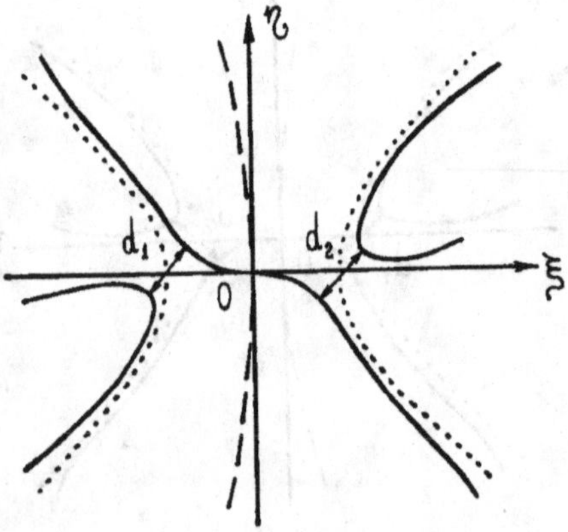

ε>0 Figure

REFERENCES *)

1. Arnol'd V.I. Reversible systems. In "Nonlinear and Turbulent Processes", Acad.Publ. New York, 1984, 1161-1174.
2. Arnol'd V.I. and Sevryuk M.B. Oscillations and bifurcations in reversible systems. In "Nonlinear phenomena in plasma physics and hydrodynamics", Edited by R.Z.Sagdeev, Mir, 1986, 31-64.
3. Devaney R.L. Reversible diffeomorphisms and flows. Trans.Am.Math. Soc., 218 (1976), 89-113.
4. Moser J.K. On the theory of quasi-periodic motions. SIAM Rev., 8, N 2 (1966), 145-172.
5. Moser J.K. Convergent series expansions for quasi-periodic motions. Math.Ann., 169 (1967), 136-176.
6. Moser J.K. Stable and random motions in dynamical systems (with special emphasis on celestial mechanics). Princeton Univ.Press, 1973.
7. Pöschel J. Integrability of Hamiltonian systems on Cantor sets. Commun. Pure Appl.Math., 35 (1982), N 1, 653-695.
8. Bibikov Yu.N. and Pliss V.A. On the existence of invariant tori in a neighbourhood of the zero solution of a system of ordinary differential equations. Differ.Equations, 3 (1967), N 11.
9. Bibikov Yu.N. The existence of invariant tori in a neighbourhood of the equilibrium position of a system of differential equations. Sov.Math.Dokl., 10 (1969), 261-265.
10. Bibikov Yu.N. The existence of conditionally periodic solutions of systems of differential equations. Differ.Equations, 7 (1971), N 8.

---

*) We refer, when possible, to translated versions of papers in Russian or French.

11. Bibikov Yu.N. Local theory of nonlinear analytic ordinary differential equations. Lect. Notes Math., 702 (1979).

12. Kolmogorov A.N. On the conservation of conditionally periodic solutions under a small perturbation of the Hamilton function. Dokl. Akad. Nauk SSSR, 98 (1954), N 4, 527-530 (in Russian).

13. Kolmogorov A.N. The general theory of dynamical systems and classical mechanics. Appendix D in Abraham R., Foundations of mechanics. Benjamin, 1967.

14. Arnol'd V.I. and Meshalkin L.D. A.N.Kolmogorov's seminar on selected problems of analysis (1958-1959). Usp.Mat. Nauk, 15(1960), N 1, 247-250 (in Russian).

15. Arnol'd V.I. The stability of the equilibrium position of a Hamiltonian system of ordinary differential equations in the general elliptic case. Sov.Math.Dokl., 2 (1961), 247-249.

16. Arnol'd V.I. Proof of a theorem of A.N.Kolmogorov on the conservation of conditionally periodic motions under a small perturbation of the Hamilton function. Russ.Math.Surv., 18 (1963), N 5, 9-36.

17. Arnol'd V.I. Small denominators and problems of stability of motion in classical and celestial mechanics. Russ.Math.Surv., 18 (1963), N 6, 85-192.

18. Arnol'd V.I. Mathematical methods of classical mechanics. New York, 1978.

19. Arnol'd V.I. Geometrical methods in the theory of ordinary differential equations. New York, 1983.

20. Arnol'd V.I. and Avez A. Ergodic problems of classical mechanics. New York, 1968.

21. Moser J.K. Lectures on Hamiltonian systems. Mem.Am.Math.Soc., 81 (1968), 1-60.

22. Siegel C.L. and Moser J.K. Lectures on celestial mechanics. Springer, 1971

23. Moser J.K. A new technique for the construction of solutions of nonlinear differential equations. Proc.Natl.Acad.Sci. USA, 47 (1961), N 11, 1824-1831.

24. Moser J.K. On invariant curves of area-preserving mappings of an annulus. Nachr.Akad.Wiss. Gött, II. Math.-Phys.Kl., 1962, Nr.1, 1-20.

25. Moser J.K. A rapidly convergent iteration method and nonlinear differential equations. I.Ann.Sc.Norm.Super. Pisa, Cl.Sci., III. Ser., 20, N 2 (1966), 265-315; II. Ann.Sc.Norm.Super.Pisa, Cl.Sci., III.Ser., 20, N 3 (1966), 499-535.

26. Lazutkin V.F. The existence of caustics for the billiard problem in a convex domain. Math.USSR, Izv., 7, N 1 (1973), 185-214.

27. Svanidze N.V. Small perturbations of an integrable dynamical system with an integral invariant. Proc.Steklov Inst.Math., 147 (1980).

28. Douady R. Une démonstration directe de l'equivalence des théorèmes de tores invariants pour difféomorphismes et champs de vecteurs. C.R.Acad.Sci., Paris, Ser. I, 295 (1982), N 2, 201-204.

29. Moser J.K. and Webster S.M. Normal forms for real surfaces in $\mathbb{C}^2$ near complex tangents and hyperbolic surface transformations. Acta Math., 150 (1983), N 3-4, 255-296.

30. Sharkovskii A.N. Differential functional equations with the finite group of argument transformations. In : "The asymptotic behaviour of solutions of differential functional equations". Kiev, 1978, 118-142 (in Russian).

31. Sharkovskii A.N. Oscillations given by autonomous difference and differential difference equations. Proc. Eighth Intern.Conf. Nonlinear Oscill., Prague, 1978, 1073-1078.

32. Lyashko O.V. Classification of critical points of functions on a manifold with a singular boundary. Funct. Anal.Appl., 17 (1983),

N 3, 187-193.

33. Roels J. Families of periodic solutions near a Hamiltonian equilibrium when the ratio of two eigenvalues is 3. J.Differ.Equations, 10 (1971), N 3, 431-447.

34. Roels J. An extension to resonant cases of Liapunov's theorem concerning the periodic solutions near a Hamiltonian equilibrium. J.Differ.Equations, 9 (1971), N 2, 300-324.

35. Henrard J. Lyapunov's center theorem for resonant equilibrium. J. Differ. Equations, 14 (1973), N 3, 431-441.

36. Malomed B.A. and Tribel'skii M.I. Bifurcations in distributed kinetic systems with aperiodic instability. Physica D, 14, N 1 (1984), 67-87.

37. Arnol'd V.I., Varchenko A.N. and Gusein-Zade S.M. Singularities of differentiable maps. Vol.1, Monographs in Mathematics, Vol.32 Birkhäuser, 1985, 1-382.

38. MacLane S. Homology. Springer, 1963.

39. Bochner S. Compact groups of differentiable transformations. Ann. Math.,II. Ser., 46, N 3 (1945), 372-381.

40. Arnol'd V.I. Instability of dynamical systems with many degrees of freedom. Sov.Math.Dokl., 5 (1964), 331-334.

41. Nekhoroshev N.N. The behaviour of Hamiltonian systems that are close to integrable ones. Funct. Anal. Appl. 5 (1971), N 4, 338-339.

42. Nekhoroshev N.N. An exponential estimate of the time of stability of nearly integrable Hamiltonian systems. Russ.Math.Surv., 32 (1977), N 6, 1-65.

43. Nekhoroshev N.N. An exponential estimate of the time of stability of nearly integrable Hamiltonian systems. II. Tr. Semin. Im. I. G.Petrovskogo, 5 (1979), 5-50 (in Russian).

SUBJECT INDEX